Sport and Exercise Psychology: International Perspectives

Sport and Exercise Psychology: International Perspectives

TONY MORRIS
Victoria University

PETER TERRY
University of Southern Queensland

SANDY GORDON
The University of Western Australia

EDITORS

Fitness Information Technology

A Division of the International Center for Performance Excellence
262 Coliseum, WVU-PE
P.O. Box 6116
Morgantown, WV 26506-6116

Library of Congress Card Catalog Number: 2007924122

ISBN: 978-1-885693-79-2

Production Editor: Matt Brann
Cover Design: 40 West Studios
Typesetter: 40 West Studios
Copyeditor: Danielle Costello
Proofreader: Val Gittings
Indexer: Val Gittings
Printed by: Data Reproductions
Cover Photos: Courtesy of MediaFocus

10 9 8 7 6 5 4 3 2 1

Fitness Information Technology
A Division of the International Center for Performance Excellence
West Virginia University
262 Coliseum, WVU-PE
PO Box 6116
Morgantown, WV 26506-6116
800.477.4348 (toll free)
304.293.6888 (phone)
304.293.6658 (fax)
Email: icpe@mail.wvu.edu
Website: www.fitinfotech.com

Table of Contents

Acknowledgments

This book would not have been completed if not for the valuable support, assistance, and advice that we have received from a number of people. We wish to express our appreciation here.

First, we want to acknowledge our colleagues Lydia Ievleva, Stephanie Hanrahan, Gregory Kolt, and Patsy Tremayne. Together with the three editors of this text, we developed the program for the XIth ISSP World Congress of Sport Psychology and worked to mount the event in collaboration with Tour Hosts, whose expertise as professional conference organizers was invaluable. Those colleagues and good friends could equally have had their names on the front of this book, but they kindly agreed to step aside in favor of us. We thank them for their generosity, after they had done so much to make the Congress, including the keynote presentations, a great success.

Next, we must express our thanks to the Managing Council of the International Society of Sport Psychology (ISSP). First, the ISSP Managing Council made the final selection of keynote presenters for the World Congress and nominated the two early career award winners, whose chapters accompany those of the keynotes in this book. Second, ISSP Managing Council endorsed the publication of the book, which undoubtedly smoothed its passage with Fitness Information Technology (FIT). We appreciate, in particular, the support of the current president, Dieter Hackfort, in this regard.

Of course, we cannot forget the contributors to the book, Hulya Aşçi, Sian Beilock, Carol Dweck, Sandy Gordon, Brad Hatfield, Daniel Landers, Franz Mechsner, Nanette Mutrie, Karl Newell, and Ken Ravizza. Their contributions to the Congress were widely appreciated and we recognize that it was a big task for them to follow that up by writing substantive chapters covering the material they presented in Sydney. That they all agreed to undertake the task and then completed it so quickly and efficiently is the single most important factor in the orderly production of the book. The quality of their chapters is a great bonus, giving us the confidence that this book contains a number of seminal contributions to the field of sport psychology. We also thank the co-authors who the keynotes invited to support them. We know they gave sterling assistance in the timely production of these quality chapters.

Our gratitude also goes to Andrew Ostrow, the director of FIT. Andy's long-time support for ISSP has been of great benefit to that organization and his backing for this book was a big boost for us, allowing the book to be published by one of the leading sport psychology publishers in the world. Andy's guidance in the production of the book proposal was most helpful. At the manuscript stage, Matthew Brann of FIT was very supportive, too. His patience and understanding, as well as his professional mode of operating, helped us to submit the manuscript in timely fashion.

Tony Morris, Peter Terry, and Sandy Gordon

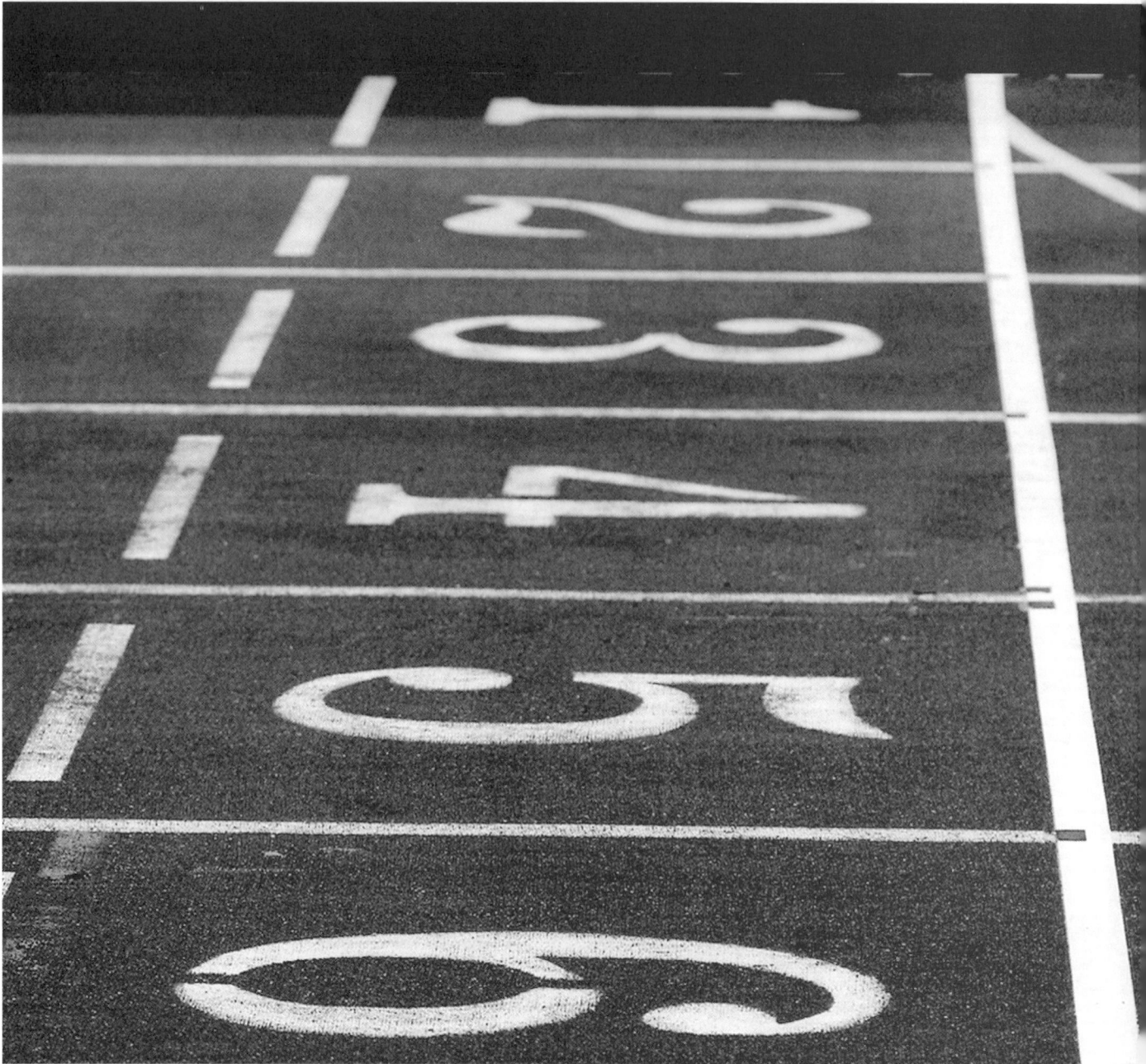

1

Introduction to *Sport and Exercise Psychology: International Perspectives*

TONY MORRIS, PETER TERRY, AND SANDY GORDON

Introduction

In August 2005, the International Society of Sport Psychology (ISSP) held its eleventh World Congress in Sydney, Australia, the Congress's first visit to the southern hemisphere. The 11th ISSP World Congress of Sport Psychology was auspicious in an even more significant sense: The year 2005 was the 40th anniversary of the occasion of the first World Congress of Sport Psychology that included the creation of ISSP.

In 1965, Feruccio Antonelli hosted the 1st World Congress of Sport Psychology in Rome, Italy. It was a large congress for its time, with around 450 delegates (Morris, Hackfort, & Lidor, 2003). Most of the delegates were doctors and psychiatrists with an interest in sport, whereas others were physical educa-

tion specialists. There were few sport psychologists present, because the profession hardly existed then. During the event, Antonelli held a business meeting in the course of which he and a colleague proposed the foundation of ISSP and Antonelli was elected its first President (Salmela, 1997).

That process of establishing ISSP brought us to the 11th ISSP World Congress of Sport Psychology in Sydney in 2005. ISSP 2005 showed the International Society as a mature organization that was able to attract almost 600 delegates—including professional sport psychologists and postgraduate students from more than 50 countries around the world—to an event with a strong scientific program. Led by eight keynote addresses presented by eminent researchers and practitioners, and three presentations invited by ISSP Managing Council to reflect its awards for achievement in the field of sport psychology, the Congress included a range of symposia, workshops, forums, free papers, and around 400 high quality posters. The Proceedings of the Congress, including nearly 600 papers, have been documented on a CD-ROM (Morris, Terry, Ievleva, Gordon, Hanrahan, Kolt, & Tremayne, 2005). Keynote papers were restricted to six pages and all other papers were given a maximum of three pages.

It is evident that six pages are not sufficient for keynote speakers and other invited presenters to fully explicate the content of 50-minute oral presentations that only summarize the noteworthy research and practice of these eminent scholars. Thus, it has become the tradition to invite the selected speakers to contribute longer papers to a volume celebrating the major presentations at the World Congress. This provides the opportunity for the delegates at the event to study those stimulating keynote addresses in more detail. It also gives all those with an interest in sport psychology the chance to read about the research and/or practical work of colleagues whose achievements merit an invitation to present a keynote address or to receive an award for their work at the premier international event in the discipline and profession of sport psychology.

This book represents the collection of the extended papers by the invited speakers, who were honored by their selection to present special addresses at the 11th ISSP World Congress of Sport Psychology. As members of the Organizing Committee of the Congress, we feel privileged to have been charged with editing this volume. Here we would like to acknowledge the other members of the Organizing Committee who placed their faith in us to carry out this duty, namely Dr Lydia Ievleva, Associate Professor Stephanie Hanrahan, Professor Gregory Kolt, and Associate Professor Patsy Tremayne. We thank them for all their hard work that contributed to the success of the World Congress.

In this introduction, we will reflect briefly on the 40-year history of ISSP and, in particular, its world congresses, acknowledging their role in the development of the discipline and profession of sport psychology. Then we will comment on the 11th ISSP World Congress before introducing the 10 substantive papers in *Sport and Exercise Psychology: Inter-* *national Perspectives,* the invited presentations at *Promoting Health and Performance for Life: The ISSP 11th World Congress of Sport Psychology.*

History of ISSP and the World Congress

Coleman Griffith, the American physical educationist and coach, has been credited as the father of sport psychology. Griffith's vision of the application of psychology to sport led him to study issues in this field as long ago as the 1920s (Morris & Summers, 2004). He published his ideas and research in two classic texts, namely *Psychology of Athletics* (Griffith, 1926) and *Psychology of Coaching* (Griffith, 1928). After Griffith's seminal work, development of the field of sport psychology experienced a long hiatus; little of note was reported until the 1960s. During that period, research did continue in motor learning, but it was largely conducted within the context of physical education. The "mother" discipline of psychology considered sport too frivolous an activity to warrant serious attention, thus missing the point that sport is a microcosm of life in which the full gamut of psychological processes can be seen, often in magnified form. On the other hand, the application of psychology was clearly central to the discipline of physical education, but those who conducted research on motor learning and psychological phenomena considered that work to be part of the physical education discipline. There certainly was a need for somebody, whether an organization or an individual, to provide a lead for the development of sport psychology as a profession and a discipline in its own right.

Ironically, it was not a sport psychologist who took the first big step in the creation of the profession of sport psychology—it was a psychiatrist or, to be more precise, two psychiatrists, Ferruccio Antonelli, from Italy, and Jose Hombravella, from Spain (Morris et al., 2003). Antonelli and Hombravella were members of the Federacion Internationale du Medecin en Sport (FIMS). Although some psychological issues were addressed within FIMS, Antonelli and Hombravella appear to have originated the idea to launch a separate worldwide sport psychology group (Morris et al., 2003). Antonelli was the front man for the bid to establish an organization, being aristocratic and diplomatic, however, Hombravella was credited as the person who came up with the idea in 1960, five years before the event at which the conception of a worldwide body came to fruition (Salmela, 1997).

As the first, and perhaps most significant, example of the influence of the World Congress of Sport Psychology on the development of the profession, Antonelli and Hombravella established the International Society of Sport Psychology (ISSP) at the "First World Congress of Sport Psychology" in Rome, Italy, in April 1965. We may note that Antonelli and Hombravella even coined the name of the event and it has persisted for at least 40 years (Morris et al., 2003). Although the event was noteworthy in itself, the fact that Antonelli and Hombravella created ISSP during the Congress must be considered the momentous achievement. They invited the 450 delegates, a very large gathering for such an event in those days, to attend a business meeting. Salmela (1997) reported that the meeting lasted for just 30 minutes. Vanek (1993), who was there, stated that the statutes were "proclaimative" (p. 154). Salmela reported that "The first MC of the ISSP was formed with Professor Venerado's proclamation: 'If you agree with this list, raise your hand. Whoever does not agree with this list, raise your hand. One. The list is approved by the vast majority!' Venerado took the Chair for the meeting, presumably because Antonelli and Hombravella were to be proposed for the senior officer positions (Salmela, 1997). Thus, there was no formal nomination process. Hombravella nominated Antonelli for President of the new body and Antonelli then proposed Hombravella for Secretary. Venerado called for a show of hands and the response was close to unanimous. Antonelli and Hombravella proposed a Managing Council, which was designed to reflect a balance of representation from around the world, in particular, ensuring that East and West were equally represented. The International Society of Sport Psychology was a reality. The next few years were to constitute a crucial period for the development of ISSP; these were times fraught with problems for the infant organization (Morris et al., 2003).

One issue that threatened the future of ISSP was that the two influential men who ran it were not sport psychologists. Vanek's (1993) view was that Antonelli, in particular, had an autocratic style of management that was often *ad hoc*. He reported

that, although the Managing Council was formally in place, Antonelli called its meetings to coincide with sessions of the group representing the Latin languages countries of FIMS. Most of the Managing Council members were not from those countries, so they did not attend and that left Antonelli and Hombravella to make decisions almost unhindered. Perhaps the biggest threat to the future of the first international organization in sport psychology, however, was the location of the 2nd World Congress of Sport Psychology and its timing.

At a time of great tension between the Eastern and Western blocs, which were then set very firmly as reflections of opposing ideologies, the 2nd World Congress was proposed for Washington, D.C., the "capital" of the West! It is not clear from documentation that has survived why this extremely contentious location was chosen, nor do we have the opportunity to ask those who made the decision. Sadly, Antonelli and Hombravella have passed away. Clearly, the siting of the 2nd World Congress in Washington made it very difficult for sport psychologists from the East to attend. Only those who had the highest level of trust were allowed to go to Washington. For example, Morris et al. (2003) reported that Ema Geron, a leading figure in the field, who was then based in Bulgaria, told them that the government did not allow her to leave the country to attend the Congress, even though she did get a visa from the USA and had a supporting letter from Antonelli. Interestingly, Geron was elected to the Managing Council in her absence.

Another problem was the timing of the 2nd World Congress. It was in 1968, only three years after Rome. This was a tumultuous year in world politics, primarily due to unrest in Czechoslovakia, which led to the appearance of Russian tanks in the streets. Based on the Russian reaction to Czech protests, tension between East and West was as high as at any time during the Cold War. Back in the world of sport psychology, the American organizers did not have much time to set up the 2nd World Congress of Sport Psychology. Salmela (1997) claimed that the North American Society for the Psychology of Sport and Physical Activity (NASPSPA) was hurriedly established in 1967 to help with the organization of the event. Not only did the American location get the eastern countries off side, but it also upset leading

French sport psychologists, because there was no translation into French at the Congress. Morris et al. (2003), citing Europeans who were involved in international sport psychology at that time, suggested that the Federation Europeenne de Psychologie des Sports et des Activites Corporelles (FEPSAC) was created as a reaction to the affront felt by the French and the Eastern bloc sport psychologists. For some time, FEPSAC and ISSP did not cooperate. Ironically, then, the major contribution of the controversial 2nd World Congress of Sport Psychology, organized by ISSP, appears not to be associated with the development of science or practice in the field. Rather, the significance of the 2nd World Congress is that it was the stimulus for the creation of two of the most successful sport psychology bodies in the world, NASPSPA and FEPSAC.

Based on their interviews with Vanek and Geron, who played a leading role in the early development of FEPSAC, as well as ISSP, Morris et al. (2003) reported that there was an uncomfortable relationship between ISSP and FEPSAC for the first few years. Despite the North American presence and its "International" tag, ISSP had a strong European leaning, which was somewhat threatening to FEPSAC. At the same time, it was not tenable to have two competing organizations both largely sustained by European sport psychologists, and FEPSAC was garnering much support from around its region. In his paper in *International Perspectives in Sport and Exercise Psychology* (Serpa, Alves, Ferreira, & Paula-Brito, 1994), the book reflecting significant contributions to the 8th World Congress of Sport Psychology, Vanek (1994) stated that he and Schilling, the incumbent President of FEPSAC at the time, agreed in 1973 that FEPSAC would be for Europe and ISSP for the rest of the world. Based on this agreement, Vanek developed the concept of ISSP as the world body, with FEPSAC and other regional/continental bodies linked to it.

With many of the sport psychologists from countries in Eastern Europe absent, not surprisingly, Antonelli and Hombravella, who represented Western Europe, were re-elected to their leading positions in ISSP. A reshaped Managing Council was still appointed based on a process of proposal by the outgoing Managing Council, rather than by individual election. Following the problems in Washington, it was difficult for the leaders of ISSP to find volunteers to host the 3rd World Congress. As a consequence, the short 3-year gap between the first two events was followed by a 5-year gap between the second and third congresses. In the end it was Hombravella's Spain that hosted the 3rd World Congress of Sport Psychology in Madrid in 1973. Salmela (1997) argued that there was another reason for the 5-year gap, namely to avoid a clash with the summer Olympic Games in 1972.

Once more, the 3rd ISSP World Congress was remarkable not for the presentation of groundbreaking scientific papers or powerful applied techniques, but for the politics. Antonelli was ousted as President by Miroslav Vanek from Czechoslovakia. In his special address to the 8th World Congress of Sport Psychology in Lisbon, Vanek (1993) claimed that this was not a "Communist putsch" (p. 156), as perceived by some Western sport psychologists at the time, because there were relatively few delegates from Eastern countries in Madrid. Vanek argued that it was a reaction to a general dislike of Antonelli's autocratic and aristocratic style. In interviews with Morris et al. (2003), past presidents and secretaries general of ISSP indicated an apparent change in the management style of ISSP, coinciding with the election of Vanek as President. This was particularly noticeable in the organization of Managing Council; meetings were now scheduled regularly, with clear and systematic procedures.

Perhaps the location of the 4th World Congress of Sport Psychology was also a political decision. The 4th World Congress was in Prague, the home of Vanek in Czechoslovakia. An alternate reason for this location choice could have been the difficult task of attracting hosts at the time. The event took place in 1977, marking the implementation of Olympic style 4-year intervals. With the support gained in his home country, not surprisingly, Vanek was re-elected President. As well as stabilizing ISSP as an organization, the next ISSP President, Robert Singer, told Morris et al. that Vanek's 12-year presidency also saw the World Congress shift to a scientific event, with its focus on the presentation of research papers. Perhaps Prague can be seen as the turning point; however, many view the 5th World Congress as the first in which the science outshone the politics.

The 5th World Congress of Sport Psychology took place in Ottawa, Canada, in 1981. The scientific quality of the event was reviewed positively by Vanek (1993). John Salmela, by then a member of ISSP Managing Council, was one of the principal organizers of the Ottawa Congress, along with Terry Orlick and John Partington. There are several factors that certainly would have contributed to a greater focus on the science and practice of sport psychology at the 5th World Congress. One was the choice of Ottawa; despite its proximity to the USA, Canada was not perceived to be strongly aligned with East or West politically, and the icy relationship between East and West had thawed, the Cold War being effectively over by this time. Canada's historical links with French culture and language—as reflected in simultaneous translation between English and French at the Congress (Salmela, 1997)—should have gotten the Francophiles on side with the World Congress for the first time. Also, because Vanek had done a good job, the political wrangling was no longer dominant. Vanek was re-elected for his third term, a clear demonstration that ISSP members perceived his contribution as valuable to the development of the world body.

The third factor that likely had a substantial impact on the shift from the political to the scholarly at the 5th World Congress was the scientific and practical development of sport psychology that took place during the 1970s, especially in western countries such as the USA, Canada, and the United Kingdom. During that period, there was a great expansion in the teaching of sport psychology as a distinct discipline, research on psychological issues related to sport performance, and the involvement of sport psychologists with sport teams (Williams, 2005). This was reflected in the first publication of the *Journal of Sport Psychology* in 1979. It was only the second journal devoted to the discipline, coming nine years after the *International Journal of Sport Psychology* was first published by Antonelli for ISSP. An applied journal, *The Sport Psychologist*, soon followed, as did the establishment of a North American organization with an applied orientation, the Association for the Advancement of Applied Sport Psychology, which held its first annual conference in 1985. By 1981 and the 5th World Congress of Sport Psychology, a substantial number of specialist sport psychologists were doing research and practicing in professional and Olympic sport, at least in North America, Europe, and Australasia.

A particularly noteworthy aspect of the 5th World Congress of Sport Psychology was that Orlick, Partington, and Salmela established the tradition of the production of a text reflecting key contributions from the event; in fact, they produced three books on sport psychology based on contributions from delegates at the Congress, under the generic title, *Mental Training for Coaches and Athletes*, in addition to the 1981 congress proceedings (Orlick, Partington, & Salmela, 1981). As far as we are aware, these were the first scholarly texts to result from a World Congress and the first to be professionally published, thus making them widely available to the international sport psychology community. The three texts focused on *Mental Training for Coaches and Athletes* (Orlick, Partington, & Salmela, 1982), *Sport in Perspective* (Partington, Orlick, & Salmela, 1982), and *New Paths of Sport Learning and Excellence* (Salmela, Partington, & Orlick, 1982). In a number of senses, the 5th World Congress of Sport Psychology signalled that sport psychology had arrived as an academic discipline.

The World Congresses since Ottawa have not been so remarkable individually. The scientific tone set at the 5th World Congress has been maintained and refined over the years. While the 6th to 10th World Congresses have not been quite as remarkable, there have been some noteworthy occurrences. At the 6th World Congress of Sport Psychology in Copenhagen, Denmark, in 1985, Vanek's long and important tenure as President of ISSP ended and American motor learning specialist Robert Singer became the third president of ISSP. Singer (1985) wrote of his hope that he would preside over a period of maturation of the young Society (Morris et al., 2003). The Congress in Copenhagen reflected an emerging pattern that at least every other World Congress would be held in Europe.

Singer was re-elected President during the 7th World Congress in Singapore in 1989. This was the first World Congress to be held outside Europe/North America. Singer (personal communication, 6th May, 2006) told us that he proposed this venue during the 1987 meeting of the ISSP Managing Council. Singer said he believed that Asia had great potential but needed a stimulus to get sport psychology established. Upon returning from a sports science conference in Singapore that was very well organized, he approached the event organizers to ask if they would be interested in running the ISSP World Congress. Singer recalled that members of ISSP Managing Council were skeptical, there being no sport psychology personnel, let alone an established sport psychology organization, in Singapore at that time. Singer reported that he won over Managing Council with his argument, based on the ISSP statutes, that ISSP's mission of developing sport psychology around the world would not be fulfilled simply by going to well-established countries and regions. Singer claimed that the 7th ISSP World Congress was the best organized he has attended and he was at every one except Rome 1965 and Sydney 2005.

The other event of note at the 7th World Congress was the establishment of the Asian South Pacific Association of Sport Psychology (ASPASP). This was a project stimulated by the ISSP Managing Council. Fujita was the Managing Council member charged to drive the process. Fujita described how Singer had proposed the idea to him in 1987 (Fujita, 2006). He gathered support at a meeting of Asian and South Pacific sport psychologists at the 1988 Pre-Olympic Scientific Congress in Seoul, Korea, another fortuitous, or perhaps symbolic, location. The statutes were presented and ASPASP became official in a meeting in Singapore during the 1989 World Congress. The juxtaposition in Asia of the Olympic Games in Seoul in 1988 and the 7th ISSP World Congress of Sport Psychology in Singapore in 1989 certainly provided the ideal opportunity to gain momentum for ASPASP at international events where a wide range of Asian and South Pacific-based scholars could attend with relative ease. The establishment of ASPASP further vindicated Singer's proposal to go to Asia at that time.

In this way, a World Congress of Sport Psychology was the stimulus and the scene for the creation of yet another important body in the discipline and the profession of sport psychology. Given that NASP-SPA has been long regarded as the regional body for North America and FEPSAC is the recognized organization for sport psychology in Europe, the establishment of ASPASP meant that the three most active regions of the world in the field of sport psychology had regional organizations linked to ISSP and generated through ISSP congresses in some way. Interestingly, South America has had regional organizations since the early days of ISSP, but the transience of its sport psychology community has caused its impetus and influence to wax and wane over the years. So far, although ISSP has recognized that sport psychologists are active in South America (indeed South American sport psychologists have periodically been elected onto ISSP Managing Council), the world body has not acted in a concerted fashion to promote a regional body in South America.

The 8th World Congress of Sport Psychology was held in Lisbon, Portugal in 1993. Here Singer stepped down as President to be replaced by Denis Glencross from Australia, perhaps a reflection of the growing international flavor of ISSP. Particularly noteworthy in Lisbon were the swan songs of Antonelli and Vanek. Showing the signs of age, especially Vanek, each made invited presentations to the Congress. It might be a reflection of their styles that Vanek (1993) submitted a written paper, which is part of the Proceedings of the event (Serpa, Alves, Ferreira, & Paula-Brito, 1993) and also wrote a longer chapter (Vanek, 1994) for the edited book that emerged from the Congress (Serpa, Alves, Ferreira, & Paula-Brito, 1994), whereas Antonelli's final address to ISSP, however memorable for those who were present, was not recorded for posterity. Although the World Congresses in Copenhagen and Singapore spawned locally edited and distributed books of proceedings, there was no professionally published book from either event. Notably, the book emanating from the 1993 World Congress (Serpa et al., 1994) was the first to be published by Fitness Information Technology (FIT). That publisher also produced Lidor and Bar-Eli's (1999) book from the 9th World Congress and is the publisher of the present collection. Perhaps we can now call FIT part of the tradition.

In 1997, the 9th World Congress of Sport Psychology took place in Netanya, Israel, at one of the better-known homes of sport science around the world, the Wingate Institute. Dramatic events had surrounded the presidency of ISSP during the previous three years. Sadly, Glencross, who was elected President in 1993, died suddenly in 1994. Past President Singer was asked to step into the breech, given his experience in the position. Examination of the statutes revealed that in such an event, the senior Vice President was supposed to take over. In 1995, Atsushi Fujita, then still President of ASPASP, became

Acting President of ISSP. In 1997, he stepped down and the 9th World Congress saw the first competitive election for the position of ISSP president since the early confrontation between Antonelli and Vanek in Madrid. After a close competition with Glyn Roberts, Gershon Tenenbaum became the fifth elected President of ISSP, perhaps another case in sport of "home advantage" for the long-time Wingate sport psychologist. The Wingate event had attracted a relatively small number of delegates, around 250. It seemed that people were wary of the location, given the regularity with which terrorist activity flared up. Nonetheless, two volumes of Proceedings were edited by Lidor and Bar-Eli (1997). They also edited a book of longer papers written by the keynote speakers (Lidor & Bar-Eli, 1998).

The new millennium started for sport psychology in Skiathos, Greece, where the Greek national sport psychology organization hosted the 10th World Congress of Sport Psychology, attracting a much bigger number of delegates to a central Mediterranean location and an attractive holiday resort setting. With around 600 delegates and as many papers, the contributions to this Congress filled five volumes of Proceedings, entitled, *In the Dawn of the New Millennium* (Pappaouannou, Goudas, & Theodorakis, 2001). Despite the large amount of material contributed to the 2001 World Congress, including contributions by 10 keynote speakers and several ISSP award winners, the organizers of the 10th World Congress decided not to produce a book. At the General Assembly in Skiathos, Tenenbaum stepped down as President, restricted by the statutes that limited the number of consecutive terms a person could be an officer of ISSP (he had been Secretary General from 1993-97). Keith Henschen, the senior Vice President, was elected President, unopposed. During the event, Bola Ikulayo, a senior Nigerian sport psychologist and Vice President of ISSP, chaired a meeting of African researchers and practitioners sponsored by ISSP to explore the possibility of creating a pan-African organization, which would become the regional body in the only area of the world without regional representation in ISSP. Attendance was "selective" but the small number of delegates who did attend supported the idea, so Ikulayo and colleagues began the process of formally establishing the African Association of Sport Psychology (AASP).

Looking back on the 10 World Congresses of Sport Psychology spanning the period from 1965 to 2001, we can see the modern history of sport psychology laid out for us. Unquestionably, the World Congresses have played a key role in the late 20th century development of sport psychology. In their early days, they provided a focus for the very tentative discipline. The quadrennial Congress acted as a vehicle for the establishment and development of ISSP, including its major business meetings, the General Assemblies, with their political wrangling, changes of statutes, and awards for distinguished contributions to the field. The Congress stimulated the development of four major regional sport psychology organizations. Over time, the event has become an ever-stronger scientific gathering, with keynote addresses by eminent scholars and practitioners, a wide range of high-quality scientific and technical communications, and an opportunity, unparalleled in the field, to meet and discuss ideas with colleagues from all parts of the world. In recent times, the Proceedings of these Congresses have become valuable documents, but there is limited space in them to allow the eminent keynote speakers to do justice to their major addresses. Thus, the tradition has emerged of the edited text, comprising of extended, significant, and high-quality papers by the keynote speakers. It is in that context that the present book has been produced from the invited presentations at the 11th ISSP World Congress of Sport Psychology, and it is appropriate to devote a little space to describing the development of that event.

11th ISSP World Congress of Sport Psychology

The fourth President of ISSP, Glencross came from Australia. Bringing the World Congress to Australia was an ambition he cherished. Had he lived, Australia might have hosted the event earlier. Ironically and perhaps surprisingly, however, Australia is the only country that can boast two nationally based Presidents of ISSP, Glencross and Tenenbaum. Tenenbaum took up a position in an Australian university, the University of Southern Queensland, the year before he was elected President of ISSP, during the 9th World Congress. He moved on to an academic post in the USA around the time he stepped down as President of ISSP, so he was based in Australia throughout his presidency. Perhaps partly due to the Glencross legacy, but also likely based on his knowledge of the status of sport psychology in Australia, Tenenbaum also became a proponent of an Australian bid to hold the world event.

Tenenbaum had a well-placed ally. Tony Morris had been elected to ISSP Managing Council (MC) at the 9th World Congress in Israel in 1997. Independently a proponent of an Australian bid, Morris was also deeply involved in the Australian College of Sport Psychologists (CoSP). When encouragement came from local convention and tourism organizations for a Sydney-based Congress, CoSP and its parent organization, the Australian Psychological Society, supported a bid. Morris led a Bid Committee supported by CoSP Chair, Sandy Gordon, along with Lydia Ievleva and Patsy Tremayne, the two senior Sydney-based sport psychologists on the CoSP Executive. Circumstances favoured the Australian bid. As had been the case with the Seoul Olympics the year before the ISSP World Congress where ASPASP was formed, the Olympic Games were to be held in Sydney in 2000. Morris and his colleagues, supported by CoSP and APS, offered to host the 2000 ISSP MC meeting immediately after the Olympics, when a number of MC members would be in Australia with their national teams. In addition to much general lobbying and the opportunity for all MC members to experience Australia and Sydney in general, two senior members of MC were designated to have a two-day tour of the intended venue of the World Congress, the proposed Congress hotel, and related facilities and attractions.

Bids for the 2005 World Congress of Sport Psychology were considered by the ISSP MC at its meeting in Skiathos, Greece, immediately prior to the 2001 World Congress. The decision was made so that it could be formally announced at the ISSP General Assembly during the Congress. The Australian team put together a polished bid, based on its history in sport psychology and ISSP, as well as the position of Sydney as one of the world's leading convention locations. In fact, at that time, Sydney had just been voted number one congress destination in the world by major tourism organizations. In terms of sport psychology, Australia had an established, internationally active research community, led by Glencross for

many years. Additionally, the role of applied sport psychology, led by Jeff Bond in the Australian sports institute system, was world-renowned and the development of the national professional organization within the country's major psychology association was also widely admired. With respect to ISSP, Australia had representation on the ISSP MC from the early years, through Geoff Jones. During the 1980s and early 1990s, Glencross had made a major contribution to the running of ISSP, culminating in his election as President in 1993. Australian sport psychologists had also hosted an ISSP Managing Council meeting in Brisbane in 1982, when Australia hosted the Commonwealth Games there. Thus, Australia had a substantial ISSP tradition, a strong professional sport psychology organization, backed by a major national psychology association, and outstanding credentials as a convention destination.

Nonetheless, the Australian bid was run close by a late bid from Morocco. Although Morocco had little history in sport psychology or ISSP, it also boasted excellent convention facilities, as well as royal support. Furthermore, it fitted with the promotion of Africa, which ISSP had prioritized at that time, despite Morocco being only a short distance from Europe. Australia's weakness was its distance from nearly everywhere. We will never know precisely what swung the vote in ISSP MC to Australia, but one additional factor was probably crucial. Although the ISSP support for the development of sport psychology in Africa was important, in 2000, there were only a handful of established sport psychologists in the whole continent. Sport psychology in Asia had been the previous focus of ISSP aims to expand the discipline. Progress had been made, but only limited numbers of Asian sport psychologists attended ISSP World Congresses. One reason for this was the distance to Europe, where the previous three events had been held (Israel is actually involved in FEPSAC *and* ASPASP, but is much closer to the hub of Europe than to the center of Asia). Singapore, in 1989, had provided impetus for the development of ASPASP, and ISSP MC met in India in 1998 and in China in 2002, but, based on the growth occurring in Asian sport psychology, there was a need for a major sport psychology congress in a location accessible to Asian colleagues. Morris, as President of ASPASP, and his Asian colleagues on ISSP MC—Fujita, Likang Chi, and

Myung Woo Han—made the case for Sydney as that location and perhaps this won the day. At the General Assembly of ISSP in Skiathos in May 2001, it was announced that the World Congress of Sport Psychology in 2005 would be in Sydney, Australia.

Morris was appointed Chair of the Organizing Committee for the 2005 World Congress. Senior sport psychologists with conference organization experience, including Stephanie Hanrahan, Jeff Bond, and Peter Terry, joined the members of the Bid Committee—Gordon, Ievleva, and Tremayne—on the larger World Congress Organizing Committee. As a signal to colleagues in New Zealand that this was an Australasian event, Morris proposed that Gregory Kolt, an Australian then in a senior position in New Zealand, should join the Organizing Committee. For the next four years, this group worked to produce the biggest and most outstanding sport psychology event ever held in Australia. The Committee also set a goal of hosting a highly professional event for the ISSP and, most importantly, for sport and exercise psychology colleagues from all around the world.

To ensure the success of the event, the Australian Organizing Committee worked with award-winning Professional Convention Manager, Tour Hosts. Together they chose the world class Sydney Convention and Exhibition Centre as the venue for the World Congress. The Organizing Committee agreed on the eight Keynote Speakers with the ISSP Managing Council, which monitored and advised throughout the process. Keynotes spanned Motivation through Carol Dweck (USA), Applied Sport Psychology through Ken Ravizza (USA) and Sandy Gordon (Australia), Exercise Psychology through Nanette Mutrie (Scotland) and Dan Landers (USA), Psychophysiology through Brad Hatfield (USA), Motor Learning through Karl Newell (USA), and Cognitive Psychology through Franz Mechsner (Germany). Although the Organizing Committee and the ISSP Managing Council aimed to select a range of speakers to provide a broad geographical spread, ultimately quality was considered to be the first priority and North America continues to be a major source of significant work in sport and exercise psychology, especially when one is looking at long-term contributions to the field.

In addition to the Keynote Addresses, there were three more invited addresses, given by the recipients of the ISSP awards for distinguished achievements. A lifetime award for a distinguished career was given to Jurgen Nitsch (Germany). Nitsch was unable to attend the event, so ISSP President, Keith Henschen, joined Dieter Hackfort, who was to replace him at the General Assembly in Sydney, to present a review of Nitsch's contribution at the Congress. Early career awards were made to two young scholars, Sian Beilock (USA) and Hülya Aşçi (Turkey), and each presented an invited paper on her work.

Featuring information on the Keynote speakers, a call for the submission of papers was widely circulated by email and by post. Although the initial response was slow, a late flood of submissions put the scientific program at least on a par with any previous World Congress, with almost 600 accepted submissions. Those submissions came from more than 50 countries, representing every inhabited continent on earth. As anticipated, both the absolute number and the proportion of papers from Asian sport psychologists were substantially larger than at previous events. There were also substantial numbers of submissions from North American and British researchers and practitioners, but the number of Australians at the event and the number of presentations they made represented by far the largest contribution to the 11th ISSP World Congress.

The submissions from all delegates reflected the range from those still studying for their master's and doctoral qualifications to the most eminent researchers and applied sport psychologists in the field. It was pleasing to note the number of previous keynote speakers who were prepared to make the long trip from North America and Europe to meet again those colleagues who had lauded them at previous world congresses. Attendance of colleagues was particularly gratifying when considering the distance traveled to join the event. Of course, Australian-based attendees pointed out that they regularly traveled long distances in order to present at such events.

The organization of the ISSP 11th World Congress of Sport Psychology was carried off with hardly the blink of a problem. The venue was set up effectively and the support staff knew their jobs very well. All the oral presenters produced a polished performance and the many posters were high quality and well displayed. Each day there were two outstanding keynote presentations, multiple concurrent oral sessions, and substantial poster sessions. There was a good balance among research in sport psychology, applied sport psychology, exercise psychology, and motor learning papers.

Immediately prior to the World Congress, there was a Denis Glencross Memorial Workshop. This is an event that had been held in 1997 and 2001, in memory of the first and only ISSP President to pass away while in office. Denis Glencross was particularly committed to the development of sport psychology through its students, and accordingly, this workshop is a two-day event, offered only to students. It was fully subscribed and well received by sport and exercise psychology students from around the world.

Despite the wide range of interesting presentations from sport psychology enthusiasts young and old, there was no doubt that the keynote presentations held the greatest interest for the delegates. Hundreds came to the large auditorium to see and hear people whose work they have often read in books and journals. Thus, it is not surprising that we consider this book to have the potential to be a valuable resource for the field of sport and exercise psychology, allowing those keynote speakers not only the opportunity to reprise their roles at the World Congress, but also to expand on their presentations in a written form that provides a permanent record of the cumulative summary of their work. It is to that work, that is, the focus of this book, that we now turn our attention.

Invited Presentations and the Structure of
Sport and Exercise Psychology: International Perspectives

As noted earlier, we invited eight eminent scholars in the broad field of sport psychology to make keynote presentations at the 11th World Congress. We also invited presentations from the two ISSP early-career awardees and the researcher who were presented with the ISSP distinguished career award. Those 11 presentations reflected a wide range of topics within the broad discipline of sport psychology. At the Congress, one keynote speaker presented in mid-morning and another presented in mid-afternoon on each of the four days. The presentation on the work of the distinguished scholar was given on the second

day, and the two early-career invited presentations formed a session on the fourth and final morning of the Congress (following the formal announcement of their awards at the General Assembly on the third afternoon).

The sequence of invited presentations at the 11th World Congress, especially the keynote topics, was determined on the basis of a variety of factors. For example, some keynotes were juxtaposed against major symposia in that subdiscipline; for instance, a keynote on physical activity near a large symposium on mood and exercise or a keynote on motor skill on the same day as several concurrent sessions on aspects of motor learning and expert performance. Others were placed so that they preceded or followed, as requested by the keynote speaker, an invited symposium or workshop on the same topic that the keynote had organized. To provide coherence to this book, we have reorganized the topics into sections reflecting different aspects of the broad field of sport psychology. These sections, in the order in which they appear in the book, are: Sport Psychology Theory and Research; Sport Psychology Practice; Psychology of Exercise; Cognitive Psychology and Psychophysiology; and Motor Skill and Expert Performance. Unfortunately, the senior members of the ISSP Managing Council, who organized the symposium on Nitsch's Action Theory at the World Congress, were not in a position to provide a full chapter elaborating on Nitsch's work, so there are 10 chapters reflecting the work of the eight keynote speakers and the two early career awardees, with two chapters falling into each section. We sanctioned contributors' selection of a co-author for their chapter, usually because the keynote or awardee wished to recognize the contribution made to their work by a colleague.

Following this introductory chapter, Section I on Sport Psychology Theory and Practice includes two chapters. In Chapter 2, entitled "Self-Theories: The Mindset of a Champion," Carol Dweck discusses theory and research that underpin a perspective on what motivates elite athletes. Dweck's work on motivation for achievement in education has been influential in the development of a major body of knowledge related to achievement goal orientations in sport. Following Dweck's work is the chapter reflecting the early career contribution of Hülya Aşçi, entitled "Physical Self: Its Examination from Cultural and Mental Well-Being Perspectives." In Chapter 3, Aşçi writes about her substantial research on physical self-concept, in which she has collaborated with leading figures to examine the psychometric properties of key measures of physical self-concept in the Turkish language. Naturally, this research focuses particularly on the cross-cultural characteristics of physical self-concept.

Section II includes two chapters addressing aspects of Sport Psychology Practice. In Chapter 4, Sandy Gordon, renowned Australia-based applied sport psychologist with national cricket teams and professional golfers and football squads, considers a concept that goes right to the heart of sport psychology practice, especially in the sphere of elite sport, namely mental toughness. While addressing the difficult issue of defining mental toughness, Gordon, Daniel Gucciardi, and Timothy Chambers focus on a particular approach to mental toughness emanating from personal construct theory. The chapter is entitled "A Personal Construct Psychology Perspective on Sport and Exercise Psychology Research: The Example of Mental Toughness." Ken Ravizza, one of the USA's longest serving and most prestigious sport psychology practitioners, with experience in professional baseball, football, basketball, and track and field, writes about key elements of his approach to the application of psychology in sport. Chapter 5, by Ravizza and Traci Statler, is entitled "Lessons Learned from Sport Psychology Consulting."

Section III of *Sport and Exercise Psychology: International Perspectives* covers topics in the area of the psychology of exercise. Nanette Mutrie contributed Chapter 6 for this book, which is entitled "Applied Exercise Psychology: Promoting Activity and Evaluating Outcomes." In this chapter, Mutrie discusses the development and examination of interventions designed to increase physical activity in real-world contexts, as opposed to laboratory exercise studies. Mutrie also addresses the vexed issue of how changes in physical activity can be reliably measured in such contexts to determine if interventions have been effective. The third section of the book is completed by Chapter 7, entitled "Exercise Relative to Other Treatments for Reduction of Anxiety/Depression: Overcoming the Principle of Least Effort," contributed by keynote speaker Dan Landers.

One of the leaders of the development of theoretical sport psychology since the 1970s, Landers' attention has, for some time, largely turned to the area of exercise psychology. In particular, in Chapter 7, Landers and Brandon Alderman discuss the research that has been conducted on the benefits of exercise for the treatment of anxiety and depression, two highly prevalent and debilitating psychological disorders. Landers and Alderman also address the fact that many people take drugs to manage problems like anxiety and depression because it is easier than doing exercise, even though exercise has many other health benefits, whereas drugs might have negative side effects.

Research on the functioning of the brain and the nervous system is featured in Section IV of *Sport and Exercise Psychology: International Perspectives*, which is called "Cognitive Psychology and Psychophysiology." In Chapter 8, keynote speaker Franz Mechsner presents his work on bimanual coordination, in a chapter entitled "A Psychological Approach to the Organization of Voluntary Movements." As the chapter title intimates, Mechsner employs the movement of fingers, such as that of a pianist, as a method of understanding how the brain handles complex movement demands. Mechsner also demonstrates how principles identified in such basic movement research can be tested in real-world contexts such as the production of sport skills. In Chapter 9, a leading exponent of research on psychophysiological processes to sport, Brad Hatfield, presents some of the key findings of this research—which stands as the meeting place of psychology and physiology—and discusses their implications for sport. In this chapter entitled "Cognitive Neuroscience Aspects of Sport Psychology: Brain Mechanisms Underlying Performance," Hatfield shows how carefully structured studies in the laboratory can help us to address complex issues that directly affect performance.

Section V of the book includes two chapters that focus on issues in the area of motor skill and expert performance. Karl Newell, a long-time leader in the field of motor learning, discusses the integration of two traditions in Chapter 10, "Issues in Motor Learning for Instructional Strategies." In this chapter, Newell and S. Lee Hong address the application to themes in motor learning of the ecological psychology approach, which has become a major perspective in the field of motor learning. Completing the chapters by invited speakers from the ISSP 5th World Congress of Sport Psychology is Sian Beilock's chapter, "Understanding Skilled Performance: Memory, Attention, and Choking under Pressure." Beilock is winner of the ISSP early-career award for her work devising new ways to examine the phenomenon of choking, to explore psychological processes that underlie choking, and to test ways of reducing choking under pressure.

Sport and Exercise Psychology: International Perspectives is completed by an Epilogue, written by the editors. In that chapter, we reflect on the major scientific event that is the source of this book, namely the ISSP 11th World Congress of Sport Psychology, considering its successes and its shortcomings. We briefly assess the contributions to the present edited text, which aims to reflect and expand on the work of the invited speakers.

Conclusion

We feel the chapters in *Sport and Exercise Psychology: International Perspectives* reflect a range of important work in sport and exercise psychology, as well as clearly demonstrating the significant impact that the contributors have had on the field. Chapters in this book are destined to become classics in the field, pulling together, as they do, substantial bodies of work by the presenters and their colleagues. We were excited and gratified to give these outstanding sport and exercise psychologists a suitable stage to present their work at the World Congress, among nearly 600 of their peers. Equally, we are honored to have the opportunity to present the work of these esteemed colleagues in more detail and for a wider audience in this book. We trust that readers will appreciate the recognition that is at the heart of the invitations to present keynote papers and to make award-winners' presentations at the ISSP World Congress. We also feel great respect for these presenters, several of whom are undoubtedly doyens of sport and exercise psychology.

References

Fujita, A. H. (2006, May). Establishment of ASPASP in the worldwide trend of sport psychology. Paper presented at the *ISN International Sports Medicine and Science Conference*, Kuala Lumpur, Malaysia.

Griffith, C. R. (1926). *Psychology of coaching*. New York: Scribner.

Griffith, C. R. (1928). *Psychology of athletics*. New York: Scribner.

Lidor, R., & Bar-Eli, M. (Eds.). (1997). *Proceedings of the 9th World Congress of Sport Psychology*. Netanya, Israel: International Society of Sport Psychology.

Lidor, R., & Bar-Eli, M. (Eds.). (1998). *Sport psychology: Linking theory and practice*. Morgantown, WV: Fitness Information Technology.

Morris, T., Hackfort, D., & Lidor, R. (2003). From Pope to hope: The First 20 years of ISSP. *International Journal of Sport and Exercise Psychology, 1*, 119-137.

Morris, T., & Summers, J. (Eds.). (2004). *Sport psychology: Theory, applications and issues*. Brisbane, Australia: Wiley.

Morris, T., Terry, P., Ievleva, L., Gordon, S., Hanrahan, S., Kolt, G., & Tremayne, P. (Eds.). (2005). *Promoting performance and health: Proceedings of the ISSP XIth World Congress of Sport Psychology*. CD-ROM. Sydney, Australia: International Society of Sport Psychology.

Orlick, T., Partington, J. T., & Salmela, J. H. (1982). *Mental training for coaches and athletes*. Ottawa, Canada: Sport in Perspective and Coaching Association of Canada.

Pappaouannou, A., Goudas, M., & Theodorakis, Y. (2001). *In the dawn of the new millennium*. Thessaloniki, Greece: Christodoulidi Publications.

Partington, J. T., Orlick, T., & Salmela, J. H. (1982). *Sport in perspective*. Ottawa, Canada: Sport in Perspective and Coaching Association of Canada.

Salmela, J. H. (1997). In R. Lidor, & M. Bar-Eli (Eds.), *The Antonelli years of the ISSP. Proceedings of the 9th World Congress of Sport Psychology* (pp. 596-598). Netanya, Israel: International Society of Sport Psychology.

Salmela, J. H., Partington, J. T., & Orlick, T. (1982). *New paths of sport learning and excellence*. Ottawa, Canada: Sport in Perspective and Coaching Association of Canada.

Serpa, S., Alves, J,. Ferreira, V., & Paula-Brito, A. (Eds.). (1993). *Sport psychology: An integrated approach*. Lisbon, Portugal: International Society of Sport Psychology.

Serpa, S., Alves, J., Ferreira, V., & Paula-Brito, A. (Eds.). (1994). *International perspectives in sport and exercise psychology*. Morgantown, WV: Fitness Information Technology.

Vanek, M. (1993). Reflections on the inception, development, and perspectives of ISSP's image and self-image. In S. Serpa, J. Alves, V. Ferreira, & A. Paula-Brito (Eds.), *Proceedings of the 8th World Congress of Sport Psychology* (pp. 154-158). Lisbon, Portugal: International Society of Sport Psychology.

Vanek, M. (1994). Reflections on the inception, development, and perspectives of ISSP's image and self-image. In S. Serpa, J. Alves, V. Ferreira, & A. Paula-Brito (Eds.). (1994). *International perspectives in sport and exercise psychology*. Morgantown, WV: Fitness Information Technology.

Williams, J. M. (Ed.). (2005). *Applied sport psychology: Personal growth to peak performance* (5th ed.). Mountain View, CA: Mayfield.

Section I
Sport Psychology Theory and Research

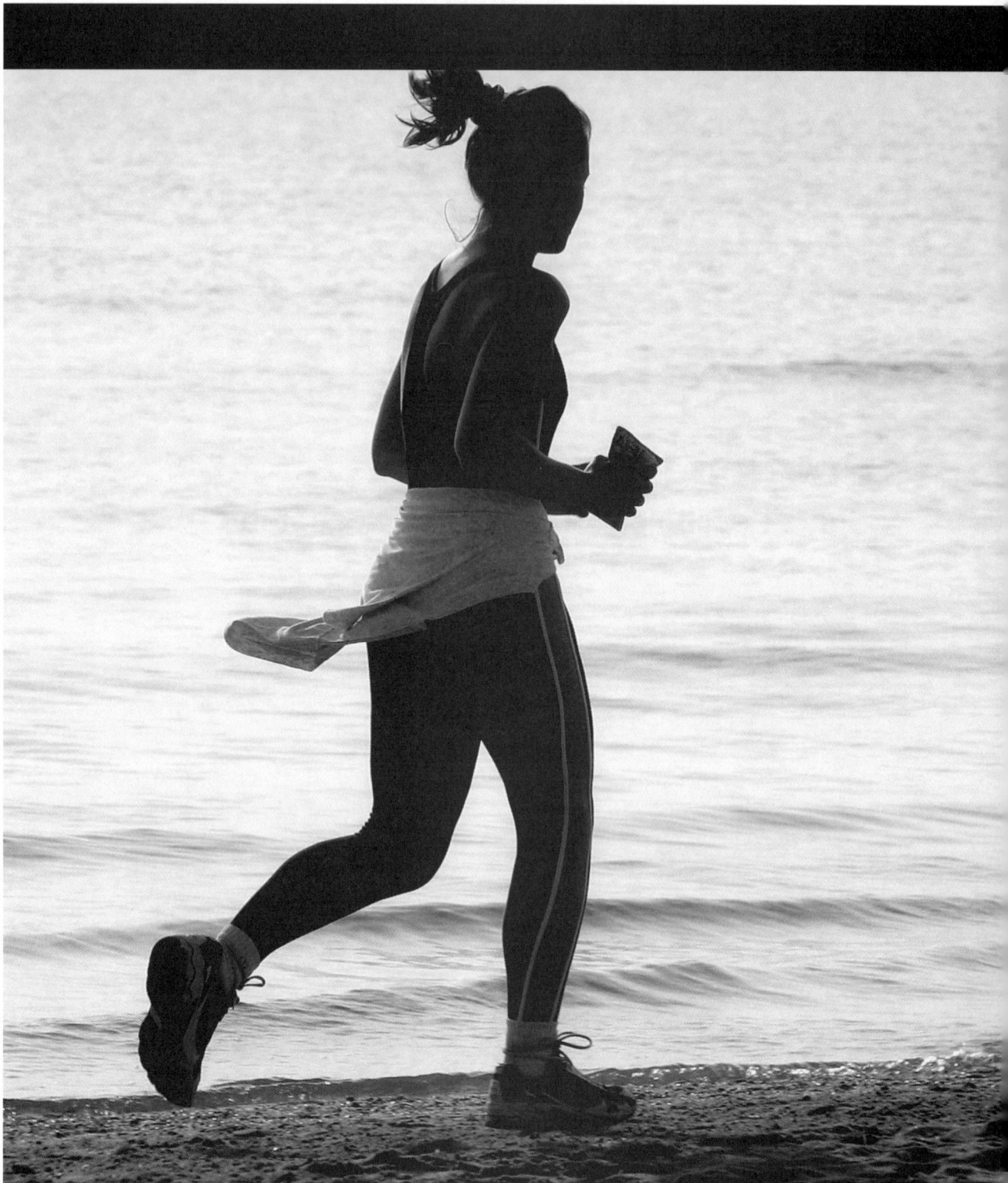

Courtesy of istockphoto.com

2

Self-Theories: The Mindset of a Champion

CAROL S. DWECK

There are things that distinguish great athletes—champions—from others. Most of the sports world thinks it's talent. I will argue that it's *mindset*. This idea is brought to life by the story of Billy Beane, told so well by Michael Lewis in the book *Moneyball* (Lewis, 2003). When Beane was in high school, he was in fact a huge talent—what they call a "natural." He was the star of the basketball team, the football team, and the baseball team. *And he was all of these things without much effort.* People thought he was the new Babe Ruth.

However, as soon as anything went wrong, Beane lost it. He didn't know how to learn from his mistakes, nor did he know how to practice in order to improve. Why? Because naturals shouldn't make mistakes or need practice. When Beane moved up to baseball's major leagues, things got progressively worse. Every at-bat was a do-or-die situation and with every out he fell apart yet again. If you're a natural, you shouldn't have deficiencies, so you can't face them and coach or practice them away.

Beane's contempt for learning and his inability to function in the face of setbacks—where did these come from? With avid practice and the right coaching he could have been one of the greats. Why didn't he seek that? I will show how his behavior comes right out of his self-theory.

Self-Theories

In my work, I have identified two theories of ability that people may hold (Dweck, 1999; Dweck & Leggett, 1988). Some hold an entity theory, in which they see abilities as fixed traits. In this view, talents are gifts—you either have them or you don't. I also call this the "fixed mindset" (Dweck, 2006).

Other people, in contrast, hold an incremental theory of ability. They believe that people can cultivate their abilities. In other words, they view talents as potentialities that can be developed through practice. It's not that people holding this theory deny differences among people. They don't deny that some people may be better or faster than others at acquiring certain skills, but what they focus on is the idea that everyone can get better over time. I also call this view the "growth mindset."

Here are some questions that are frequently asked about self-theories:

Which theory is correct? Psychologists have advocated both theories, but, with respect to the trait of intelligence, it is interesting to note that Alfred Binet (the inventor of the IQ test) held a radical incremental theory (Binet, 1909/1973). Without denying individual differences, he believed that the most basic ability to think and learn could be transformed through education. It is also true, in line with this, that modern neuroscience is revealing the great plasticity of the human brain throughout life (see, for example, Kass, 2001).

Which theory is most popular? When we examine people's theories about intelligence or personality, we find that both theories are just about equally popular. It seems that both messages are available in our culture.

Do people hold the same theories with respect to different traits? Not necessarily. People can hold one theory about intelligence and another about sports ability. Moreover, whichever theory they hold in a given area will guide their motivation in that area.

Are people's theories related to their level of ability in the area? No, at least not at first. People with all skill levels can hold either theory, but over time those with the incremental theory appear to gain an advantage (Aronson, Fried, & Good, 2002; Blackwell, Trzesniewski, & Dweck, 2006; Good, Aronson, & Inzlicht, 2003; Robins & Pals, 2002).

Are self-theories fixed or can they be changed? Self-theories are fairly stable beliefs, but they are beliefs, and beliefs can be changed. Later on, I will discuss interventions that altered self-theories and had a real effect on motivation and performance.

Self-Theories and Goals

We have found in our research that people's theories or mindsets set up completely different motivational systems (Molden & Dweck, 2006). The fixed theory, in which you have only a certain amount of a valued talent or ability, leads people to put a premium on "performance goals." A performance goal is the goal of proving that you have an admirable amount of that talent or ability. Not surprisingly, when people are focused on performance goals, they try to highlight their proficiencies and hide their deficiencies (Rhodewalt, 1994). In fact, we have found, they will often reject valuable learning opportunities if these opportunities hold the risk of unmasking their shortcomings (Dweck & Leggett, 1988; Hong, Chiu, Dweck, Lin, & Wan, 1999; Mueller & Dweck, 1998).

Doesn't everyone have shortcomings? Isn't that what learning is for—to overcome them? Of course. However, the fixed mindset does not give people the leeway to expose and remedy their weaknesses because any weakness can indicate a permanent lack of ability.

In contrast, the incremental theory, in which ability can be developed, leads people to want to do just that. It leads them to put a premium on "learning goals" (see Duda, 1998). This difference in goal-seeking is starkly demonstrated in a study I conducted with Ying-yi Hong, C.Y. Chiu, Derek Lin, and Wendy Wan (1999). We recruited entering students at the University of Hong Kong, an elite university where everything—classes, textbooks, term papers, exams—is in English. However, not all incoming students are proficient in English. We assumed they would be eager to improve their skills and asked how many of them would take a remedial English class if it were offered. Students with an incremental theory of intelligence were eager for this course. It could help them master the very skills they needed. However, students with an entity theory were not enthusiastic. Because they did not want to expose their deficiency, they were not willing to put their college career in jeopardy.

In another study (Mueller & Dweck, 1998), we've seen students in a fixed mindset lie about their deficiencies. Students performed some very challenging sets of problems and then were asked to write about their experiences to students in another school—students they would never meet. There was a place on the sheet where they were asked to report their scores. Almost 40% of the students in the fixed mindset, perhaps feeling that their poor scores were a reflection of their permanent ability, lied about their scores. Only 10% of those in the growth mindset saw fit to falsify their performance. Like Billy Beane, those in the fixed mindset didn't think they should make mistakes.

We have also studied the brain to examine the impact of self-theories on people's attention to performance-relevant information or to learning-relevant information (Dweck, Mangels, & Good, 2004). Here, college students came to the EEG lab, where an electrode cap was placed on their heads, and recordings were made from the parts of the brain that reflected attentional processes as they performed a highly difficult task. Each time they answered a question on the task, they were told whether their answer was correct or incorrect, and then a little later were told the correct answer. What we found was eye-opening.

Students who held an incremental theory of intelligence paid close attention to the performance-relevant feedback *and* the learning-relevant feedback, because both are actually important for future learning. In contrast, the students who held an entity theory of intelligence, paid attention only to the performance-relevant information. Once they knew whether their answer was right or wrong, they had little further interest in learning the right answer. Thus, their interest in performance took strong precedence over their interest in learning. In later research, we showed that this significantly hurt their subsequent performance on a re-test of the material (Mangels, Butterfield, Lamb, Good, & Dweck, 2006).

By the way, it's clear that both performance and learning goals are important in a sports setting. It's equally important to validate ability through high quality performance as it is to cultivate skill over time. The problem with an entity theory is twofold. First, any lapse in performance is a threat to people's sense of their underlying ability, and hence, their sense of their future. Secondly, great concern with ability tends to drive out learning goals, often when they are most needed. It's hard to see how people can thrive in the world of sports if they don't have strong learning goals.

Self-Theories and Effort

As we have seen, people in the fixed mindset feel measured by setbacks and mistakes. They also feel measured by the very fact of exerting effort. They believe, like Billy Beane, that if you have ability, you shouldn't need effort (Blackwell, Trzesniewski, & Dweck, 2007). Things come easily, they say, to people who are true geniuses. Yet, there is no important endeavor in life—certainly not in the sports world—that can be accomplished without intense and sustained effort. A mindset of fixed ability, however, interprets effort as a sign that talent or ability is lacking.

In contrast, people in the growth mindset understand that effort is the way that ability is brought to life and allowed to reach fruition. Far from indicating a lack of talent, they believe that even geniuses need great effort to fulfill their promise. In other words, they subscribe to Thomas Edison's formula: Genius is 1% inspiration and 99% perspiration. By the way, Edison should know. He was not a born genius laboring in solitude (Israel, 1998). In fact, he had a large, state-of-the-art lab with many scientists and technicians, and he labored for years to build his skills and arrive at his great discoveries.

Incremental theorists not only believe in the *power* of effort, they hold effort as a *value*. Ian Thorpe, the illustrious Australian swimmer, feels that as long as he's tried his best, he's been victorious. "For myself, losing is not coming second. It's getting out of the water and knowing you could have done better. For myself, I have won every race I've ever been in" (www.brainyquote.com/quotes/quotes/i/ianthorpe167157.html).

Self-Theories and Mastery-Oriented Coping

It will come as no surprise that the self-theories, with their different emphases on learning and effort, lead to different ways of coping with difficulty. Basically, the entity theory often leaves people few good ways of reacting to setbacks. In one study (Blackwell, et al., 2007), we compared students with an entity theory to those with an incremental theory of intelligence, and found that those with entity theory were more likely to say that if they did poorly on a test—even if it were in a new course and one they liked a lot—they would study *less* in the future and would seriously consider cheating. This is how people cope when they think setbacks mean they lack permanent ability. In contrast, those students with an incremental theory said they would study more or study differently. They planned to take charge of the situation and work to overcome the setback.

When the going gets rough, people in the incremental/learning framework not only take charge of improving their skills, they take charge of their *motivation* as well (Grant, 2004). Despite setbacks—or even because of them—they find ways to keep themselves committed and interested. On the other hand, students with an entity/performance framework lose interest as they lose confidence. As the difficulty mounts, their commitment and enjoyment go down. Since all important pursuits in life involve setbacks sooner or later (more likely, sooner *and* later), it is a serious liability to lose interest and enjoyment simply because greater effort is required.

Thus, an entity theory framework leads people to value looking good over learning, to disdain and to fear effort, and to abandon effective strategies when they are needed the most. An incremental framework, on the other hand, leads people to seek challenges and learning, to value effort, and to persist effectively in the face of obstacles. What's more, it allows people to sustain their enjoyment even when the going gets rough.

Billy Beane, over time, actually came to recognize that these incremental ingredients—the ability to see setbacks as a natural part of learning, to improve through effort, and to sustain enjoyment and commitment—were keys to success in the sports world (Lewis, 2003). With this knowledge, as general manager of the Oakland Athletics, he led his team to several seasons of almost record-breaking wins on one of the lowest budgets in baseball.

Naturals Revisited

But aren't there people who *are* true naturals? Michael Jordan? Babe Ruth? Wasn't Babe Ruth this out-of-shape guy who dragged his paunch to the plate and belted out his home runs? An examination of almost any of the greats will reveal people who practiced like fiends and honed their skills over many years. The story of Babe Ruth's development as a home-run king is surprising (Creamer, 1974/1983). Ty Cobb argued that it was Ruth's career as a pitcher that helped him become a great hitter. No one ex-

pected a pitcher to hit well, so Ruth could experiment with his big swing, seeing what worked and what didn't. When it didn't work, nobody cared. After all, he was the pitcher. Over time, he learned more and more about how to control his swing, so that when he became an outfielder, he was ready to hit. And hit he did.

Any "natural" you can name—Jackie Joyner-Kersee, Mia Hamm, Muhammad Ali—just look more closely and you can see the discipline, perseverance, and commitment that went into their success. Sure, they had talent, but they also had the right mindset.

Self-Theories and Confidence

Isn't motivation just a matter of confidence? To some extent, yes; however, one of the most fascinating findings in all of my research is the fact that within the incremental framework, with its focus on growth, it is far easier to sustain confidence (Blackwell, et al., 2007; Grant & Dweck, 2003; Mueller & Dweck, 1998; see also Jourden, Bandura, & Banfield, 1991; Martocchio, 1994; Wood & Bandura, 1989). In the entity framework, with its focus on proving ability, a poor performance casts doubt on deep-seated ability and can undermine confidence. Someone else's good performance can undermine your confidence: "Maybe they have more talent than I do" (Butler, 2000). Even needing effort and practice can undermine your confidence—so it's a constant battle to stay confident in the face of inevitable challenges.

Within the incremental framework, making mistakes or even having an obvious deficit doesn't mean you aren't good at something or won't be good at it in the future. It's simply an occasion for learning. Moreover, a wagon-load of confidence isn't needed to embark on learning. The real necessity is a belief in improvement over time.

Some years ago, I received a letter from a competitive swimmer who had come across my work. She told me she had always had a confidence problem. Coaches told her to believe in herself 100%—never to doubt herself—but she couldn't do it. Every time she posted a disappointing time or lost a meet, she fell into self-doubt. However, thinking from the perspective of a learning framework, where setbacks are just information about what you need to do in the future, allowed her to maintain confidence in those very same situations. The setbacks simply meant: Get back to work.

The Idea of Potential

Many of the scouts in the sports world scout for naturals, for people who look like superstars, that is, are shaped like superstars and move like superstars (Lewis, 2003). If they don't look the part, they aren't recruited. Yet Ben Hogan, one of the greatest golfers of all time, did not have the grace of a natural golfer. Muhammad Ali actually did not have the build of the natural boxer. He did not have a champion's fists, reach, chest expansion, and heft. People gave him no chance against Sonny Liston, who seemed to have it all (Dennis & Atyeo, 2003). Mugsy Bogues at 5'3" or the little quarterback Doug Flutie—anyone could look at them and tell you they were not naturals and by that they would mean they did not have the potential to make it.

Given the nature of the entity theory framework of fixed traits, it is easy to (incorrectly) assess potential. You just look at the person's gifts right now and project them into the future. Talented now equals talented in the future. Not talented now equals not talented in the future.

Yet, within an incremental framework, potential is difficult to judge. Sure "natural talent" buys you a lot, and if you're accomplished now, you've got a leg up on others. But after that you cannot know where someone might end up with years of passion, discipline, and commitment—and good instruction.

The most dramatic example of how hard it is to judge potential from current ability is contained in the book *Drawing on the Right Side of the Brain* (Edwards, 1999). The author, Betty Edwards, is an art professor who leads workshops for people who wish to learn to draw better. In her book, she shows the self-portraits drawn on Day 1 by the students in one of her workshops. Some of the self-portraits are excellent and others are the equivalent of stick figures—primitive, childish, and completely devoid of talent. She then shows the self-portraits done by these same people five days later at the end of the workshop. *All* of them are amazing—detailed, dramatic, professional. What's more is that those who started out better did not necessarily end up better.

Now, drawing is often considered to be one of those "natural" talents; you either have it or you don't. Yet Edwards' students' before-and-after pictures demonstrate the striking fact that diagnosing people's talent at Time 1 does not tell you their ability at Time 2. When people don't do well without instruction, it does not tell you that they will still lag behind others when they do have instruction.

Self-Theories in Sport

Recently, Stuart Biddle and his colleagues (Biddle, Wang, Chatzisarantis, & Spray, 2003; Sarrazin, Biddle, Famose, Cury, Fox, & Durand, 1996) and Yngvar Ommundsen (2001, 2003) have taken self-theories directly into the domain of sports. Biddle and his colleagues (Sarrazin, et al., 1996) have created a questionnaire that assesses young people's entity and incremental theories about their sports ability. For example, belief in an entity theory is represented by statements like:

"You have a certain level of ability in sport and you cannot really do much to change that level."

"Even if you try, the level you reach in sport will change very little."

"To be good at sport you need to be naturally gifted."

An incremental theory and a learning approach are represented by statements like:

"How good you are at sport will always improve if you work at it."

"If you put enough effort into it, you will always get better at sport."

*To be successful in sport you need to learn techniques and skills and practice them regularly."

This questionnaire has produced many interesting findings, and here is a sampling:

Goals: First, entity and incremental beliefs predict different goals and views of success, with entity theorists saying they feel most successful when they beat out others (a common and legitimate, yet limiting view of success in sports), but incremental theorists saying they feel most successful when they improve and master new things (a view that will serve best in the long haul). Indeed, *many* top athletes (like Ian Thorpe and Tiger Woods) and coaches (like the legendary coach John Wooden) stress that they care less about the win *per se* than the knowledge that they have given all and stretched themselves.

Enjoyment: An incremental view also predicted the extent to which participants said they enjoyed sports. Incremental athletes like Michael Jordan and Tiger Woods love their sport, but entity athletes like John McEnroe, although as talented as they come, did not. McEnroe was so focused on winning and so anxious about looking good that he lost any zest for the game that he might have had when he started out (McEnroe, 2002). (By the way, by his own admission, his tantrums were designed to cover up the fact that he was losing his grip on a match. Such defensiveness, in place of perseverance, is yet another symptom of the entity framework.)

Here are some findings from the work of Ommundsen (2001, 2003):

Goals: Indicative of incremental theorists' learning stance was their willingness to ask for help (instead of hiding their deficiencies).

Enjoyment vs. Anxiety: Ommundsen found, as well, that holding an entity theory directly gave rise to increased levels of anxiety and reduced satisfaction in physical education classes, as indicated by agreement with the following statements:

Anxiety: "Before I compete, I worry about not performing well."

Satisfaction: "When taking part in PE, I usually wish the class would end quickly."

As opposed to:

"I usually enjoy taking part in PE lessons."

"I usually find that time flies when I am taking part in PE activities."

Helpless vs. Mastery-Oriented Reactions: In his research, Ommundsen also found that an incremental theory predicted a mastery-oriented, persistent, analytic stance toward sports:

"If the activities or exercises are difficult to understand, I change the way I approach them."

As opposed to:

"When the activities or exercises are difficult, I give up or take on the easy ones."

Finally, Ommundsen found that an entity theory predicted self-handicapping, a defensive strategy designed to protect people's view of their ability even as it sabotages their chances for success. Specifically, holding an entity theory was positively related to (and holding an incremental theory was negatively related to) the tendency to recognize oneself in the following statements:

"Some pupils fool around the night before a test in PE so that if they don't do as well as they hoped, they can say that is the reason."

"Some pupils let their friends keep them from paying attention in PE classes or from practicing. Then if they don't do well they can say that is the reason."

Thus, this work, which takes self-theories directly into the world of sport, provides exciting support for the view that passion and excellence in sport are guided by people's self-theories about their sports abilities.

Where Do Self-Theories Come From?

More and more we are finding that self-theories are fostered by the kind of feedback students get from the people who evaluate them: their parents, their teachers, and presumably, their coaches. Specifically, the self-theories are fostered by a focus on *traits* (e.g., talent or ability) as opposed to a focus on *process* (e.g., effort or learning) (Dweck & Lennon, 2001; Kamins & Dweck, 1999; Mueller & Dweck, 1998).

First, we have found that when adults evaluate youth on their traits (like intelligence or goodness)—even when the adult offers praise for these traits—it promotes an entity theory framework (Kamins & Dweck, 1999; Mueller & Dweck, 1998). For example, in one set of studies (Mueller & Dweck, 1998), we gave children some problems to solve from a nonverbal IQ test and then, in one condition, lauded their performance and praised them for their intelligence. These children

- now favored an entity theory of intelligence (compared to a group that was praised for their effort),

- rejected an opportunity to learn a new task in favor of a chance to look smart again,

- lost interest in the task when it became harder, and

- performed poorly on the trial that followed the difficult problems.

These are the children who lied about their performance when asked to report about the task and their scores to students in another school.

In contrast, students who were praised for the *process* they engaged in—in this case, their effort—rather than for their traits:

- now expressed a more incremental theory of intelligence,

- overwhelmingly went for the task that would give them a chance to learn,

- maintained their interest when the task became harder, even when it exceeded their abilities, and

- performed exceedingly well on the trial that followed the difficult problems.

Further, we have found that adolescents who endorse an entity theory report that their parents tend to give them feedback that focuses on their underlying traits, whereas adolescents who have an incremental theory report that their parents focus on giving them feedback about their *process*—learning, studying, effort, strategies (Dweck & Lennon, 2001). We are now following up on this by studying groups of parents and their children over time (Pomerantz & Dweck, 2006.)

It would be fascinating to look at this with coaches too. The illustrious John Wooden, who coached the UCLA basketball team to 10 NCAA championships, constantly focused on his players' learning and improvement (Wooden, 1972, 1997). Although he recognized that some players had more talent than others, he was committed to developing each player's ability to the fullest.

As an example, he recruited another player the same year that he recruited the great Bill Walton. He informed this player, who played the same position as Walton, that he might get very little playing time in actual games, but he assured him that he would be offered a professional contract when he graduated. True to Wooden's promise, this player not only got a pro contract, but was also named rookie of the year in his league.

Moreover, Wooden tells countless stories about players who arrived at UCLA seeming like sorry (even hopeless) raw material, but eventually blossomed into top players on his championship teams. By focusing on process and learning, Wooden seemed to imbue his players with a belief in their own development, a belief that paid good dividends.

Can Self-Theories Be Changed?

Can an incremental theory be taught and will people reap benefits from learning it? In four studies to date—two from my laboratory (Blackwell, et al., 2007; Blackwell, Trzesniewski, & Dweck, 2006) and two by Joshua Aronson, Catherine Good, and their colleagues (Aronson, Fried, & Good, 2002; Good, Aronson, & Inzlicht, 2003)—workshops have been developed to teach an incremental theory. In these workshops, students (from junior high through college, depending on the study) learned that the brain was a dynamic, malleable organ and that every time they learned something, their brain formed new connections. Over time, these proliferating connections would make them smarter. Students were also shown how this idea could be applied to their schoolwork. These interventions were relatively modest but had immediate and striking effects.

In every one of these studies, students who learned the incremental theory of intelligence showed significant gains in grades and/or achievement test scores. In some studies, these gains were made relative to control groups that were also given noteworthy interventions, such as training sessions in study skills.

In one of our studies (Blackwell et al., in press), teachers singled out the students who had been in the incremental intervention and noted clear changes in their motivation (even though these teachers were blind to the intervention condition). Here are some of the things they said:

> "L., who never puts in any extra effort and often doesn't turn in homework on time, actually stayed up late working for hours to finish an assignment early so I could review it and give him a chance to revise it. He earned a B+ on the assignment (he had been getting C's and lower)."

> "Lately I have noticed that some students have a greater appreciation for improvement … R. was performing below standards … He has learned to appreciate the improvement from his grades of 52, 46, and 49 to his grades of 67 and 71 … He valued his growth in learning Mathematics."

"M. was far below grade level. During the past several weeks, she has voluntarily asked for extra help from me during her lunch period in order to improve her test-taking performance. Her grades drastically improved from failing to an 84 on the most recent exam."

"Positive changes in motivation and behavior are noticeable in K. and J. They have begun to work hard on a consistent basis."

"Several students have voluntarily participated in peer tutoring sessions during their lunch periods or after school. Students such as N. and S. were passing when they requested the extra help and were motivated by the prospect of sheer improvement."

These findings brought home the idea that motivation and love of learning are always lurking there, right beneath the surface. No one ever lives happily ever after with the idea that they're stupid or incapable of learning. As L., the young man in the quote above, said as we introduced the incremental theory, "You mean I don't have to be dumb?" The incremental theory allows people to open up to the possibility of growth and improvement, a possibility that may have seemed closed to them before.

It would be fascinating to see how an incremental intervention works in the domain of sport, to see the impact that it has on the desire to practice, the enjoyment of sport, and the ability to cope effectively with setbacks, especially for those who have been turned off the joy of sport.

It would also be fascinating to look at the impact of such interventions on elite athletes as well. Would it help "naturals" to develop the incremental attitudes and habits that would allow them to fulfill their potential, rather than going the way of Billy Beane?

Finally, it would be fascinating to see what an incremental intervention does for teamwork. Instead of each player vying to be the most talented star, always trying to look better than his or her teammates, would an incremental theory foster a more cooperative, learning-together environment?

Conclusion

Without denying the importance of that thing called "talent," I have tried to show that something else—an athlete's mindset—can be equally important. I have described one mindset, built around a belief in fixed traits, that limits athletes' ability to fulfill their potential. It does so by making them prize looking good over learning, by making their confidence vulnerable in the face of setbacks, and by fostering defensive strategies over perseverance and commitment.

And I have described another mindset, built around the belief in expandable skills, that can foster athletes' ability to fulfill their potential by making them prize learning, by making confidence (in improvement) easier to maintain, and by fostering effective strategies and sustained effort in the face of difficulty.

Even more important, this mindset can be learned.

References

Aronson, J., Fried, C., & Good, C. (2002). Reducing the effects of stereotype threat on African American college students by shaping theories of intelligence. *Journal of Experimental Social Psychology, 38*, 113-125.

Biddle, S .J .H., Wang, J., Chatzisarantis, N., & Spray, C. M. (2003). Motivation for physical activity in young people: Entity and incremental beliefs about athletic ability. *Journal of Sports Sciences, 21*, 973-989.

Binet, A. (1909/1973). *Les idees modernes sur les enfants* [Modern ideas on children]. Paris: Flamarion.

Blackwell, L. S., Trzesniewski, K., & Dweck, C. S. (in press). Implicit theories of intelligence predict achievement across an adolescent transition: A longitudinal study and an intervention. *Child Development.*

Blackwell, L. S., Trzesniewski, K., & Dweck, C. S. (2006). A computer-based intervention for teaching students about the brain, learning, and theories of intelligence. Unpublished data, Columbia University.

Butler, R. (2000). Making judgments about ability: The role of implicit theories of ability in moderating inferences from temporal and social comparison information. *Journal of Personality & Social Psychology, 78*, 965-978.

Creamer, R. W. (1974/1983) *Babe: The legend comes to life.* New York: Penguin Books.

Dennis, F., & Atyeo, D. (2003). *Muhammad Ali: The glory years.* New York: Hyperion.

Duda, J .L. (Ed.). (1998). *Advances in sport and exercise psychology measurement.* Morgantown, WV: Fitness Information Technology.

Dweck, C. S. (1999). *Self-theories: Their role in motivation, personality, and development.* Philadelphia: Psychology Press.

Dweck, C. S. (2006). *Mindset.* New York: Random House.

Dweck, C. S., & Leggett, E .L. (1988). A social-cognitive approach to motivation and personality, *Psychological Review, 95,* 256-273.

Dweck, C. S., & Lennon, C. (April, 2001). *Person vs. process-focused parenting styles.* Symposium paper presented at the Meeting of the Society for Research in Child Development. Minneapolis, MN.

Dweck, C. S., Mangels, J., & Good, C. (2004). Motivational effects on attention, cognition, and performance. In D.Y. Dai & R. J. Sternberg (Eds.), *Motivation, emotion, and cognition: Integrated perspectives on intellectual functioning.* Mahwah, NJ: Erlbaum.

Edwards, B. (1999). *The new drawing on the right side of the brain.* New York: Tarcher/Putnam.

Good, C. Aronson, J., & Inzlicht, M. (2003). Improving adolescents' standardized test performance: An intervention to reduce the effects of stereotype threat. *Journal of Applied Developmental Psychology, 24,* 645-662.

Grant, H. (2004). *Goal orientations influence both knowledge and use of self-regulated learning strategies.* Unpublished data, New York University.

Grant, H. & Dweck, C. S. (2003). Clarifying achievement goals and their impact. *Journal of Personality and Social Psychology, 85,* 541-553.

Hong, Y., Chiu, C., Dweck, C. S., Lin, D., & Wan, W. (1999) Implicit theories, attributions, and coping: A meaning system approach. *Journal of Personality and Social Psychology, 77,* 588-599.

Israel, P. (1998). *Edison: A life of invention.* New York: Wiley.

Jourden, F. J., Bandura, A., & Banfield, J. T. (1991). The impact of conceptions of ability on self-regulatory factors and motor skill acquisition. *Journal of Sport and Exercise Psychology, 13,* 213-226.

Kamins, M. & Dweck, C. S. (1999). Person vs. process praise and criticism: Implications for contingent self-worth and coping. *Developmental Psychology, 35,* 835-847.

Kass, J. H. (Ed.). (2001). *The mutable brain: Dynamic and plastic features of the developing and mature brain.* Amsterdam: Harwood.

Lewis, M. (2003). *Moneyball: The art of winning an unfair game.* New York: Norton.

McEnroe, J. (with Kaplan, J.).(2002). *You cannot be serious.* New York: Berkley.

Mangels, J. A., Butterfield, B., Lamb, J., Good, C.D., & Dweck, C.S. (2006, in press). Why do beliefs about intelligence influence learning success? A social-cognitive-neuroscience model. *Social, Cognitive, and Affective Neuroscience.*

Martocchio, J. J. (1994). Effects of conceptions of ability on anxiety, self-efficacy, and learning in training. *Journal of Applied Psychology, 79,* 819-825.

Molden, D. C., & Dweck, C. S. (2006). Finding "meaning" in psychology: A lay theories approach to self-regulation, social perception, and social development. *American Psychologist, 61,* 192-203.

Mueller, C. M. & Dweck, C. S. (1998). Intelligence praise can undermine motivation and performance. *Journal of Personality and Social Psychology, 75,* 33-52.

Ommundsen, Y. (2001). Pupils' affective responses in physical education classes: The association of implicit theories of the nature of ability and achievement goals. *European Physical Education Review, 7,* 219-242.

Ommundsen, Y. (2003). Implicit theories of ability and self-regulation strategies in physical education classes. *Educational Psychology, 23,* 141-157.

Park, C. L., & Folkman, S. (1997). Meaning in the context of stress and coping. *Review of General Psychology, 1,* 115-144.

Pomerantz, E., & Dweck, C. S. (2006). *The impact of parents' judgment vs. process feedback on children's self-theories.* Research in progress, University of Illinois.

Rhodewalt, F. (1994). Conceptions of ability, achievement goals, and individual differences in self-handicapping behavior: On the application of implicit theories. *Journal of Personality, 62,* 67-85.

Robins, R. W. & Pals, J. L. (2002). Implicit self-theories in the academic domain: Implications for goal orientation, attributions, affect, and self-esteem change. *Self and Identity, 1,* 313-336.

Sarrazin, P., Biddle, S. J. H., Famose, J. P., Cury, F., Fox, K., & Durand, M. (1966). Goal orientation and conceptions of the nature of sport ability in children: A social cognitive approach. *British Journal of Social Psychology, 35,* 399-414.

Wood, R., & Bandura, A. (1989). Impact of conceptions of ability on self-regulatory mechanisms and complex decision making. *Journal of Personality and Social Psychology, 56,* 407-415.

Wooden, J. (with Jamison, S.). (1997). *Wooden: A lifetime of observations and reflections on and off the court.* Lincolnwood, IL: Contemporary Books.

Wooden, J. (with Tobin, J.). (1972). *They call me coach.* Waco, TX: World Books.

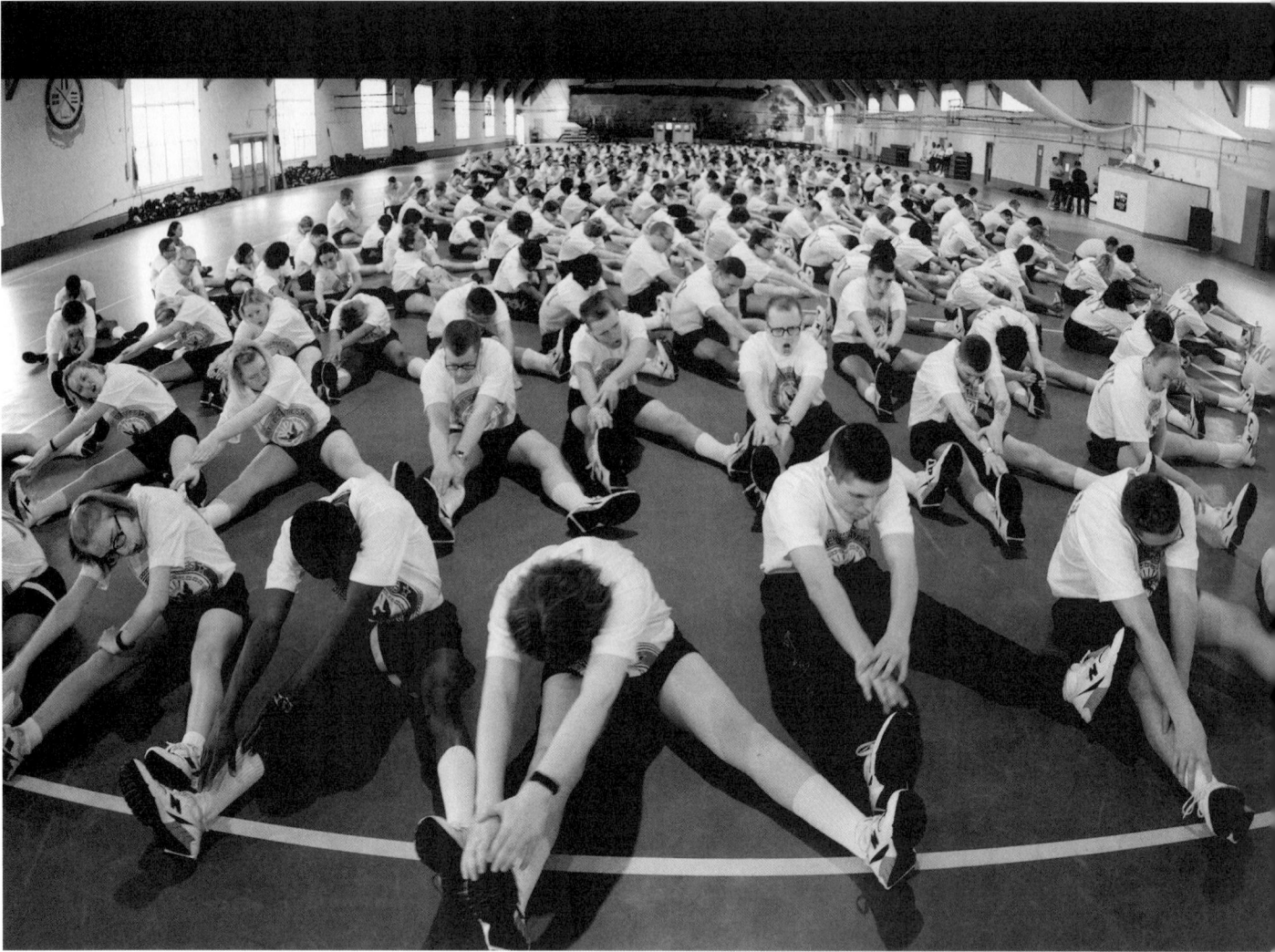

Courtesy of U.S. Navy

3

Physical Self:
Its Examination from
Cultural and
Mental Well-Being
Perspectives

F. HÜLYA AŞÇI

During the past decade there has been a re- surgence of interest in the self that has fo- cused on the study of individual differences as well as developmental change. Much of this work can be subsumed under the general rubric of *self-concept,* or under the more specifically evaluative component of self-concept referred to as *self-esteem*, or (synonymously as) *self-worth*. This proliferation of interest has been largely stimulated by the emerging important dual role that self-esteem has been shown to play as both a human mental health and as a mo- tivational variable (Fox, 1990; Harter, 1990; Marsh, 1993a). Research has shown that self-esteem is asso- ciated with many positive achievements and social related behaviors, including leadership ability, satis- faction, decreased anxiety, and improved academic and physical performance (Fox, 1992). Additionally, "interest in self-esteem stems from its recognition as a valued outcome in itself, the assumption that the improvements of self-esteem may facilitate improve- ments in other areas" (Marsh, Smith, Barnes, Butler, 1983, p. 772). Fox (1988, 1990) believed that much of what we do, whether conscious or not, is directed towards maximizing our chances of feeling good about ourselves: We learn to avoid situations that call our confidence into question and expose us to our inadequacies and we are attracted to those that provide us with success. Therefore, the issue of self-esteem is central to our understanding of human motivation and human behavior.

Positive self-esteem is widely posited to be a desirable outcome to explain overt behaviors and other constructs in many areas of psychological research. Despite the theoretical and practical significance of self-esteem, like many other personality constructs, reviews of the research typically identify the poor quality of measurement instruments used to assess it, along with a lack of theoretical models to define and interpret the constructs (Marsh & Jackson, 1986; Wells & Marwell, 1976; Wylie, 1974, 1979). In an attempt to remedy this problem, researchers shift the focus from studying self-concept as a broad global construct to self-concept as a multifaceted, hierarchical construct (Marsh, 1993a, 1994; Marsh & Jackson, 1986). Recognition of the multidimensionality of the self has led to a more detailed study of the composition and psychological importance of its components—one of which has been the physical subdomain (Fox 1990, 1992, 1997). Self in the physical domain is viewed as an important contributor to overarching, global perceptions of self-worth in the multidimensional, hierarchical models of self-esteem (Marsh & Sonstroem, 1995). In this chapter, firstly, the concept of self in the physical domain (physical self) is discussed and then the recent research in the physical self will be summarized. Self-concept and self-esteem will be considered to be synonymous throughout this chapter because the clarification among these constructs has not been clearly established (Byrne, 1996; Sonstroem, 1997).

Physical Self

Physical self is considered to be an important psychological outcome, correlate, and antecedent of physical activity behavior (Fox, 1997) and is viewed as an important contributor to overarching, global perceptions of self-worth in multidimensional, hierarchical models of self-esteem (Marsh & Sonstroem, 1995). According to Fox (2000), "the physical self

has occupied a unique position in the self-esteem system because the body, through its appearance, attributes, and abilities, provides the substantive interface between individuals and the world" (p. 230). It has also been noted that the physical self affects social communication and interaction (Fox, 2000) and is associated with aspects of life adjustment such as depression, mood, and reported physical and psychological health (Sonstroem & Potts, 1996). Indeed, a highly valued perception of the physical self has emerged as particularly important to global self-esteem development (Heine, Lehman, Markus, & Kitayama, 1990) and is potentially an influential factor on physical activity behavior patterns (Hagger, Ashford, & Stambulova, 1998).

This important psychological construct—physical self—is defined as an individual's perception of himself/herself in aspects of physical domains such as strength, endurance, sport ability, and physical appearance (Fox & Corbin, 1989). A review of early self-esteem measures in relation to physical self concluded that most either ignored physical self-esteem completely or treated physical self-esteem as a relatively unidimensional domain incorporating characteristics such as fitness, health, appearance, grooming, sporting competence, body image, sexuality, and physical activity into a single score (Marsh, 1997). With the establishment of multidimensionality, the physical self became systematically measurable as part of comprehensive models alongside perceived competence or adequacy in other life domains. For example, physical self was represented by two short subdomains in Harter's Self-Perception Profiles (Harter, 1985, 1988) and Marsh's Self-Description Questionnaires (Marsh, 1992). However, these subscales do not provide sufficient detail to address research questions about the physical self, which warranted more comprehensive and systematic study. This concern led to the development of new instruments for measuring self in the physical domain. Thus, an integral part of the research of the last two decades has been the development of instrumentation for the measurement of physical self.

In exercise sciences, Fox and Corbin (1989) used a combination of qualitative and quantitative methods to identify key subcomponents of physical self-perceptions, and to test their validity as part of the newly proposed multidimensional and hierarchical

Figure 1: Heirarchical organization of physical self

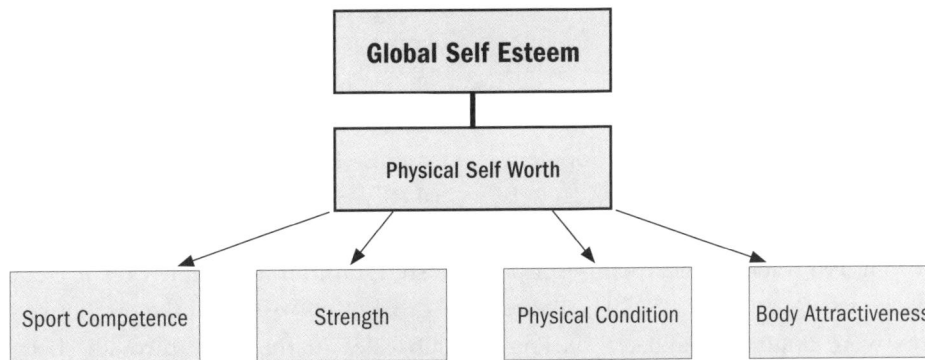

K. R. Fox & C. B. Corbin (1989). The Physical Self-Perception Profile: Development and Preliminary Validation. *Journal of Sport and Exercise Psychology, 1,* p. 414.

conceptualization of self-esteem. Specifically, they developed and validated the Physical Self-Perception Profile (PSPP) as a questionnaire with scales for measuring global physical self-esteem, and four subdomain areas—body attractiveness adequacy, sport/athletic competence, strength competence, and physical condition adequacy. In the hypothesised hierarchical model, global self-esteem is placed as a superordinate domain above more specific but global domains—such as physical self-worth—which, in turn, are hierarchically above the more differentiated subdomains. In the PSPP model, illustrated in Figure 1, global physical self-worth is proposed to mediate the relationship between specific (subdomain) physical self-perceptions and general (global) feelings of self-esteem (Fox, 1990). Further, these subdomains were viewed as specific and changeable aspects of the self, with perceptions becoming more general and enduring the higher the level of the hierarchy (Fox, 1997).

More recently, another well-validated multidimensional and hierarchical instrument consistent with the basic assumption of Shavelson, Hubner, and Stanton (1976), the Physical Self-Description Questionnaire (PSDQ; Marsh, Richards, Johnson, Roche, & Tremayne, 1994) has been developed to provide a comprehensive self-perception profile of the physical aspects of the self. The PSDQ is designed to measure nine specific components of physical self (strength, body fat, physical activity, endurance/fitness, sport competence, coordination, health, appearance, and flexibility), along with global physical self-worth and

global self-esteem. The theoretical rationale for the PSDQ is based on the Marsh/Shavelson self-concept model and some previous research by Marsh (1990, 1992) on the Self-Description Questionnaire (SDQ). The PSDQ reflects scales from an earlier version of the measure presented by Marsh and Redmayne (1994) and scales of SDQ such as physical ability, physical appearance, and esteem. The PSDQ also reflects the parallel component of physical fitness identified in Marsh's (1993b) study. In the PSDQ, there is a hierarchical ordering in which general self-esteem is at the apex, global physical self-esteem is at the next level, and specific components of physical self-esteem are at the third level (Marsh, 1996a).

In summary, in the past two decades, great steps forward in the measurement of physical self have been achieved from both multidimensional and hierarchical perspectives. These advancements in physical self-measurement have produced much richer profiles of characterising groups or individuals, provided links between the physical self and related behaviors, and allowed more precise reports on self-perception change (Fox, 1997). In addition, researchers and practitioners are better able to (a) study psychometric properties of physical self instruments in other cultures; (b) examine the cross-cultural generalizability of physical self measurement, theory, and models across different cultures; and (c) investigate physical self as an important outcome variable in exercise interventions. In the following section, studies on the physical self construct will be discussed based on the above categories.

Psychometric Properties of Physical Self Instruments in Different Cultures

Recently, the greatest step forward in physical self research has been facilitated by the development of multidimensional and hierarchical physical self instruments of the Physical Self-Perception Profile (PSPP, Fox & Corbin, 1989) and Physical Self-Description Questionnaire (PSDQ, Marsh et al., 1994). These two instruments were originally validated on English-speaking populations and Western cultures with a strong emphasis on individualism (Fox & Corbin, 1989; Marsh et al., 1994). Heine et al. (1990) argued that much of what we apparently know about self-concept is based substantially on a North American perspective that cannot be assumed to generalize to other social and cultural settings. In physical self research and sports sciences more specifically much support for the psychological instruments and theoretical models has been based largely on responses of students from English-speaking countries. Although there has been some research in other countries, it is important to evaluate rigorously the responses of instruments that have been carefully translated, and to test the theoretical predictions in cross-cultural settings.

Translation of instruments into other languages offers the opportunity to study the construct validity of the questionnaire in different cultures and assess the generalizability of its factor structure. However, it is well known among test developers that the use of a test in a culture other than the one in which it was developed requires evidence of the test's reliability and validity in the new setting. Nowadays, there is an increasing attempt to test the psychometric properties of the physical self instruments in non-English speaking nations and cultures other than those in developed Western European nations. For example, Aşçi, Aşçi, and Zorba (1999) investigated the psychometric properties of PSPP and provided support for its validity and reliability specifically among Turkish University students. The four-factor structure of PSPP was supported and the obtained reliability evidence was acceptable. Zero order and partial correlation analysis also supported the hierarchical structure of the Turkish version of PSPP. In addition, the PSPP was validated with college students in the United Kingdom (Page, Ashford, Fox, & Biddle, 1993), and among Flemish adults (Van de Vliet et al., 2002). The PSPP has been found to have good cross-cultural validity in a number of other countries including Canada (Crocker, Eklund, & Kowalski, 2000), Spain (Atienza, Balaguer, Moreno, & Fox, 2004) and Portugal (Ferreira & Fox, 2003).

The predictive validity of the PSPP was also tested in different countries. For example, Fox and Corbin (1989) assessed the predictive validity of the subscales in the PSPP through their relationships with both degree and type of physical activity involvement among American university students. The analysis indicated that the four PSPP subscale scores differentiated between active and non-active American university students (percent correctly classified for females was 70.7% and for males 70.4%). For both American females and males, the *physical condition* scores were the most important determinant of physical activity participation. Page et al. (1993) evaluated the predictive validity of PSPP for British University students and reported that the four PSPP subdomains could correctly classify 74.1% of subjects as low and 83.3% as high in physical activity. Similar to American University students, the physical condition scores were the dominant variable in physical activity prediction. Recently, Aşçi, Çağlar, and Karaca (2003) tested the predictive validity of a Turkish version of the PSPP on 879 university students. The discriminant analysis using the four PSPP subscale scores to differentiate between active and non-active Turkish University students indicated that the PSPP could correctly classify 59% of males and 61.3% of females. The physical condition variable for males and the sport competence variable for females were the most important in their respective discriminant functions.

Besides studies on the psychometric properties of PSPP, some researchers have examined the psychometric properties of the PSDQ for different cultures. For instance, Aşçi (2000) conducted a study on the psychometric properties of PSDQ in the Turkish culture and reported that PSDQ is a psychometrically sound instrument for measuring physical self of Turkish university students. In addition, Nigg, Norman, Rossi, and Benisovich (2001) tested the internal validity of the PSDQ factor structure in a North American sample of young adults and examined the multidimensional hierarchical structure of physical self. CFA results provided clear support for the 11 theoretical constructs of the PSDQ for American university students. Klomsten also validated the PSDQ among Norwegian populations, and the results supported the *a priori* structure of the PSDQ (Klomsten, Skaalvik, & Espnes, 2004). Stille, Marsh, Richards, and Alfermann (2003) used the construct validation approach to test the psychometric properties of PSDQ for elderly Australians and sound psychometric properties were found. Recently, Stille and Alfermann (2005) tested the German version of PSDQ for adolescents and young adults (16 - 28 year olds) and found support for 11 components of the German version of the PSDQ.

The Children and Youth Physical Self-Perception Profile (CY-PSPP) is another physical self instrument for assessing perceptions of children in the psychomotor domain. Whitehead (1995) published a version of the PSPP that was modified for children and youth (the CY-PSPP). This modification was developed with the assumption that, because self-esteem is becoming differentiated in childhood and adolescence, the CY-PSPP content would be the same as for the college students' PSPP, but would, perhaps, be less factorially distinct in subdomains. However, the same four-factor structure and hierarchical model was supported, and further evidence of construct validity was found. Similar results were reported by Welk, Corbin, and Lewis (1995) using the CY-PSPP with a sample of athletes. Subsequently, Eklund, Whitehead, and Welk (1997) examined the factorial validity and the hierarchical global-to-specific domain structure of the CY-PSPP using confirmatory factor analysis (CFA) and supported the initial evidence of reliability and validity published by Whitehead (1995). An exploratory study by Welk, Corbin, Dowell, and Harris (1997) and a recent confirmatory study by Welk and Eklund (2005) supported the utility of the CY-PSPP model on elementary school children.

Like the PSPP and PSDQ, the psychometric properties of CY-PSPP have been tested in different cultures. For example, Aşçi, Eklund, Whitehead, Kirazci, and Koca (2005) recently reported evidence supporting the factorial validity and reliability of the CY-PSPP for Turkish children and youth. Furthermore, Raustorp, Stahle, Gudasic, Kinnunen and Mattsson (2005) validated the Swedish translation of the CY-PSPP and reported good concurrent and content validity and test-retest reliability.

In summary, these studies have provided strong support for the utility of physical self instruments in various cultural settings. Specifically, the findings revealed acceptable psychometric properties of physical self instruments in non-English speaking nations and cultures other than those in developed Western European nations. In the literature, however, it is possible to find studies that have used different methodological approaches for testing the validity of physical self-instruments in different cultures. In the following sections these studies will be briefly summarzied under three subheadings: multitrait multimethod analysis, relations of physical self instruments with external criteria, and known group differences.

Multitrait Multimethod (MTMM)
Comparison of Physical Self Instruments

Reviewers of self-concept measurement (e.g., Marsh, 1990; Shavelson et al., 1976; Wylie, 1974, 1979) emphasize the central role of MTMM in full first-time analyses in the construct validation of self-concept responses. In this approach, multidimensional self-concept instruments purporting to measure the same or substantially overlapping scales are administered to the same group of respondents. The approach consists of a systematic evaluation of correlations between scales from different instruments that are posited to be matching (the same or similar content) and nonmatching. In this approach, convergent validity is supported by large correlations between matching scales from different instruments, and discriminant validity is supported when convergent validities are larger than other correlations.

The first MTMM study of multidimensional physical self instruments was conducted by Marsh et al. (1994). In this study, students completed three physical self-concept instruments: the PSDQ, PSPP, and Richard's Physical Self Concept (PSC) scale. Based on the evaluation of the content to the 11 PSDQ, 7 PSC, and 5 PSPP scales, Marsh and colleagues predicted which scales from different instruments would be most highly correlated. Correlations (convergent validities) among scales from the three instruments predicted to be matching were systematically larger than those among nonmatching scales. PSDQ convergent validities were higher than those involved in the other two instruments. These results supported the convergent and discriminant validity of PSDQ responses for Australian high school students.

Another MTMM analysis was conducted on the responses of Turkish university students to the PSDQ and PSPP (Marsh, Aşçi, & Tomas, 2002). Marsh et al. (2002) compared the content of items from 16 scales (11 PSDQ, 5 PSPP) and predicted which scales from different instruments were most correlated. Based on this, 55 correlations relating to 11 PSDQ and 5 PSPP scales were classified into three categories: (a) three convergent validities in which scales were most closely matched; (b) four convergent validities in which scales were ambiguously or less closely matched; and (c) nonmatching correlations (hetero-trait-heteromethod). Strength, sport competence, and global physical self-worth scales of the PSPP were most logically related to the PSDQ strength, sport competence, and general physical self-concept scales. All three of these convergent validities were very large and larger than correlations with other PSDQ factors: Strength (.84), sport (.86), and general physical self-worth (.76). The other four convergent validities—PSPP body with PSDQ physical appearance (.69), PSPP condition with PSDQ endurance (.76), and PSDQ physical activity (.65)—were substantial with the possible exception of .34 between PSDQ body fat and PSPP body attractiveness. These expected convergent validities were systematically higher than those among nonmatching scales. This provides good support for convergent and divergent validities of the PSDQ among Turkish university students.

Recently, MTMM evaluation of three physical self measures was conducted by Richards, Marsh, Bar-Eli, and Zach (2005), who compared MTMM responses of two samples of Israeli university students with Australian high school students on three physical self instruments. Consistent with previous MTMM studies (Marsh et al., 1994, 2002), content of items from scales of three instruments were compared to predict which scales from different instruments would be most correlated. The results supported the predictions that convergent validities were consistently large and larger than correlations among non-matching factors.

In summary, these three MTMM studies provide evidence for the utility of using physical self instru-

ments in Australian, Turkish, and Israeli cultures. The MTMM analysis supported both the convergent and discriminant validity of the PSDQ and, to a lesser extent, the PSPP in different cultural settings.

Relations to External Criteria

Most of the research with the PSPP and the PSDQ has generally focused on the within-network concerns (internal or structural), emphasizing tests of hypothesized factor structures underlying PSPP and PSDQ responses. Despite the support for the internal and factor structure of the PSPP and PSDQ, there have been few attempts to study the construct validity of the PSPP and PSDQ using between-network designs or external criteria. In addition, less evidence for the construct validity of the PSPP and PSDQ using external criteria on different cultures has been provided. For example, Marsh (1996a) related PSDQ responses of Australian high school students to 23 external validity criteria: measures of body composition, physical activity, endurance, strength, and flexibility. Each criterion was predicted to be most highly correlated to one of the PSDQ scales.

Like Marsh (1996a), Guerin, Marsh, and Famose (2004) tested between-construct validity of PSDQ responses in relation to a multidimensional profile of fitness measures in French high school students. Guerin et al. (2004) related PSDQ responses with external measures of body mass index, physical activity, and 10 field exercises selected from the Eurofit European test battery of physical fitness; Marsh's (1996a) PSDQ between-construct study; and Fleishman's fitness tests (cited in Marsh, 1993). The relationship between 13 external criteria and the PSDQ subscales was tested by both bivariate correlation and structural equation analysis. Both bivariate and structural equation analysis revealed similar patterns of correlations, and all of the 13 external criteria of physical fitness were strongly and highly correlated with corresponding PSDQ scales. Guerin et al. classified obtained correlations into three categories. Thirteen correlations were classified as primary convergent validities in which scales were most closely matched. Six correlations were classified as secondary convergent validities in which scales were less closely matched. The remaining correlations fell into the discriminate validities category. Based on these classifications, Guerin et al. obtained good support for primary and secondary convergent validities and also discriminant validities.

Aşçi (2005) also examined the construct validity of two well-accepted physical self-instruments—the PSPP and PSDQ—for Turkish university students by relating the PSPP and PSDQ scores to objective measures of physical fitness (body composition, body mass index, aerobic endurance, muscular endurance, back and leg strength, flexibility). For the PSPP, the expected seven primary convergent validities were significant, with the exception of body mass index and body attractiveness. However, only three convergent validities were larger than correlations of external criteria with uncorresponding PSPP scales. In addition, strength measures (back and leg strength, sit-ups) were significantly correlated with PSPP strength scales, but these measures were highly correlated with PSPP sport competence and physical condition. For the PSDQ, Aşçi expected nine primary convergent validities in which nine external criteria were most closely related to corresponding PSDQ subscales. All of the obtained nine primary convergent validities were significant and larger than the remaining correlations of fitness parameters with other PSDQ subscales.

Aşçi (2005) also conducted partial correlation analysis by controlling for gender. The partial correlations provided clear support for the expected convergent validities of the PSPP. Unlike the zero order correlation results, all of the expected seven primary convergent validities of PSPP were significant and each of the seven external criteria had higher correlations with corresponding PSPP scales than other scales, except body mass index and sit-up (.16 to .42, $M = .27$). Discriminant validity was supported, in that all of the obtained convergent validities (except body mass index and sit-up) were higher than the remaining correlations (.00 to .30; $M = .11$). Gender had little effect on either size or pattern of correlations between nine external criteria and nine PSDQ scales (.25 to .50, $M = .37$). There was clear support for the convergent and discriminant validity of the PSDQ physical activity and strength scales. In general, the findings of this study (Aşçi, 2005) indicated that the objective measures of physical fitness were highly related to the corresponding PSPP and PSDQ scales. This provides initial support for the construct validity of Turkish university students responses to

PSPP and PSDQ in relation to external criteria.

The above between-construct validity studies, conducted in Australia, France, and Turkey, indicate that the original and translated versions of physical self instruments are psychometrically sound and useful for research in different cultures. These studies also extend earlier findings on Western cultures cross-culturally.

Known Group Differences

It is possible to find some known group difference studies in the literature for testing the psychometric qualities of physical self instruments. These studies were carried out on sample groups from different nations. For example, Marsh (1998) compared two elite athlete groups with non-athletes. He found that PSDQ responses were much higher for the two elite athlete groups (Australian Institute of Sport and sports high school) than for two non-elite groups (non-athletes at sports high school and non-sport high school). Similar comparisons among Turkish athletes and non-athletes were investigated by Aşçi (2004a), who compared 329 elite athlete responses to the PSPP with 429 non-athlete university student responses. Results indicated that elite athletes had higher scores on the perceived sport competence, physical condition, and strength subscales than non-athletes.

In addition, Çağlar and Aşçi (2006) and Aşçi (2004b) compared the physical self scores of high and low physically active Turkish university students by using the PSPP and PSDQ, respectively. The findings of these studies revealed that high physical activity groups scored higher than low physical activity groups in almost all subscales of the PSPP and PSDQ. Van de Vliet et al. (2002) examined the discriminant validity of the PSPP among Flemish adults by comparing the PSPP scores of non-clinical samples with a psychiatric sample. Significant differences in physical self-perceptions between psychiatric patients and normal adults, as well as the successful categorization of normal individuals and psychiatric patients, provided evidence for the discriminant validity of the Flemish version of the PSPP.

In summary, known group difference studies have provided some evidence for the discriminant validity of the PSPP and PSDQ across different nations.

Cross-cultural Examination of Physical Self and Physical Self Instruments

Despite the construct validation of physical self instruments in different cultures, few attempts have been made to examine the appropriateness and generalizability of models and instruments across cultures. Such studies provide an opportunity to study the construct validity of questionnaires across cultures and help to assess the generalizability of its factor structure. Theoretically, the generalizability of the overall form or pattern of a model across cultures is expected based on research that has identified the self as a universal trait (etic) construct as opposed to a culture specific trait (emic) or state-like construct (Tafarodi & Swann, 1996). In addition, the extension of research on physical self measurement and theory from a cross-cultural perspective integrating social value system exhibits the differences in physical self between individualist versus collectivistic cultural orientation (Markus & Kitayama, 1991).

One difficulty with the cross-cultural study of models is that replication of the factor pattern or overall form of the self-esteem model in other cultures does not on its own imply the universality of the proposed model (Hagger, Biddle, Chow, Stambulova, & Kavussanu, 2003). As a result, some researchers (Bond & Smith, 1996; Kohn, 1987; Watkins 2000) have emphasized the inclusion of at least three countries in the evaluation of self-esteem models. Marsh, Marco, and Aşçi (2002) reported that this approach facilitates comparisons based on cultural dimensions and enables researchers to examine cross-cultural differences in self-esteem by triangulation. Specifically, Marsh et al. (2002) suggested that the cross-cultural evaluation of hierarchical multidimensional models of physical self-esteem should be conducted simultaneously across at least three samples from different cultures to test the similarity of factor structure, the invariance of structural parameters such as invariance of factor loading, factor correlations, factor variance, and the similarity of measurement error.

Based on the above suggestions, some cross-cultural studies were conducted to examine the adequacy of physical self instruments by using multiple samples. For example, Marsh et al. (2002) compared PSDQ responses of Australian high school students with those of Spanish high school students and Turkish university students. The overarching purpose of their study was to evaluate cross-cultural generalizability of the factor structure and psychometric properties underlying responses to the PSDQ in Spanish, Australian, and Turkish cultures. Samples of 986 Australian and 986 Spanish high school students and 1137 Turkish university students completed the PSDQ. In evaluating the invariance of factor structures across different groups, researchers were able to fit the data subject to the constraint that any one, any set, or all parameter estimates were equal in the multiple groups. Based on the root mean square error of approximation (RMSEA), the *a priori* model provided a good fit to the data based on responses from Australia (RMSEA = .042), Spain (RMSEA = .044), and Turkey (RMSEA = .047). Consistent with expectations, the fit of this *a priori* model is somewhat better in the Australian sample, but differences between countries were smaller than anticipated. The success of the *a priori* model with Turkish university students supported the appropriateness of the instrument with older respondents. In addition, the researchers tested the model based on the invariance of factor loadings, factor correlations, and factor variances, and then subsequent tests of uniqueness.

These detailed comparisons of invariance provided support for the generalizability of the PSDQ from an Australian setting where it was developed in two very different settings that involved the translation of the instruments into new languages and responses by students from different cultures. Marsh et al. (2002) also tested the models by freeing the parameters from each of the three countries. Freeing parameters had little effect on the goodness of fit, and RMSEA values ranged from .045 to .049. In general, freeing parameters for Turkish university students indicated greater improvement of fits and slightly more positive effect on goodness of fit. This indicated that the factor structures based on responses by the Australian and Spanish high school students were found to be more similar to each other than to the factor structure based on responses by Turkish university students.

Hagger, Aşçi, and Lindwall (2004) examined the cross-cultural validity of the hierarchical model of the PSPP across three nations that represented diverse multiregional cultures; namely, Turkey, Great Britain, and Sweden. Hagger et al. also examined the mean differences in the levels of the PSPP constructs across these three diverse cultures. The factor structure of PSPP and the hierarchical relationship among PSPP subdomains were supported for each of the three nations. The single and multiple sample analysis supported the replicability and generalizability of the PSPP factor structure and provided evidence of a higher-order physical self-worth factor to explain the covariance between four subdomains of the PSPP for each nation and across nations. Some latent mean differences in PSPP subdomains were reported and findings demonstrated that PSPP scales were rated more highly in British university students with the exception of the physical condition subscale, which was rated more highly among Swedish and Turkish university students. Hagger et al. concluded that discrepancy in the meaning of some individual items was evident and physical self-esteem in general, and aspects relating to sport prowess and appearance specifically, were highly valued in predominantly individualist societies, while aspects relating to fitness were highly valued in cultures with high collectivist norms.

The PSPP model has also been evaluated cross-culturally on children. Hagger and his colleagues (Hagger et al. , 1998, 2003) have evaluated the generalizability of PSPP models and mean differences in physical self-perception across different nations. In the first study (Hagger et al., 1998), the factor stucture of the PSPP-C for British and Russian children and mean differences in PSPP-C subdomains between these two nation groups were investigated. Results supported the factor structure of the PSPP-C across Russian and British children, and four PSPP-C subdomains were distinguishable between children with high and low levels of physical activity. Variable discrimination analyses revealed that perceived physical condition was more relevant for Russian girls and boys but perceived sport competence and strength were most important for British boys and girls, respectively. In another study, based on triangulation methodology, Hagger et al. (2003) confirmed the appropriateness and generalizability of Fox and Corbin's (1989) hierarchical multidimesional model of physical self-perceptions across adolescents from Great Britain, Hong Kong, and Russia. Results revealed lower PSPP-C scores for Hong Kong Chinese and Russian adolescents, which is consistent with the results of the study that examined differences in physical self-esteem among Brtitish, Swedish, and Turkish university students (Hagger et al., 2004). Together these findings suggest a tendency of individualist cultures to endorse the physical self more than collectivist cultures. In general, the findings of these studies indicate cross-cultural generalizability and utility of physical self-instruments across different nations.

Summary Evidence of Cultural Studies

The psychometric and cross-cultural studies of physical self generally provide supportive evidence on the cross-national and cross-cultural generalizability of physical self measurement, theory, and research. The psychometric studies increase the normative data available for the scales and provide important information on the applicability of instruments. The cross-cultural studies with the inclusion of three countries provide a much richer basis for cross-cultural comparison and indicate the relevancy of the individualistic phenomenon of self to collectivist culture and extend the findings of previous studies to other cultural contexts. In addition, these studies clearly demonstrate the replication of Western hierarchical and multidimensional models in collectivist cultures.

Exercise Interventions and Physical Self

Physical activity or exercise has become increasingly popular in recent years and much research describing the psychological benefits of fitness has emerged from a variety of settings. Physical educators, exercise physiologists, psychologists, rehabilitation counselors, psychiatrists, and physicians have all addressed this issue (Folkins & Sime, 1981). Participation in physical activity or exercise is not only associated with physiological improvement in aerobic capacity, cardiovascular functioning, muscular strength, flexibility and body composition, but it also provides psychological benefits including decreased anxiety, increased self-confidence, improved mood, and increased self-esteem (Caruso & Gill, 1992).

Several researchers (Fox, 2000; Leith, 1994;

Sonstroem, 1984; Sonstroem & Morgan, 1989) have identified self-esteem as the psychological variable with the most potential to reflect psychological benefits as a result of regular participation in physical activity/exercise. With the recognition of the multidimensionality of the self and development of new instruments to measure the unique and specific aspects of self-esteem, researchers began to examine the role of exercise interventions on specific aspects of self-esteem such as physical self. Fox (2000) emphasized the mental health properties of physical self and indicated that physical self may be worthy of consideration as a legitimate and practically important outcome variable in exercise interventions as far as mental well-being is considered and should be used as a key target of exercise programs. From this perspective many researchers, as illustrated in Table 1, have examined the physical self construct

Authors	Date	Subjects	Exercise Mode	Length	Instruments	Results
Caruso & Gill	1992 (first study)	34 female university students; 15 (aerobic), 13 (strength), 6 (control)	Strength training and aerobic exercise	10 weeks	PSPP	Improvement of PSPP subdomains after strength and aerobic exercise, but these improvements were not significant.
Caruso & Gill	1992 (second study)	37 males and 28 females; 42 (strength), 23 (different physical activities)	Strength training and varieties of physical activities (volleyball, golf, fencing, basketball)	10 weeks	PSPP	No significant changes in physical self-perception scores.
Page, Fox, Armstrong, & McAndle	1993	18 females	20 min aerobic exercise on bicycle ergometer	8 weeks	PSPP	Significant improvements in strength, physical condition, and physical self-worth subscales, but no significant changes in sport competence and body attractiveness scores.
McAuley, Mihalko & Bane	1997	Middle-aged sedentary adults	Exercise program	20 weeks	PSPP	Improvement in perceived physical condition, body attractiveness, global physical self-worth, and global self-worth.
Aşçı, Kin, & Koşar	1998	45 female university students 15 (aerobic dancing), 15 (step dancing), & 15 (control)	Aerobic and step dance program	8 weeks	PSPP	Improvement in all subscales of PSPP but this improvement did not depend on type of activities.
Aşçı	1998	40 female university students 10 (physical fitness training), 10 (group counseling), 10 (group counseling and physical fitness training), 10 (control)	Physical fitness training, group counseling	10 weeks	PSDQ	The physical activity, sport competence, coordination, and strength scores of experimental groups increased more than control group.
Daley & Buchanan	1999	113 girls, 15-16 years old	Physical education class and PE class with aerobic dance	5 weeks	PSPP	The sport competence, physical condition, strength, and global physical self-worth scores of girls significantly improved after participating in physical education with aerobic dancing.

as an outcome variable in exercise interventions by using specific physical self instruments.

In this regard, there are randomized trial studies that have compared both the effects of different exercise programs on the physical self and the effects of exercise versus no exercise or even no activity on the physical self. For example, Caruso and Gill (1992) studied the effects of 10 weeks of aerobic exercise, strength training, and physical activities on the physical self-perception of 34 female undergraduates and reported that physical self-perception changed over the 10-week period; however, improvements in physical self-perception occurred independent of exercise/activity group. In the second aspect of their study, Caruso and Gill compared the effects of weight training and physical education activities (non-fitness activities) on the physical self-perception and body image of 37 males and 28 females. Results

Authors	Date	Subjects	Exercise Mode	Length	Instruments	Results
Shaw, Ebbeck, & Snow	2000	44 females, 50-75 years old	Strength training	9 months	Not reported	Low self-esteem groups improved physical appearance scores.
Alfermann & Stoll	2000	24 female and male adults (experimental group), 13 females and males (control group)	Physical fitness program (endurance, strength, coordination & flexibility)	6 months	Physical Self Scales (31 items)	Experimental group decreased negative physical self-worth and concern about physical attractiveness scores.
Aşçı	2001	73 female & 65 male university students	Step dance	10 weeks	PSDQ	Females and males in the experimental group improved their physical self scores more than control group.
Aşçı	2002	73 female & 65 male university students	Step dance	10 weeks	PSPP	Experimental group improved more on all subdomains of PSPP than control groups, and females and males had similar gains.
Van Vorst, Buckworth, & Mattern	2002	139 university students	Strength training	9 weeks	PSDQ	Improvement in physical self scores.
Daley	2002	1,130 girls and boys, 14-15 years old	Extracurricular activities	-	CY-PSPP	Changes in body atttractiveness and global physical self-worth scores.
Aşçı	2003	40 female university students 20 (physical fitness training), 20 (control)	Physical fitness training (aerobic and step dance)	10 weeks	PSDQ	PSDQ physical activity, coordination, sport competence, and flexibility scores improved more in experimental group than in control group.
Ransdell, Detling, Taylor, Reel, & Shultz	2004	20 mother-daughter pairs	University-based and home-based exercise	-	PSPP	Both experimental groups improved body attractiveness and sport competence scores over time.
Lindwall & Lindgren	2005	110 non-physically active Swedish girls	Exercise intervention program ($n = 56$) and control group ($n = 54$)	6 months	PSPP	No significant improvement in PSPP subdomains.

Table 1: Interventional Studies on Physical Self

revealed no significant changes in physical self-perception over the 10-week program. Alfermann and Stoll (2000) conducted two studies on the effects of exercise on the physical self. In the first study, the effects of a 6-month physical exercise program on the physical self of 24 female and male participants were compared with a wait-list control group who had no exercise or any other supervised activity over six months. Alfermann and Stoll concluded that the exercise group improved significantly in terms of physical self. In their second study, they investigated the effects of different exercise programs (jogging and fitness) on the physical self by comparing these effects with different control conditions (relaxation and training for strengthening back muscles). Results indicated that participants improved in terms of perceived physical fitness and their perceived negative physical self-worth decreased regardless of the kind of intervention program involved.

As mentioned previously, there are studies that have investigated the effects of exercise on the physical self by comparing exercise effects with no exercise or no activity. For instance, Aşçi, Kin, and Koşar (1998) used the PSPP to examine the effects of an 8-week aerobic dance and step aerobics program on the physical self-perception of female university students and reported that the improvement in the mean scores of physical self-perception were independent from the group. In additon, Aşçi (2003) has conducted another study and again compared the effects of a 10-week physical fitness program on the physical self, measured by the PSDQ, with no exercise and reported that participants in the experimental group demonstrated significant improvement in physical activity, coordination, sport competence, and flexibility subscales of the physical self in contrast to the no-exercise lecture control group. Recently, Magnus and Lindgren (2005) examined the effects of a 6-month exercise intervention program on physical self-perceptions of 110 non-physically active adolescent Swedish girls. No post-intervention changes were evident in PSPP subdomains.

Some studies have examined the role of exercise programs on physical self specifically without the use of a control group. For example, Page, Fox, McManus, and Armstrong (1993) investigated the impact of an 8-week aerobic exercise program using bicycle ergometers on the physical self-perception of adolescent females. Significant improvement was evident in group mean scores for the physical condition, strength, and physical self-worth subscales of the PSPP. Other studies (e.g. Daley & Buchanan, 1999; Ransdell, Detling, Taylor, Reel, & Shultz, 2004) compared different types of exercise programs to each other without control groups and reported changes in some aspects of physical self-perception.

Furthermore, in recent studies, gender differences in physical self-perception changes through exercise have been investigated. For instance, Aşçi (2002) examined gender differences in the effects of step dance on the physical self-perception of 73 female and 65 male university students between 18 and 27 years old. Participants were randomly assigned to step dance and control groups while maintaining gender balance in each group. The experimental group attended step dance sessions for 50 minutes per day, 3 days per week for 10 weeks, while subjects in the control group did not participate in any regular physical activity. Participants in the experimental group improved more on all subdomains of the PSPP than participants in the no exercise control group, while male and female participants did not develop differently on physical self-perception throughout 10 weeks of the step dance program. Aşçi (2001) also addressed gender differences in physical self by using another well validated physical self instrument, the PSDQ. Her findings indicated that participants who attended the step dance program improved their PSDQ scores more than the control group, and no gender differences in the physical self scores were obtained over a 10-week program except in the physical activity and self-esteem subscales of the PSDQ.

Summary evidence of interventional studies. The effects of different exercise interventions on physical self using specific self scales in the psychomotor domain—the PSPP and more recently the PSDQ—have been examined extensively in the last two decades. The research has demonstrated that different modes of exercise such as step dance, aerobic dancing, and physical fitness programs that emphasize cardiovascular and aerobic conditioning have positive effects on the physical self. In general, interventional studies have reported significant changes in almost all subdomains of physical self, although strength, physical condition/endurance, and sport competence were the subdomains of physical self mostly affected. The research provides evidence that males and females have similar gains from exercise intervention, although it is important to note that findings should be carefully interpreted due to the limited number of studies in this area, small sample sizes, and a reliance on university sample groups. Nevertheless, the evidence shows clearly that exercise helps people feel better about their physical abilities and personal characteristics. These findings may be practically and clinically important as there is evidence that physical self is directly linked to mental well-being. As a consequence physical self constructs, which are important aspects of global self-esteem and mental well being, should be considered as target outcomes of interventions based on physical activity and exercise programs.

Final Comments

Understanding the physical self is important for researchers and practitioners in the field of health promotion as well as sport and exercise psychology. Physical self plays a unique role in the self system and is a powerful indicator of a person's global self-esteem and mental and emotional well-being. The increased interest in physical self research from cultural perspectives clearly demonstrates the generalizability of the physical self construct across cultures and the role of cultural values and aspirations on the physical self. Although cultural studies show similarity in the structure of physical self among different cultures, results reflect how social value systems influence the important construct of physical self. Interventional research suggests that physical activity can influence the development of the physical self. Research shows that physical self constructs are more likely to be sensitive to changes in mental well-being resulting from exercise, and such changes may contribute to a participant's sense of well-being and overall self-evaluation. These findings indicate that health professionals should consider physical self as a significant element of health promotion and should actively promote participation in physical activity/ exercise.

References

Alfermann, D., & Stoll, O. (2000). Effects of physical exercise on self-concept and well being. *International Journal of Sport Psychology, 30,* 47-65.

Aşçi, F. H. (1998). The effects of physical fitness training and group counseling on self-concept and physical self-concept of female university students. Unpublished doctoral dissertation. Middle East Technical University, Ankara, Turkey.

Aşçi, F. H. (2000). Reliability and validity of physical self-description questionnaire for Turkish university students. In *Proceedings of the VIth International Sport Sciences Congress* (pp. 122-123). Antalya, Turkey: Sport Sciences Association.

Aşçi, F. H. (2001). Gender differences in psychological effects of exercise. In A. Papaioannou, M. Goudas, & Y. Theodorakis (Eds.), *Proceedings of the International Society of Sport Psychology 10th World Congress* (pp. 292-295). Thessaloniki, Greece: Christodoulidi Publications.

Aşçi, F .H. (2002). The effects of step dance on physical self-perception of female and male university students. *International Journal of Sport Psychology, 33,* 431-442.

Aşçi, F. H. (2003). The effects of physical fitness training on trait anxiety and physical self-concept of female university students. *Psychology of Sport and Exercise, 4,* 255-264.

Aşçi, F. H. (2004a). Physical self-perception of elite athletes and non-athletes: A Turkish sample. *Perceptual and Motor Skills, 99,* 1047-1052.

Aşçi, F. H. (2004b). Comparison of physical self-perception with regard to gender and physical activity level. *Hacettepe Journal of Sport Sciences, 15,* 39-48.

Aşçi, F. H. (2005). Construct validity of two physical self-concept measures: An example from Turkey. *Psychology of Sport and Exercise, 6,* 659-669.

Aşçi, F .H., Aşçi, A., & Zorba, E. (1999). Cross-cultural validity and reliability of Physical Self-Perception Profile. *International Journal of Sport Psychology, 30,* 399-406.

Aşçi, F. H., Çağlar, E., & Karaca, A. (2003). The predictive and construct validity of physical self-perception profile. In R. Stelter (Ed.), *Proceedings of the XIth European Congress of Sport Psychology* (p.24). Copenhagen, Denmark: ECSS.

Aşçi, F. H., Eklund, R. C., Whitehead, J. R., Kirazci, S., & Koca, C. (2005). Use of the CY-PSPP in other cultures: A preliminary investigation of its factorial validity for Turkish children and youth. *Psychology of Sport and Exercise, 6,* 33-50.

Aşçi, F. H., Kin, A., & Kosar, N. (1998). Effect of participation in an 8 week aerobic dance and step aerobics program on physical self-perception and body image satisfaction. *International Journal of Sport Psychology, 29,* 366-375.

Atienza, F. L., Balaguer, I., Moreno, Y., & Fox, K. R. (2004). Physical self-perception profile: Psychometric properties of the Spanish version, and validity of the physical self-perception hierarchical structure. *Psicothema, 16,* 461-467.

Bond, M. H., & Smith, P. B. (1996). Cross-cultural social and organizational psychology. *Annual Reviews of Psychology, 47,* 205-235.

Byrne, B. M. (1996). Measuring self-concept across the lifespan: Issues and instrumentation. Washington, DC: American Psychological Association.

Çağlar, E., & Aşçi, F. H. (2006). Gender and physical activity level differences in physical self-perception of university students: A case of Turkey. *International Journal of Sport Psychology, 37,* 58-74.

Caruso, C. M., & Gill, D. L. (1992). Strengthening physical self-perceptions through exercise. *Journal of Sports Medicine and Physical Fitness, 32,* 416-427.

Crocker, P. R. E., Eklund, R. C., & Kowalski, K. C. (2000). Children's physical activity and physical self-perceptions. *Journal of Sports Sciences, 18,* 383-394.

Daley, A. J. (2002). Extra-curricular physical activities and physical self-perception in British 14-15 year old male and female adolescents. *European Physical Education Review, 8,* 37-50.

Daley, A. J., & Buchanan, J. (1999). Aerobic dance and physical self-perceptions in female adolescents: Some implications for physical education. *Research Quarterly for Exercise and Sport, 70,* 196-200.

Eklund, R. C., Whitehead, J. R., & Welk, G. J. (1997). Validity of children and youth physical self-perception profile: A confirmatory factor analysis. *Research Quarterly for Exercise and Sport, 68,* 249-256.

Ferreira, J. P., & Fox, K. R. (2003). Evidence of cross-cultural validity and reliability of Portuguese version of the physical self-perception profile. In R. Stelter (Ed.), *Proceedings of the XIth European Congress of Sport Psychology* (p.58). Copenhagen, Denmark: ECSS.

Folkins, C. H., & Sime, W. E. (1981). Physical fitness training and mental health. *American Psychologist, 36,* 373-389.

Fox, K. R. (1988). The child's perspective in physical education. The self-esteem complex. *British Journal of Physical Education, 19,* 247-252.

Fox, K. R. (1990). *The physical self-perception profile manual* (PRN monograph). Dekalb, IL: Northern Illinois University Office for Health Promotion.

Fox, K. R. (1992). Physical education and development of self-esteem in children. In N. Armstrong (Ed.), *New directions in physical education* (pp. 33-54). Champaign, IL: Human Kinetics.

Fox, K. R. (1997). The physical self and process in self-esteem development. In K. R. Fox (Ed.), *The physical self: From motivation to well being* (pp.111-139). Champaign IL: Human Kinetics.

Fox, K. R. (2000). Self-esteem, self-perceptions and exercise. *International Journal of Sport Psychology, 31,* 228-240.

Fox, K. R., & Corbin C. B. (1989). The Physical Self-Perception Profile: Development and preliminary validation. *Journal of Sport and Exercise Psychology, 11,* 408-430.

Guerin, F., Marsh, H. W., & Famose, J-P. (2004). Generalizablity of the PSDQ and its relationship to physical fitness: The European French connection. *Journal of Sport and Exercise Psychology, 26,* 19-38.

Hagger, M. S., AsÁi, F. H., & Lindwall, M. (2004). A cross-cultural evaluation of a multidimensional and hierarchical model of physical self-perceptions in three national samples. *Journal of Applied Social Psychology, 34,* 1075-1107.

Hagger, M., Ashford, B., & Stambulova, N. (1998). Russian and British children's physical self-perceptions and physical activity participation. *Pediatric Exercise Science, 10.* 137-152.

Hagger, M. S., Biddle, S. J. H., Chow, E. W., Stambulova, N., & Kavussanu, M. (2003). Physical self-perceptions in adolescence. Generalizability of a hierarchical multidimensional model across three cultures. *Journal of Cross-Cultural Psychology, 34,* 611-628.

Harter, S. (1985). *Manual for the Self-Perception Profile for Children.* Denver, CO: University of Denver.

Harter, S. (1988). *Manual for the Self-Perception Profile for Adolescents.* Denver, CO: University of Denver.

Harter, S. (1990). Causes, correlates, and the functional role of global self-worth: A lifespan perspective. In J. Kolligian & R. Sternberg (Eds.), *Perceptions of competence and incompetence across the life span* (pp. 67-97). New Haven, CT: Yale University Press.

Heine, S. H., Lehman, D. R., Markus, H. R., & Kitayama, S. (1990). Is there a universal need for positive self-regard? *Psychological Review, 106,* 766-794.

Klomsten, A. T., Skaalvik, E. M., & Espnes, G. A. (2004). Physical self-concept and sports: Do gender differences still exist? *Sex Roles, 50,* 119-127.

Kohn, M. L. (1987). Cross-national research as an analytic strategy. *American Sociological Review, 52,* 713-731.

Leith, L. M. (1994). *Foundations of exercise and mental health.* Morgantown, WV: Fitness Information Technology.

Magnus, L., & Lindgren, E. C. (2005). The effects of a 6 month exercise intervention programme on physical self-perceptions and social physique anxiety in non-physically active adolescent Swedish girls. *Psychology of Sport and Exercise, 6,* 643-658.

Markus, H. R., & Kitayama, S. (1991). Culture and the self: Implications for cognition, emotion and motivation. *Psychological Review, 98,* 224-253.

Marsh, H. W. (1990). A multidimesional, hierarchical self-concept: Theoretical and emprical justification. *Educational Psychology Review, 2,* 77-172.

Marsh, H. W. (1992). Self-Description Questionnaire II: Manual. Macarthur, NSW: Publication Unit, Faculty of Education, *University of Western Sydney.*

Marsh, H. W. (1993a). Physical fitness self-concept: Relations of physical fitness to field and technical indicators for boys and girls aged 9-15. *Journal of Sports and Exercise Psychology, 15,* 184-206.

Marsh, H. W. (1993b). The multidimensional structure of physical fitness: Invariance over gender and age. *Research Quarterly for Exercise and Sport, 64,* 256-273.

Marsh, H. W. (1994). The importance of being important: Theoretical models of relations between specific and global components of physical self-concept. *Journal of Sport and Exercise Psychology, 16,* 306-325.

Marsh, H. W. (1996a). Construct validity of Physical Self-Description Questionnaire responses: Relations to external criteria. *Journal of Sport and Exercise Psychology, 18,* 111-131.

Marsh, H. W. (1996b), Physical Self-Description Questionnaire: Stability and discriminant validity. *Research Quarterly for Exercise and Sports, 67,* 249-264.

Marsh, H. W. (1997). The measurement of physical self-concept: A construct validation approach. In K. R. Fox (Ed.), *The physical self: From motivation to well being* (pp. 27-58). Champaign, IL: Human Kinetics.

Marsh, H. W. (1998) Age and gender effects in physical self-concepts for adolescent elite athletes and non-athletes: A multi-cohort-multioccasion design. *Journal of Sport and Exercise Psychology, 20,* 237-259.

Marsh, H. W., AsÁi, F. H., & Tomas, M. I. (2002). Multi-trait multi-method analyses of two physical self-concept instruments: A cross-cultural perspective. *Journal of Sport and Exercise Psychology, 24,* 99-119.

Marsh, H. W., & Jackson, S. A. (1986). Multidimensional self-concepts, masculinity and femininity as a function of women's involvement in athletics. *Sex Roles, 15,* 391-416.

Marsh, H. W., Marco, I. T. , & AsÁi, F. H. (2002). Cross-cultural validity of the Physical Self-Description Questionnaire: Comparison of factor structures in Australia, Spain and Turkey. *Research Quarterly for Exercise and Sport, 73,* 257-270.

Marsh, H. W. & Redmayne, R. S. (1994). A multidimensional physical self-concept and its relation to multiple components of physical fitness. *Journal of Sport and Exercise Psychology, 16,* 43-55.

Marsh, H. W., Richards, G. E., Johnson, S., Roche, S., & Tremayne, P. (1994). Physical Self-Description Questionnaire: Psychometric properties and a multitrait-multimethod analysis of relations to existing instruments. *Journal of Sport and Exercise Psychology, 16,* 270-305.

Marsh, H. W., Smith, I. D., Barnes, J., & Butler, S. (1983). Self-concept: Reliability, stability, dimensionality, validity and the measurement of change. *Journal of Educational Psychology, 75,* 772-790.

Marsh, H. W., & Sonstroem, R. J. (1995). Importance ratings and specific components of physical self-concept: Relevance to predicting global components of self-concept and exercise. *Journal of Sport and Exercise Psychology, 17,* 84-104.

McAuley, E., Mihalko, S. L., & Bane, S. M. (1997). Exercise and self-esteem in middle aged adults: Multidimensional relationships and physical fitness and self-efficacy influences. *Journal of Behavioral Medicine, 20,* 67-83.

Nigg, C. R., Norman, G. J., Rossi, J. S., & Benisovich, S. V. (2001). Examining the structure of physical self-description using an American sample. *Research Quarterly for Exercise and Sport, 72,* 78-83.

Page, A., Ashford, B., Fox, K., & Biddle, S. (1993). Evidence of cross-cultural validity for the Physical Self-Perception Profile. *Personality and Individual Differences, 14,* 585-590.

Page, A., Fox, A., McManus, A., & Armstrong, N. (1993). Profiles of self-perception change following an eight week aerobic training programme. In *UK Sport: Partners in Performance. Book of Abstracts.* Manchester, UK: Sports Council.

Ransdell, L. B., Detling, N. J., Taylor, A., Reel, J., & Shultz, B. (2004). Effects of home and university based programs on physical self-perception in mothers and daughters. *Women and Health, 39,* 63-79.

Raustorp, A., Stahle, A., Gudasic, H., Kinnunen, A., & Mattsson, E. (2005). Physical activity and self-perception in school children assessed with the children and youth physical self-perception profile. *Scandinavian Journal of Medicine and Science in Sports, 15,* 126-134.

Richards, G. E., Marsh, H. W., Bar-Eli, M., & Zach, S. (2005). A mutitrait-multimethod evaluation of three physical self-concept measures: A cross national comparison of Australian and Israeli responses. In T. Morris, P. Terry, S. Gordon, S. Hanrahan, L. Ievleva, G. Kolt, & P. Tremayne (Eds.), *Promoting Health and Performance for Life: Proceedings of the ISSP 11th World Congress of Sport Psychology* [CD-ROM]. Sydney: International Society of Sport Psychology.

Shavelson, R. J., Hubner, J. J., & Stanton, G. C. (1976). Self-concept: Validation of construct interpretations. *Review of Edu-*

cational Research, 46, 407-441.

Shaw, J. M., Ebbeck, V., & Snow, C. M. (2000). Body composition and physical self-concept in older women. *Journal of Women and Aging, 12,* 59.

Sonstroem, R. J. (1984). Exercise and self-esteem. *Exercise and Sport Science Reviews, 12,* 123-155.

Sonstroem, R. J. (1997). The physical self-system: A mediator of exercise and self-esteem. In K. R. Fox (Ed.), *The physical self: From motivation to well-being* (pp. 3-26), Champaign, IL: Human Kinetics.

Sonstroem, R. J., & Potts, S. A. (1996). Life adjustment correlates of physical self-concepts. *Medicine and Science in Sports and Exercise, 28,* 619-624.

Sonstroem, R. J., & Morgan, W. P. (1989). Exercise and self-esteem: Rationale and model. *Medicine and Science in Sports and Exercise, 21,* 329-337.

Stille, J., & Alfermann, D. (2005). Testing a German version of the physical self-description questionnaire. In T. Morris, P. Terry, S. Gordon, S. Hanrahan, L. Ievleva, G. Kolt, & P. Tremayne (Eds.), *Promoting Health and Performance for Life: Proceedings of the ISSP 11th World Congress of Sport Psychology* [CD-ROM]. Sydney: International Society of Sport Psychology.

Stille, J., Marsh, H. W., Richards, G. E., & Alfermann, D. (2003). Measuring physical self-concept in the elderly. *Proceedings of the XIth European Congress of Sport Psychology* (pp. 164). Copenhagen, Denmark: ECSS.

Tafarodi, R. W., & Swann, W. B., (1996). Individualism-collectivism and global self-esteem: Evidence for a cultural trade-off. *Journal of Cross-Cultural Psychology, 27,* 651-672.

Van de Vliet, P., Knapen, J., Onghena, P., Fox, K., Van Coppenolle, H., David, A., et al. (2002). Assessment of physical self-perceptions in normal Flemish adults versus depressed psychiatric patients. *Personality and Individual Differences, 32,* 855-863.

Van Vorst, J. G., Buckworth, J., & Mattern, C. (2002). Physical self-concept and strength changes in college weight training classes. *Research Quarterly for Exercise and Sport, 73,* 113-117.

Watkins, D. (2000). The nature of self-conception: Findings of a cross-cultural research program. In R. G. Craven & H. W. Marsh (Eds.), *Self-concept theory, research and practice: Advances for the new millennium. Collected papers of the inaugural Self-concept Enhancement and Learning Facilitation (SELF) research centre international conference* (pp. 108-117). Sydney, Australia: SELF Research Centre.

Welk, G. J., Corbin, C. B., Dowell, M. N., & Harris, H. (1997). The validity and reliability of two different versions of children and youth physical self-perception profile. Measurement in *Physical Education and Exercise Science, 3,* 163-177.

Welk, G. J., Corbin, C. B. & Lewis, L. A. (1995). Physical self-perceptions of high school athletes. *Pediatric Exercise Science, 7,* 152-161.

Welk, G. J., & Eklund, R. C. (2005). Validation of the children and youth physical self-perceptions profile for young children. *Psychology of Sport and Exercise, 6,* 51-66.

Wells, L. E., & Marwell, G. (1976). *Self-esteem: Its conceptualization and measurement.* London: Sage.

Whitehead, J. R. (1995). A study of children's physical self-perceptions using an adapted physical self-perception profile questionnaire. *Pediatric Exercise Science, 7,* 132-151.

Wylie, R. C. (1974). *The self-concept: A review of methodological consideration and measuring instrument.* Lincoln: University of Nebraska Press.

Wylie, R. C. (1979). *The self-concept: Theory and research on selected topics* (Rev. ed.). Volume II. Lincoln: University of Nebraska Press.

Section II
Sport Psychology Practice

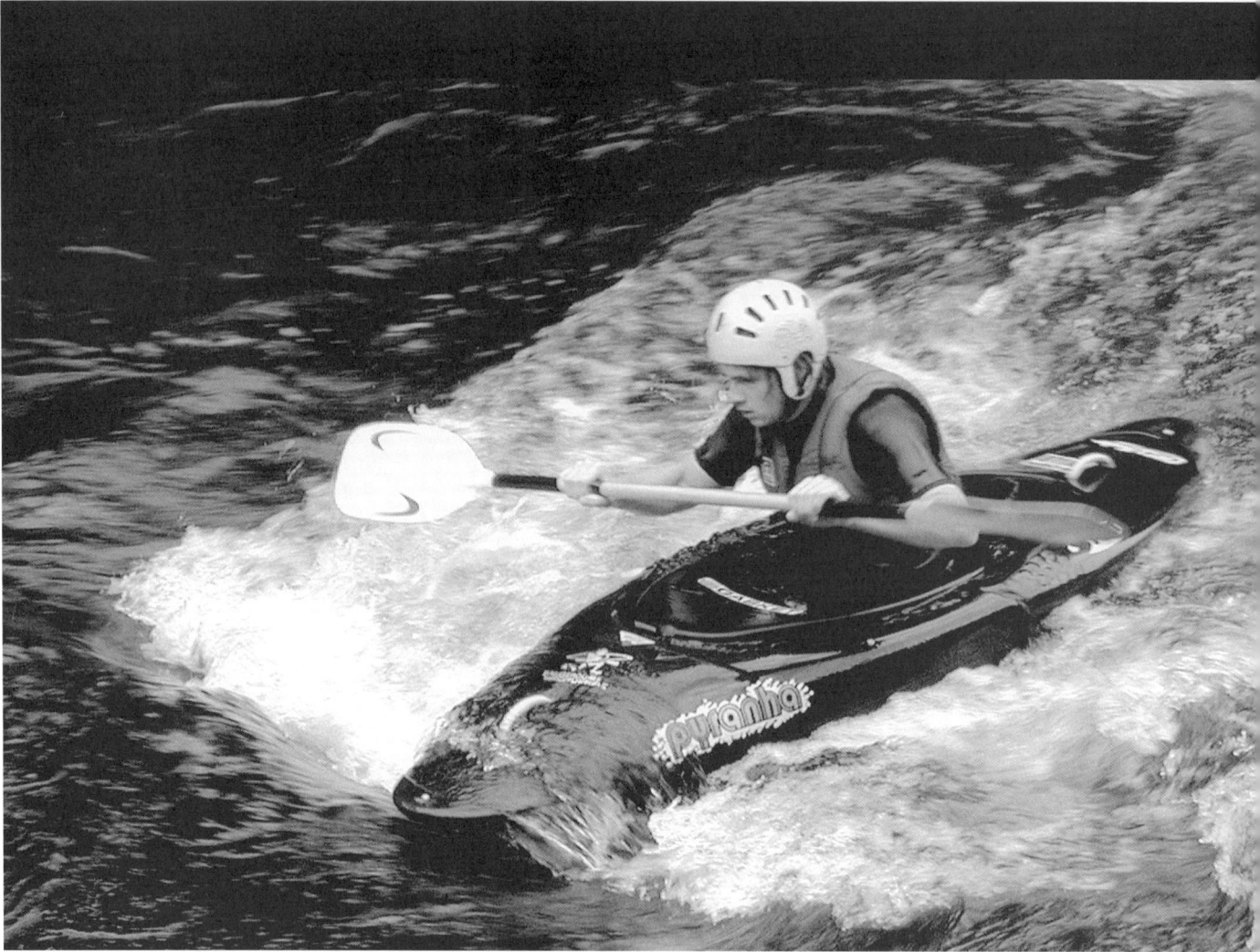

4

A Personal Construct Psychology Perspective on Sport and Exercise Psychology Research: The Example of Mental Toughness

SANDY GORDON, DANIEL GUCCIARDI, AND TIMOTHY CHAMBERS

Personal Construct Psychology (PCP) (Kelly, 1955) is a theory that, rather than telling us *what to think*, tells us *how* we can go about understanding what we think. It presents a framework within which we, as researchers, practitioners, and people, can understand and appreciate how other people theorize about their worlds; it is a theory about theories. Over the years, PCP has been applied extensively to a range of areas subject to psychological inquiry, including clinical settings (Winter, 1992), nursing (Costigan, Ellis, & Watkinson, 2003), education (Pope & Denicolo, 2001), forensics (Horley, 2003) and politics (Stojnov, 2003). However, with the exception of investigations involving Butler's (1991) performance profiling technique, researchers in sport and exercise psychology have largely ignored PCP. The main purpose of this chapter, therefore, is to provide a PCP framework for studying psychological variables in sport and exercise settings. In doing so, we hope to illustrate the usefulness of PCP as a framework for the design of empirical research in sport and exercise settings, and provide a PCP theoretical base for interpreting the data from such research. The example of mental toughness was chosen as the illustrative example for this paper because the research to date on this topic has not been linked to any theoretical framework. While Jones, Hanton, and Connaughton (2002) mentioned that their research was based on a general framework of PCP, no clear link was presented to specifically demonstrate how the theory guided their research.

Following a brief overview of mental toughness research in sport, both the repertory grid and performance profiling techniques are discussed, and a model of the PCP experience cycle is described. The chapter concludes with an illustration of how PCP can be employed for understanding and developing any psychological phenomenon in sport and exercise settings. The essential components of PCP, presented in Table 1, are discussed throughout the paper, highlighting their relevance to the research agenda.

Mental Toughness in Sport

Within scientific and coaching communities, mental toughness is acknowledged as being one of the most important psychological attributes in achieving performance excellence (Bull, Shambrook, James, & Brooks, 2005; Fourie & Potgieter, 2001; Goldberg, 1998; Gould, 2002; Jones et al., 2002; Middleton, Marsh, Martin, Richards, & Perry, 2004a). Most individuals use the term implicitly, and accordingly scientific literature contains a plethora of widely differing definitions of mental toughness; without a general consensus as to its meaning, the term serves to complicate rather than clarify discussion (Jones et al., 2002). Moreover, until several recent qualitative investigations (Bull et al., 2005; Fourie & Potgieter, 2001; Gould, Dieffenbach, & Moffett, 2002; Jones et al., 2002; Middleton et al., 2004a; Thelwell, Weston, & Greenlees, 2005), much of what was known about mental toughness was based on anecdotal reports.

Studies by Jones et al. (2002) and Middleton et al. (2004a) were specific attempts to elucidate an understanding of mental toughness within their given cohorts. These investigations with athletes and coaches provided some insight into the complexity of the concept and provided definitions of, and characteristics essential to, mental toughness. Jones et al. (2002) provided this definition:

> Mental toughness is having the natural or developed psychological edge that enables you to: Generally, cope better than your opponents with the many demands (competition, training, life style) that sport places on the performer. Specifically, be more consistent and better than your opponents in remaining determined, focused, confident, and in control under pressure (p. 209).

They also identified 12 attributes as keys to mental toughness: an unshakeable self-belief to achieve competition goals; an unshakeable self-belief in their unique qualities that make them better than the rest; an insatiable desire to succeed; the ability to bounce back from set-backs; to thrive on pressure; to accept anxiety as inevitable; to not be affected by performances of others; to remain focused despite personal issues; to switch sport focus on and off as required; to remain focused despite competition issues; to push physical and emotional pain boundaries while maintaining technique and effort; and to regain psychological control following unexpected or uncontrollable competitive events (Jones et al., 2002).

Middleton et al. (2004a), however, asserted that the Jones et al. (2002) definition was inadequate as it only described the outcomes of being mentally tough and did not define mental toughness itself. Based on their qualitative research, these authors concluded that mental toughness is "an unshakeable perseverance and conviction towards some goal despite pressure or adversity" (p. 6). They also identified 12 key mental toughness characteristics, which included *self-efficacy* in your ability to achieve in a chosen sport; a strong and positive *mental self-concept* with regards to dealing with adversity; believing in your own *potential* and capacity for growth and development; *task-specific attention* whilst being able to block out distracting or negative thoughts; *perseverance* in the face of adversity; *task familiarity* and understanding adversity; intrinsically motivated

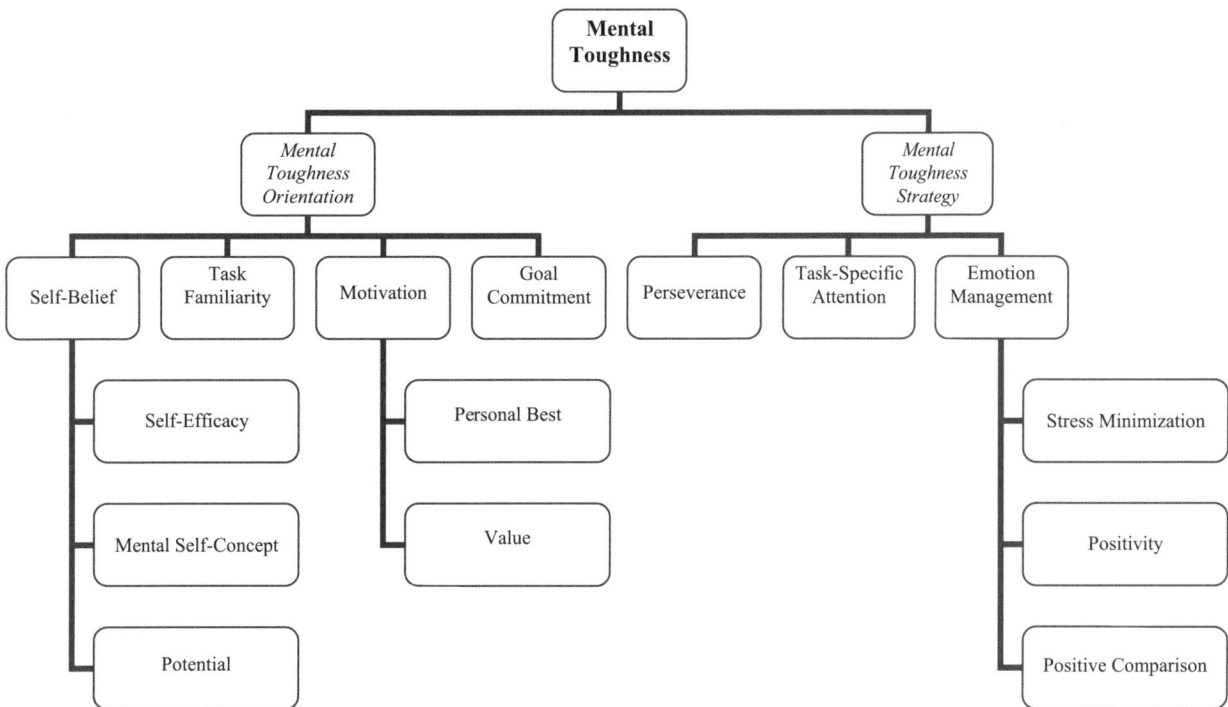

to achieve personal bests; *task value* in the quality and success of performance; intellectual and emotional goal commitment; *positivity* when faced with adversity; *stress minimisation* when under pressure or adversity; and *positive comparisons* with your opponents in coping better with adversity. Middleton et al. went one step further and proposed a model of mental toughness (Figure 1) that is both multidimensional and hierarchical, attempting to capture the complexity of this concept with greater specificity. This model separates mental toughness into *orientation* and *strategy*, with further distinctions emphasizing factors that are actions (coping strategies, focusing of attention) and personal characteristics (self-beliefs, motivations). The authors argued that their definition and model illustrate not only what mental toughness is, but also what the actions of mental toughness are (e.g., emotion management, perseverance, and task focus), together with the role of some of the factors that orient individuals to be mentally tough (e.g., self-belief, determination, commitment, attitude, and task familiarity).

Middleton and colleagues have also developed a Mental Toughness Inventory (MTI) based on their definition and model, which encompasses 13 factors in total. These include the 12 components of mental toughness mentioned previously, plus a global mental toughness measure (Middleton, Marsh, Martin, Richards, & Perry, 2004b). The inventory was piloted at a specialist sports school in Sydney, Australia, with 279 male and 200 female athletes between 12 and 19 years old. The MTI showed good reliability and the measurement model was supported in a confirmatory factor analysis.

Research by Bull et al. (2005) focused specifically on mental toughness in elite cricket. They sought to gain a better understanding of how mental toughness is conceptualized in that sport, and to determine how players developed the qualities of mental toughness. Twelve English cricketers identified by 101 coaches as being among the mentally toughest during the previous 20 years were interviewed. Analysis of their 1:1 interview transcripts identified four themes, which were subsequently used to disseminate findings among England's cricket coaching and playing population. The first theme, *environmental influence,* provides the foundation for the development of mental toughness. In the formative years, parental influence and childhood background were identified as the primary contributors together with secondary factors such as needing to "earn" success, having opportunities to survive early setbacks, and being exposed to foreign cricket. Having a *tough character* was the first of three themes focusing on the individual player, and included common personality characteristics such as resilient confidence, independence, self-reflection, and competitiveness with oneself as well as others. The third theme of *tough attitudes* was considered an important component for the successful exploitation of tough character. These attitudes include a never-say-die mindset, a go-the-extra-mile mindset, thirst for competition, a belief in making a difference, exploiting learning opportunities, a willingness to take risks, a belief in quality preparation, the determination to make the most of ability, and the tendency to self-set challenging targets. The final theme of *tough thinking* relates to cognitions most desirable in and around competitive events, such as clear thinking (e.g., good decision-making, keeping perspective, honest self-appraisal) and robust self-confidence (e.g., overcoming self-doubts, feeding off physical conditioning, maintaining self-focus).

The most recently published research into mental toughness was conducted by Thelwell et al. (2005), who focused on professional soccer and aimed to confirm the definition of, and attributions for, mental toughness identified by Jones et al. (2002). In Study 1, interviews with six international soccer players suggested general consensus with the Jones et al. definition. The sole variation was that mentally tough soccer players should always cope better than their opponents with the demands of soccer rather than generally cope better. The attributes of the mentally tough soccer player, identified in Study 1, also closely resembled those provided by Jones et al. In Study 2, 43 male professional players with first team playing experience ranked the 10 attributes associated with mental toughness in descending order: Having total self-belief at all times that you will achieve success; wanting the ball at all times (when playing well and not so well); having the ability to react to situations positively; having the ability to hang on and be calm under pressure; knowing what it takes to grind yourself out of trouble; having the ability to ignore distractions and remain focused; controlling emotions throughout performance; having a presence that affects opponents; having everything outside of the game in control; and enjoying the pressure associated with performance.

As the first published sport-specific research on mental toughness, the previous two studies represent significant contributions toward achieving a context-rich understanding of the phenomenon. At a practical level they also provide some useful insights into how to develop mental toughness among young cricketers and soccer players. Clearly, however, the conceptual ambiguities acknowledged by all previously mentioned researchers still exist. In other words, mental toughness in sport remains an intuitively attractive yet poorly understood concept that requires considerably more research attention.

Personal Construct Psychology (PCP): The Experience Cycle

The root metaphor that Kelly (1955) employed for his theory of personal constructs was "man-the-scientist" (p. 4). He saw human beings as "forms of motion" (p. 48) constantly engaged in actively describing and evaluating the phenomena they experience by developing and maintaining internal representations (called *personal constructs*) so that they may anticipate and predict what will happen in the future. *Construing* is the term Kelly coined to represent this interpretive process and Kelly refers to the dual process where we abstract recurring themes and their contrasts from the succession of events we experience throughout our lives. The PCP emphasis on the role in behavior of viewing the future distinguishes the Kellyan approach in psychology. Kelly, in fact, saw anticipatory processes or personal construing as the source of all psychological phenomena. The theory of PCP is comprised of a fundamental postulate and 11 subsequent corollaries, presented in Table 1, which elaborate on the fundamental postulate and provide greater specificity by describing the nature of construing.

The fundamental postulate epitomizes what Kelly (1955) envisioned human behavior to entail

PCP Component	Kelly's (1955) Words	Our Words
Fundamental Postulate	A person's processes are psychologically channelized by the ways in which he anticipates events (p. 46).	Interactions with our external environment lead us to operate (psychologically) by developing, maintaining, and modifying descriptive and evaluative internal representations of the phenomena we experience in an attempt to actively anticipate and predict what will happen in the future.
Construction Corollary	A person anticipates events by construing their replications (p. 50).	People develop personal meaning by recognizing regularities and recurring patterns in their experiences.
Individuality Corollary	Persons differ from each other in their construction of events (p. 55).	People develop their individuality through a unique and different approach to construing similar events.
Organization Corollary	Each person characteristically evolves, for his convenience in anticipating events, a construction system embracing ordinal relationships between constructs (p. 56).	Each person develops a unique hierarchical system where some constructs are more important (superordinate) than others (subordinate) to reduce the chaos of the external world so that consistent predictions can be made.
Dichotomy Corollary	A person's construct system is composed of a finite number of dichotomous constructs (p. 59).	Constructs are reference axes, with one personally relevant pole describing the similarities between two events and a contrasting pole implying the distinction between two similar events and another event.
Choice Corollary	A person chooses for himself that alternative in a dichotomised construct through which he anticipates the greatest possibility for elaboration of his system (p. 64).	By expressing preference for one pole of a construct, people aim to increase the accuracy of their predictions and anticipations, thus allowing extension and definition of their system of processes.
Range Corollary	A construct is convenient for the anticipation of a finite range of events only (p. 68).	A personal construct does not apply to everything it encompasses like a concept, and will only account for the anticipations known to that individual.
Experience Corollary	A person's construction system varies as he successively construes the replication of events (p. 72).	People are consistently engaging in experiments (events of their lives) with their hypotheses (constructs) and the result of these experiments (confirm/disconfirm) leave their constructs open to amendment in light of those events.
Modulation Corollary	The variation in a person's construction system is limited by the permeability of the constructs within whose ranges of convenience the variants lie (p. 77).	Some personal constructs are more accommodating (permeable) of new or novel events within their range of convenience.
Fragmentation Corollary	A person may successively employ a variety of constructions subsystems that are inferentially incompatible with each other (p. 83).	The meaning generated through the elaboration of a person's system can be inferentially incompatible with an existing subsystem of constructs.
Commonality Corollary	The extent that one person employs a construction of experience which is similar to that employed by another, his processes are psychologically similar to those of the other person (p. 90).	People are not similar because they encounter similar events or behave similarly, but rather because they construe events similarly.
Sociality Corollary	To the extent that one person construes the construction process of another he may play a role in a social process involving the other person (p. 95).	Any attempt to construe what another person is also construing of the situation influences our own construction of that event.

Table 1. The Essential Components of PCP and Their Meaning.

and states: "*A person's processes are psychologically channelized by the ways in which he anticipates events*" (p. 46). Interactions with our external environment lead us to operate (psychologically) by developing, maintaining, and modifying descriptive and evaluative internal representations (*personal constructs*) of the phenomena we experience. This whole process operates through a structured network of pathways (i.e., the construct system) and the fundamental postulate highlights that people are not reactive, but rather, proactive, in trying to make sense of what may seem an otherwise chaotic world of events.

The experience cycle, illustrated in Figure 2, is based on the experience corollary, and explains how the assertions of PCP are integrated into a cyclical process. *Anticipation* initiates this cycle—without it, individuals would have no knowledge of their experiences and no understanding of their future (Landfield & Leitner, 1980). *Inferences* are the assumptions we abstract from the investment process and represent an individual's hypotheses or predictions formulated from each construct within their system regarding the likelihood of future events (Kelly, 2003). Once a choice has been made about which alternative in a construct best permits elaboration of their system, the individual can hypothesise possible outcomes of events incorporating similar elements. The *event* (encounter) marks the stage in the experience cycle where individuals test the anticipations and predictions they have ascribed to the chosen construct. In Kelly's (1955) words, "The constructions one places upon events are working hypotheses, which are about to be put to the test of experience" (p. 72). In keeping with Kelly's "man-the-scientist" metaphor, the encounter would be considered as analogous to the running of an experiment for the scientist. Subjective and objective feedback (or data) from the encounter allows people to determine if they correctly anticipated the event.

According to Kelly (1955), *validation* "represents the compatibility (subjectively construed)

Figure 2. Experience Cycle. Adapted with permission from Middleton et al.'s (2004a) proposed Model of Mental Toughness.

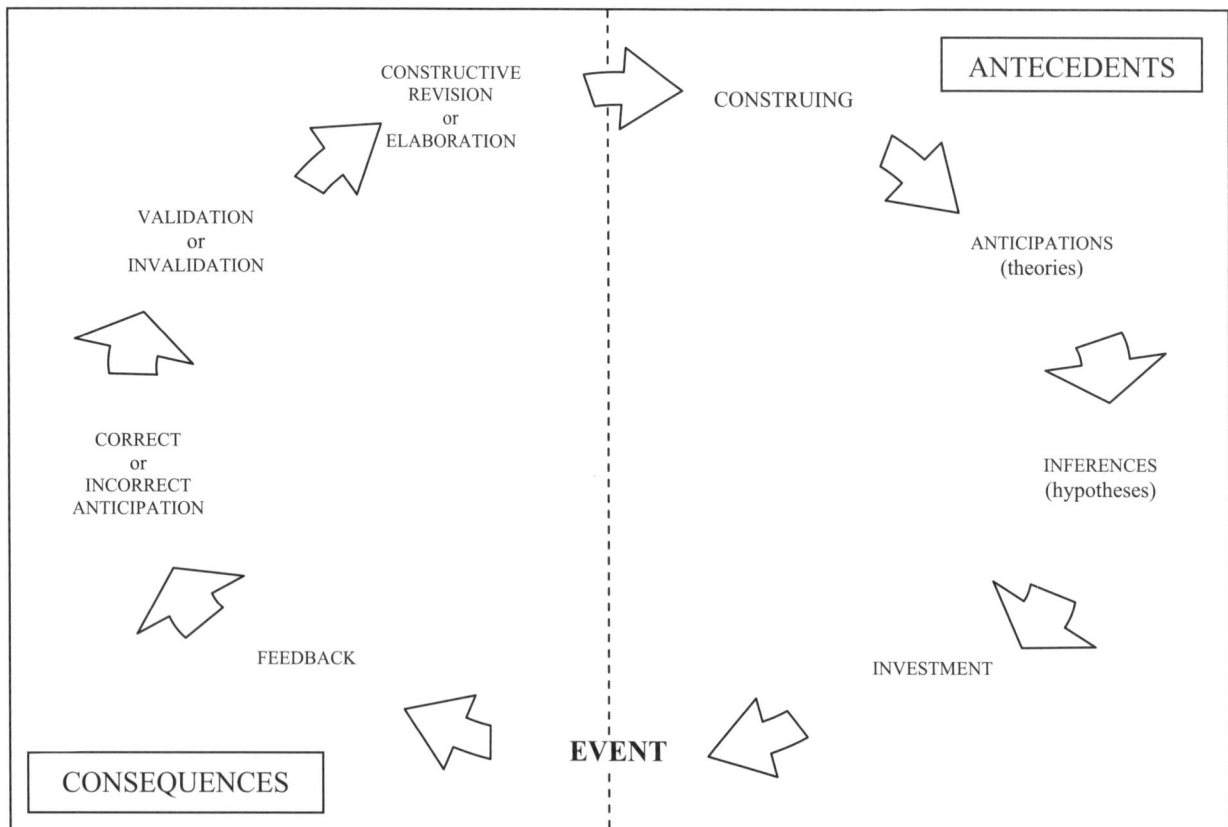

between one's predictions and the outcome he observes. Invalidation represents incompatibility (subjectively construed) between one's predictions and the outcome he observes [sic]" (p. 158). In other words, both subjective and objective feedback may either confirm or disconfirm an individual's hypotheses about a particular event, which will either lead to retainment of that construct or constructive revision. Thus, the validational stage of the experience cycle is where individuals subjectively assess their commitment made during the encounter, the feedback received from the encounter, and whether the resulting evidence confirmed or disconfirmed their anticipations. Both the validation and invalidation of a construct can lead individuals to revise their construct in the final phase of the cycle. Generally, we retain a belief when a construct has been validated by the feedback from the encounter.

One personal construct that an individual may consider useful for mental toughness, for example, is that of *team-focused* versus *individual-focused*. Let us consider John, who, involved in a team sport, employs the personally relevant team-focused pole to anticipate (theorize about) certain future events for which he considers this construct useful (e.g., competition). Based on these anticipations, John will make inferences (hypotheses) about what he believes will eventuate from an event when employing this construct (e.g., fluent passing of the ball, more blocks for team-mates). John invests himself in the event and receives feedback from what happens. This feedback is used as data to determine if he correctly anticipated the event. In the event that the data validate the usefulness of the construct (e.g., fluent passing, more blocks), John may simply retain that belief or revise that construct to include other elements previously not considered as part of that construct. On the other hand, the data may disconfirm the usefulness of the construct (e.g., scrappy passing, no blocks), which may encourage John to search for more information to revise the construct.

PCP Repertory Grids and Performance Profiling

Probably the most frequently used technique to explore personal construing is the *repertory grid*, which has flourished to the point where it has almost become synonymous with PCP. There are other PCP techniques such as laddering, pyramiding, self-characterization sketches, bow-ties, illuminative incident analysis, snakes and rivers, and the lying game, but these are much less prominent techniques than repertory grids. (For a more in-depth discussion of both these techniques and the repertory grid technique, the reader is referred to Fransella, Bell, & Bannister, 2004). Whereas traditional methods (i.e., tests and questionnaires) measure an individual on *a priori* constructs, the repertory grid enables the researcher or practitioner to elicit what is important to the individual by identifying the structure and content of meaning (Fransella et al., 2004). This gives the individual freedom to personally pursue meaningful constructs, as opposed to forcing responses to predetermined measures.

There are a number of techniques that can be employed for construct elicitation and the most commonly used include triadic or dyadic comparisons of a concept in 1:1 interviews, during which participants elicit their own set of constructs to describe the similarities and differences associated with the object of study. After the constructs have been elicited a grid is drawn up, with elements listed horizontally and constructs listed vertically.

There are several studies within sport (Clarke, 1994, 1995; Cripps, 1999; Feixas, Marti, & Villegas, 1989; Russell & Salmela, 1992) and exercise (Furnham, Titman, & Sleeman, 1994: Jones & Harris, 1996; Jones, Harris, & Walter, 1998) settings that have employed grid methodology. Feixas et al. (1989) employed the repertory grid to understand various perspectives of the manager, individual team members, and the whole team among a Spanish football team. Two grids were administered, one elicited by individual team members and a second containing common constructs elicited from interviews. They identified two clusters of constructs relating to professional characteristics (e.g., hard-working, responsible) and personal characteristics (e.g., introverted, talkative). Additionally, a discrepancy was revealed in one element (the player "Andres") that helped the manager explore reasons for this discrepancy (i.e., his public criticisms of this player). The authors concluded that the information gained through grid methodology provided insight into the manager's and players' construction patterns, which could expand the manager's understanding of the players' construals, thus allowing meaningful role relationships between them, as asserted by the *sociality corollary*.

Nearly a decade later, Jones et al. (1998) demonstrated the usefulness of grid methodology for eliciting the expectations of people with regard to an exercise program. Participants were interviewed prior to the commencement of a 10-week exercise program during which they completed repertory grids designed to elicit constructs about exercise-related change. Three individual case studies illustrated the diversity and often over-optimistic expectations of change with regard to the program. Results indicated that those participants who held modest expectations were more likely to complete the program. Moreover, those who completed the program demonstrated less discrepancy between current views of themselves and views of how they would like to be. It was concluded that having realistic aims and an understanding of the outcomes of a brief exercise program are important predictors of success.

The most prominent use of a PCP-based technique in sport is *performance profiling*, which is "a natural application of Kelly's 1955 Personal Construct Theory to sport psychology" (Butler & Hardy, 1992, p. 254). Using this technique, the researcher or practitioner elicits constructs or qualities that an individual perceives as essential to achieving personal performance excellence. After these constructs have been elicited, the athlete self-rates his or her own achievement or current status for each of the constructs, which are presented as a visual profile. Subsequently, the performer's coach adds his or her rating of the individual on this profile, which enables the performer to learn more about how the coach construes the performer (Butler, Smith, & Irwin, 1993). Consistent with PCP's *sociality corollary*, this proposes to lead to the development of more effective and more meaningful coach-athlete relationships and, in turn, this partnership also enhances the athlete's ability to extend his or her personal construct system.

From a team perspective, performance profiling may be employed to create an open, non-judgmental atmosphere for athlete/teammate/coach communication, in turn facilitating team goals and cohesion. Dale and Wrisberg (1996) presented a case study illustrating the effectiveness of performance profiling with a Division I women's volleyball team. Performance profiles were conducted pre-season, mid-competitive season, and at the end of the competitive season. It was revealed that both athletes and coach agreed that the profiling process resulted in a more open communication medium, through which athletes expressed appreciation for their role in the decision-making process regarding training programs and goal setting. These qualitative results were paralleled with significant improvements by each athlete, the coach, and the team on one or more characteristics of the performance profile.

PCP Retrospective Interview

Despite the currency of repertory grids in PCP research and limited use of performance profiling research in sport research, we believe that much more attention should be given to examining the effectiveness of a PCP interview methodology as a research tool. To both identify and understand the phenomena associated with mental toughness in sport, we propose an adaptation of Kelly's (1955) psychotherapy retrospective interview, which is illustrated in Table 2. Interestingly, in talent development research among elite performers, Côté, Ericsson, and Law (2005) have also recommended the retrospective interview as an important research tool:

> As long as we are not able to predict accurately which young athlete will eventually reach the highest level, these outstanding athletes can only be distinguished after the fact. Consequently, retrospective interviews with such outstanding athletic performers will remain one of the primary sources of information on the acquisition of the highest levels of performance for the foreseeable future (p. 15).

Prior to considering each question in Table 2, there are two tenets of PCP that bear the stamp of

Kellyan thinking and guide the interview methodology. First, the *credulous approach* means the interviewer must not disregard anything recorded at any time. Second, interviewers need to establish each interviewee's constructions in terms of *bipolar* or *dichotomous constructs*. In PCP, understanding the meaning of anything becomes possible only by understanding a sense of its opposite.

Q1. Please describe what you consider mental toughness to be for your sport. Can you offer a definition, phrase, or quote to describe it? (individuality corollary)

Q2. In your sport, what do you think are the situations that require an individual to be mentally tough and those situations that do not? (events)

Q3. Having identified situations that require mental toughness, what do you think are the characteristics that distinguish mentally tough individuals from mentally weak individuals? What attitudes and/or beliefs do you consider to be the contrast of each of these characteristics? (dichotomy corollary)

Q4. In your opinion, what do you consider to be the role(s) or purpose(s) of each of these characteristics? (behaviors)

Q5. Of all of the characteristics that you have mentioned, please rank these characteristics in order of importance for mental toughness. (organization corollary)

Q6. Now that you have identified these characteristics, please list all the situations to which these characteristics apply. (range corollary)

Q7. Please put yourself in your coach's shoes and describe what he or she would consider mental toughness to be. Again, what would he or she contend to be characteristics of a mentally tough individual and what is the role of each characteristic? (sociality corollary)

Q8. Are there any significant others (e.g., coach, team-mates, parents, etc.) who you feel have played a crucial role in the development of your mental toughness? What have these individuals done to help? What have they not done? Are there any techniques or methods that you have experienced that you feel have influenced the development of mental toughness? (sociality corollary)

Q9. Please think of someone you know whom you would characterize as being mentally tough. How do you think they have developed their mental toughness? (sociality corollary)

Table 2. Proposed Personal Construct Psychology Interview Protocol for Understanding Sport-Specific Mental Toughness.

The following series of questions is based on an interview protocol that the second author is currently using for his doctoral research, in an effort to identify and understand mental toughness and how it can be developed among Australian Rules footballers. In presenting this retrospective interview schedule, we hope to illustrate how several simple ideas derived from the fundamental postulate and its associated corollaries can inform researchers wishing to explore the personal construing process.

Q1. Please describe what you consider mental toughness to be for your sport. Can you offer a definition, phrase or quote to describe it? (individuality corollary)

The *individuality corollary* emphasises that we always have our own individual anticipations of certain events and even identical events can be construed differently from person to person. So, the credulous approach (Kelly, 1955), which encourages the interviewer to see the interviewee's world through the interviewee's eyes, starts here and is maintained throughout the interview in an attempt to arrive at a value-free understanding of another's construal and behaviour.

Q2. In your sport, what do you think are the situations that require an individual to be mentally tough and those situations that do not? (situations)

Situations and *people* are the most frequently employed elements in PCP research. Initially, we ask the interviewee about those situations that do and do not require mental toughness to encourage the interviewee to place himself or herself in these situations and identify salient features of these personal experiences. Moreover, by identifying situations that do and do not require an individual to be mentally tough, it is possible to gain an insight into possible event simulations that are useful when designing interventions for developing mental toughness.

Q3. Having identified situations that require mental toughness, what do you think are the characteristics that distinguish mentally tough individuals from mentally weak individuals? What attitudes and/or beliefs do you consider to be the contrast of each of these characteristics? (dichotomy corollary)

There will always be people regarded as mentally tough and those who are not, and interviewees will import characteristics of these people from their encounters with them. So, elaborating on Q2, we ask about the characteristics that distinguish mentally tough people from mentally weak people in the situations identified previously. In the *construction corollary*, the regularities and inconsistencies of situations and people come to represent the characteristics or constructs of those phenomena that they experience. The *dichotomy corollary* extends this notion to the extent that wherever there is a personally-relevant consistency pole there will also be a contrasting pole that implies some distinction or inconsistency.

Q4. In your opinion, what do you consider to be the role(s) or purpose(s) of each of these characteristics? (behaviors)

Having identified constructs ascribed to mentally tough individuals, we now try to identify what the interviewee considers to be the roles or behaviors of these constructs. By identifying which behaviors are inferred from the constructs, we not only learn how a mentally tough individual behaves but also get insights into possible techniques for facilitating the development of mental toughness (e.g., coping and/or stress reduction strategies).

Q5. Of all the characteristics that you have mentioned, please rank these characteristics in order of importance for mental toughness. (organization corollary)

According to the *organization corollary*, personal constructs are arranged into a hierarchical system with some constructs being more personally important than others. PCP suggests that the purpose of this organization is to reduce the chaos of the external world for people and provide them with clearer avenues to infer understanding from experiences. We ask the interviewee to rate the constructs in order of importance in an attempt to identify and understand the organization of personal superordinate and subordinate constructs.

Q6. Now that you have identified these characteristics, please list all the situations to which these characteristics apply. (range corollary)

Elaborating on Q5, and further strengthening our understanding of the organizational properties of an individual's personal construct system, we ask the interviewee to list all the situations to which each superordinate and subordinate construct applies.

When a construct has a higher range of perceived utility, more inferences can be made regarding its significance across a variety of situations. A construct with a higher range of utility would be considered more superordinate than a construct that has a lower range of utility.

Q7. Please put yourself in your coach's shoes and describe what he or she would consider mental toughness to be. Again, what would he or she contend to be characteristics of a mentally tough individual and what is the role of each characteristic? (sociality corollary)

When a psychological phenomenon like mental toughness involves more than one individual's construing (called the *commonality corollary*) and it seems necessary to understand the construing of others (e. g., in team sport settings), the sociality corollary is required. Using the *sociality corollary*, we simply ask the interviewee to consider another individual and to describe the characteristics this individual might believe represents mental toughness. By taking the perspective of another individual, interviewees are being encouraged to go beyond their own idiosyncrasies and further explore how others conceptualize mental toughness. The purpose is to gain more explicit and in-depth information about mental toughness from the interviewee.

Q8. Are there any significant others (e.g., coach, team-mates, parents, etc.) who you feel have played a crucial role in the development of your mental toughness? What have these individuals done to help? What have they not done? Are there any techniques or methods that you feel have influenced your mental toughness? (sociality corollary)

Researchers have yet to investigate formally how mental toughness can be developed. So the final two questions, which are also influenced by the sociality corollary, examine development ideas and avenues that might be explored. The sociality corollary extends the interviewee's personal construct system by obliging an understanding of how others give meaning to the interviewee's world.

Q9. Please think of someone you know whom you would characterize as being mentally tough. How do you think they have developed their mental toughness? (sociality corollary)

Finally, we ask the interviewee to construe how others might develop mental toughness.

In a sport-specific sample of interviewees, we are likely to find commonality in the meanings ascribed to different events. These meanings represent a certain similarity in the psychological processes in those individuals. However, it is important to remember that people are not similar because they experience similar events—they are similar because of the commonalities in their construing of events.

PCP Research Template

In the previous section we explained how the components of PCP can be employed to design an interview protocol for understanding mental toughness. The PCP research template illustrated in Figure 3 separates the research agenda into an *understanding* and a *developing* phase, with further distinctions identifying the essential characteristics of each phase.

PCP emphasizes that if we are to gain an accurate understanding of any psychological phenomenon we need to identify the content, structure, and organization of meaning among our research cohorts. At this early stage in the research process, we can also probe individuals about certain methods for changing or developing specific psychological attributes among people. More importantly, we can design an interview protocol that addresses each of these categories and adheres to the essential proponents of PCP.

Regarding the development of mental toughness, PCP also presents researchers with the repertory grid that has been extended to sport and exercise settings in the form of the performance profile (Butler, 1989). Subsequently, a profile instrument that incorporates the key characteristics of mental toughness could be employed to assess and monitor changes in its development, which is a necessity for evaluating any intervention program designed to enhance a psychological attribute. In addition, based on an understanding of mental toughness and in conjunction with the assertions postulated by PCP, intervention programs

Figure 3. Personal Construct Psychology template for identifying, understanding, and developing a psychological attribute.

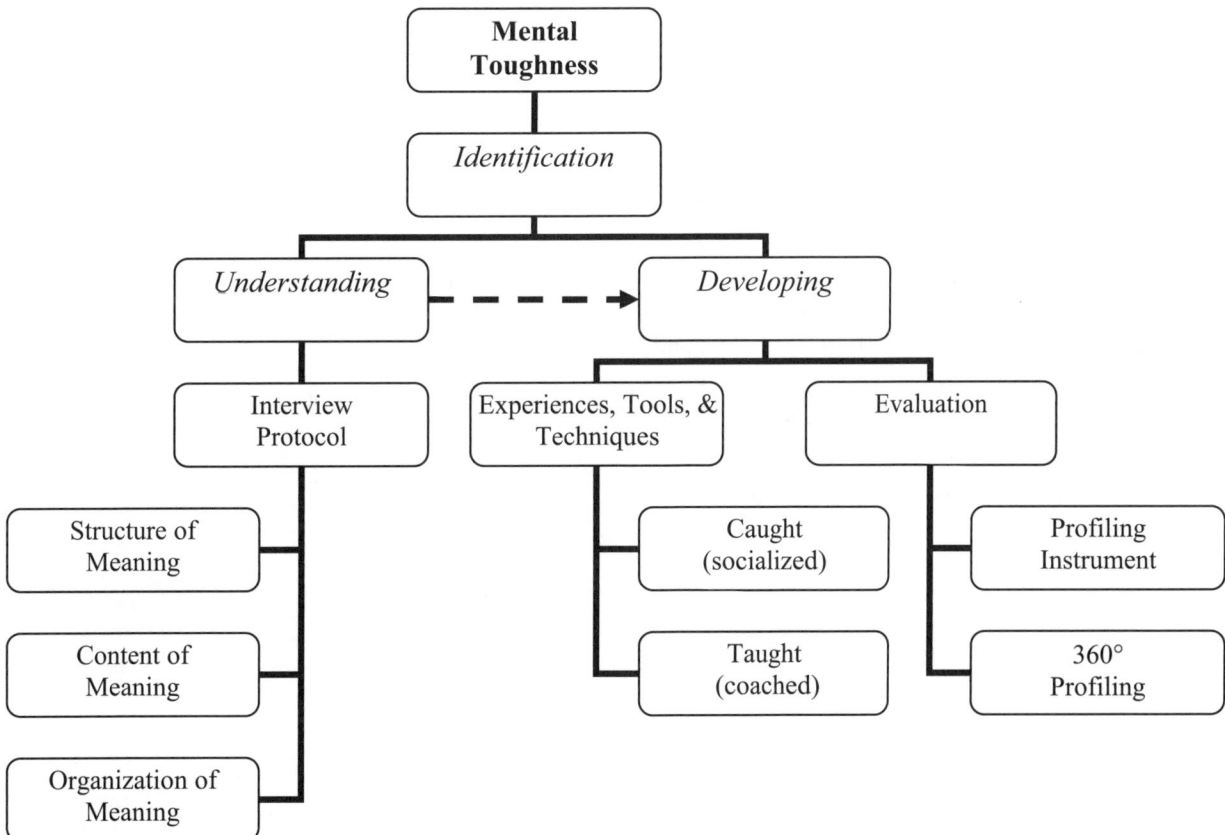

that might include exposure to certain experiences as well as mental skills training could be designed specifically to develop mental toughness.

Using a PCP framework, we can envisage athletes as in a continual cycle of construing that enables them to generate an elaborate theory of their physical and psychological condition as to direct their behavior (see Figure 2). Applying the PCP approach in sport and exercise, therefore, involves trying to understand how an individual's unique interpretation of the world contributes to the development and maintenance of his/her behavior. So, if we want to identify and understand mental toughness among athletes, the first phase in the experimental project would entail qualitative research methodologies, such as retrospective interviewing, to enable researchers to examine different levels of meaning. This research would be aimed at gaining an understanding of the meanings athletes and coaches ascribe to the concept of *mental toughness*. Such an approach appropriately places the individual at the center of knowledge. We are aiming to elicit information about individual construct systems by encouraging interviewees to explore and explicitly communicate what comes implicitly to them, which usually occurs at a low level of awareness (Ravanette, 1977).

Summary

The main objective of this chapter was to introduce a PCP research framework for researchers engaged in trying to identify, understand, and develop any psychological attribute associated with sport and exercise performance. The template provides sport and exercise psychology researchers with an understanding of the pertinent theoretical assertions of PCP that can guide the design of both qualitative and quantitative research methods. The theoretical framework proposes qualitative techniques, such as retrospective interviewing, as an essential starting point for investigating any psychological attribute that is not clearly understood. This foundational knowledge can be extended to develop valid and reliable performance profiling measures associated with a particular psychological attribute. Subsequently, these profiles can be employed to evaluate intervention programs designed to enhance and develop the psychological attribute.

References

Bull, S. J., Shambrook, C. J., James, W., & Brooks, J. E. (2005). Towards an understanding of mental toughness in elite English cricketers. *Journal of Applied Sport Psychology, 17,* 209-227.

Butler, R. J. (1989). Psychological preparation of Olympic boxers. In J. C. Kremer, & W. Crawford (Eds.), *The psychology of sport: Theory and practice* (pp. 74-84). Leicester, England: British Psychological Society.

Butler, R. J. (1991). *The performance profile: Developing elite performance.* London: British Olympic Association Publishing.

Butler, R. J., & Hardy, L. (1992). The performance profile: Theory and application. *The Sport Psychologist, 6,* 253-264.

Butler, R. J., Smith, M., & Irwin, I. (1993). The performance profile in practice. *Journal of Applied Sport Psychology, 5,* 48-63.

Clarke, P. T. (1994). *Professional soccer coaches' perceptions of coaching attributes.* Paper presented at the XV Commonwealth Games Conference, University of Victoria, BC, Canada.

Clarke, P. T. (1995). The perception of coaching qualities held by professional soccer players. In H. F. Fu, & M. Ng (Eds.), *Sport psychology: Perspectives and practices toward the 21st century* (pp. 273-284). Hong Kong: Hong Kong Baptist University.

Costigan, J., Ellis, J. M., & Watkinson, J. (2003). Nursing. In F. Fransella (Ed.), *International handbook of personal construct psychology* (pp. 427-430). Chichester, England: Wiley.

Côté, J., Ericsson, K. A., & Law, M. P. (2005). Tracing the development of athletes using retrospective interview methods: A proposed interview and validation procedure for reported information. *Journal of Applied Sport Psychology, 17,* 1-19.

Cripps, B. (1999). Constructing the athlete's world. In H. Steinberg, & I. Cockerill (Eds.), *Sport psychology in practice: The early stages* (pp. 8-15). Leicester, England: British Psychological Society.

Dale, G. A., & Wrisberg, C. A. (1996). The use of a performance profiling technique in a team setting: Getting the athletes and coach on the "same page." *The Sport Psychologist, 10,* 261-277.

Feixas, G., Marti, J., & Villegas, M. (1989). Personal construct assessment of sport teams. *International Journal of Personal Construct Psychology, 2,* 49-54.

Fourie, S., & Potgieter, J. R. (2001). The nature of mental toughness in sport. *South African Journal for Research in Sport, Physical Education and Recreation, 23,* 63-72.

Fransella, F., Bell, R., & Bannister, D. (2004). A manual for repertory grid technique. (3rd ed.). Chichester, England: Wiley.

Furnham, A., Titman, P., & Sleeman, E. (1994). Perception of female body shapes as a function of exercise. *Journal of Social Behaviour and Personality, 9,* 335-352.

Goldberg, A. S. (1998). *Sports slump busting: 10 steps to mental toughness and peak performance.* Champaign, IL: Human Kinetics.

Gould, D. (2002). Sport psychology in the new millennium: The psychology of athletic excellence and beyond. *Journal of Applied Sport Psychology, 14,* 247-248.

Gould, D., Dieffenbach, K., & Moffett, A. (2002). Psychological characteristics and their development in Olympic champions. *Journal of Applied Sport Psychology, 14,* 172-204.

Horley, J. (2003). *Personal construct perspectives on forensic psychology.* London: Bruner-Routledge.

Jones, G., Hanton, S., & Connaughton, D. (2002). What is this thing called mental toughness? An investigation of elite sport performers. *Journal of Applied Sport Psychology, 14,* 205-218.

Jones, F., & Harris, P. (1996). The use of repertory grid technique in exercise psychology. In C. Robson, B. Cripps, & H. Steinberg, (Eds.), *Quality and quantity: Research methods in sport and exercise psychology* (pp. 3-9). Leicester, England: British Psychological Society.

Jones, F., Harris, P., & Waller, H. (1998). Expectations of an exercise prescription scheme: An exploratory study using repertory grids. *British Journal of Health Psychology, 3,* 277-289.

Kelly, G. A. (1955). *The psychology of personal constructs.* New York: Norton.

Kelly, G. A. (2003). A brief introduction to personal construct theory. In F. Fransella (Ed.), *International handbook of personal construct psychology* (pp. 3-20). Chichester, England: Wiley.

Landfield, A. W., & Leitner, L. M. (1980). Personal construct psychology. In A. W. Landfied, & L. M. Leitner (Eds.), *Personal construct psychology* (pp. 3-17). New York: Wiley.

Middleton, S. C., Marsh, H. W., Martin, A. J., Richards, G. E., & Perry, C. (2004a, July). *Developing the mental toughness inventory* (MTI). Paper presented at the 3rd International Biennial SELF Research Conference, Berlin, Germany.

Middleton, S. C., Marsh, H. W., Martin, A. J., Richards, G. E., & Perry, C. (2004b, July). *Discovering mental toughness: A qualitative study of mental toughness in elite athletes.* Paper presented at the 3rd International Biennial SELF Research Conference, Berlin, Germany.

Pope, M., & Denicolo, P. (2001). *Transformative education: Personal construct approach to practice and research.* London: Whurr Publications.

Ravenette, A. T. (1977). *PCT: An approach to the psychological investigation of children and young people.* London: Academic Press.

Russell, S. J., & Salmela, J. H. (1992). Quantifying expert athlete knowledge. *Journal of Applied Sport Psychology, 4,* 10-26.

Stojnov, D. (2003). Moving personal construct psychology to politics: Understanding the voices with which we disagree. In F. Fransella (Ed.), *International handbook of personal construct psychology* (pp. 191-198). Chichester, England: Wiley.

Thelwell, R., Weston, N., & Greenlees, I. (2005). Defining and understanding mental toughness within soccer. *Journal of Applied Sport Psychology, 17,* 326-332.

Winter, D. A. (1992). *Personal construct psychology in clinical practice: Theory, research and applications.* London: Routledge.

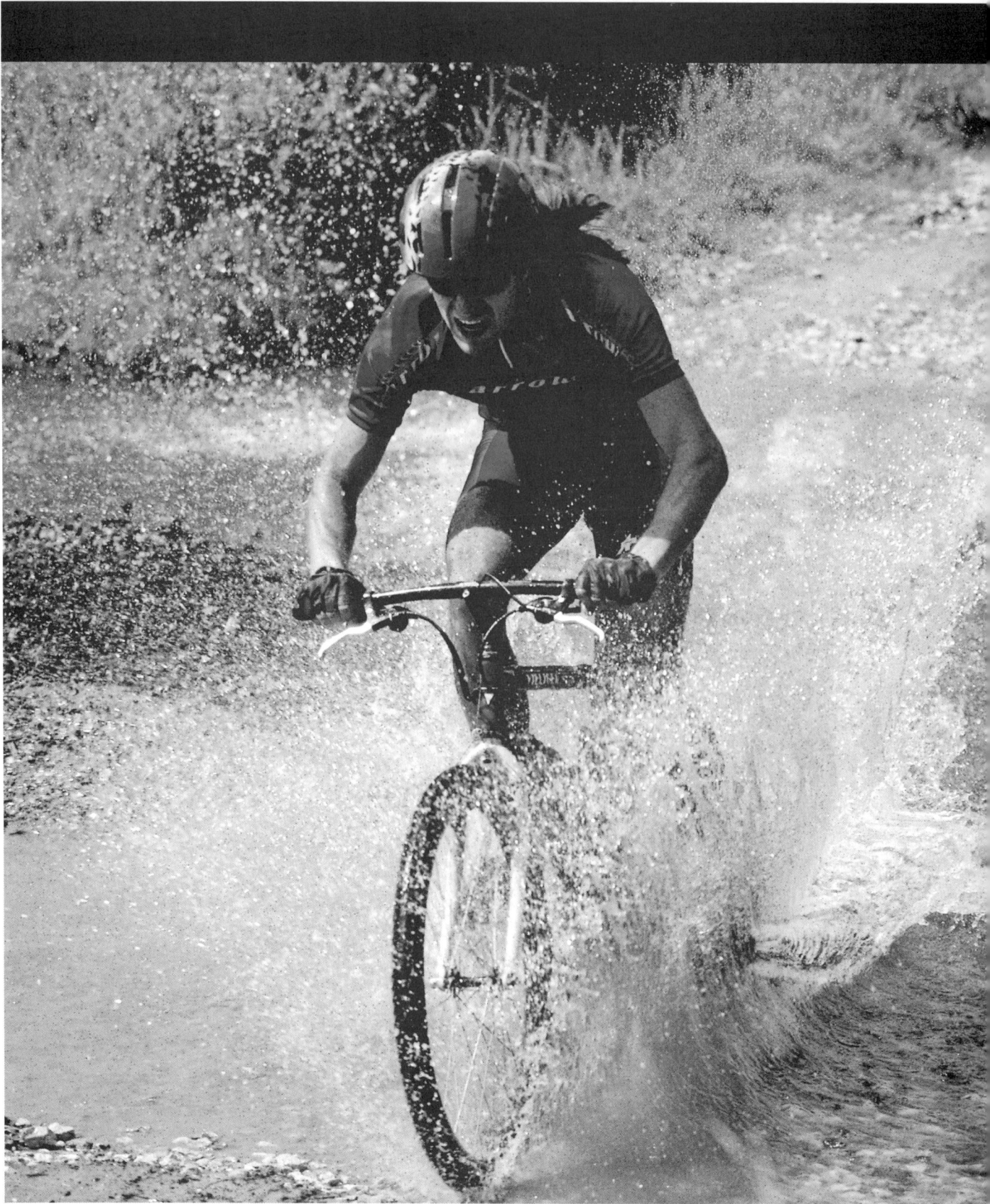

Courtesy of MediaFocus

5

Lessons Learned from Sports Psychology Consulting

KENNETH H. RAVIZZA AND TRACI A. STATLER

As sport psychology consultants working with teams on a season-long basis, we are all performers similar to the athletes with whom we work. Just as the athlete strives to perform to his or her potential, we as consultants must have a similar focus, especially if we are to be effective throughout the entire season and during pressure situations. The mental skills that we teach athletes and coaches to enhance their performances are skills that we should regularly use to enhance our own performances. For many of us, this pressure occurs most often in the "Gaining Entry" phase (Ravizza, 1988). During the selection process (with coaches and management) as well as before the introductory presentation to a team, we still feel the "butterflies." We expect that we will always have these feelings and sensations because we are excited about the op-

portunity and want to do well. Like the athlete, we set high expectations for ourselves, and it is completely natural and appropriate to employ techniques that improve our performance. This is an opportunity to practice what we preach and use skills like breathing and relaxation to calm ourselves and maintain a present focus.

Early in the lead author's career he was invited by a professional baseball team to give a presentation on the "Importance of Sport Psychology to Enhance Performance." If the presentation was well received, he would be given the opportunity to develop and deliver a program for the team. He was given a 30-minute time period and would have to get 75% of the players to indicate that they wanted more. They would vote "yes" or "no" on his return right after the talk. This was your classic "sport psychology sell job." If he didn't get 75% of the players to vote "yes," then he would not be given an opportunity to work with the team. For the consultant, there was definitely pressure. Even the coaches recognized that in this situation, he had only one chance to make a favorable impression, while their players have far more opportunities to show their potential.

He gave the presentation in the back of the locker room, where the hot water heater was located. In the midst of the talk, the water heater turned on and made a loud, continuous roaring sound. He was either so focused or so nervous that he didn't even hear it. After the 30-minute presentation, which was well received, 90% of the players voted "yes." Many of the players said they were so impressed with the way he handled the noise distraction that they figured that they had something they could learn from him about focus.

We as sport psychology consultants are models for the mental skills that we teach, and applying them in our own work, allows us to continuously refine and develop them for our own application and to educate others. In this paper, we will address some of the major issues and skills that we discuss with teams and how we can use them ourselves in our consulting performance. This should not, by any means, be considered an exhaustive list, but your ability to incorporate these techniques will take you a long way in establishing a successful relationship with a sports team. The issues we will discuss include: cultivating a clear understanding of one's personal philosophy and why we choose to work as sport psychology consultants; knowing and understanding one's personal strengths and weaknesses as a consulting professional; the realities and expectations of peak experiences in the consulting setting; the value of preparation as a consultant; approaching the consultancy as a performance, and incorporating performance routines; the need to maintain present focus when working with others; the necessity and value of performance evaluation; long-term strategies for taking care of oneself; and finally, the need to keep learning.

Philosophy: Why Do You Do Sport Psychology Consulting?

One of the first issues that we discuss with athletes is why they are involved in their sport. Athletes' clarity about their purpose provides a foundation for their passion. The passion provides direction and fuels the motivation to achieve performance excellence. The pursuit of excellence in sport is a love/hate relationship with one's sport. Similarly, sport psychology consulting brings up many questions and challenges. Being on the road away from one's family and the daily routines is not always a positive thing. It is important to know why you choose to do sport psychology consulting. What do you love about it? What is your purpose in being involved in this area of sport? There are as many reasons as there are consultants, and each consultant must find his or her own meaning. For some, it is about furthering the profession; for others it is about the joy of teaching, one athlete at a time. For us, enjoyment comes from working with highly committed people, teaching and learning from athletes and coaches, effectively collaborating with coaches and the total staff, the immediate feedback that sport provides, and the creativity and flexibility that is required to deliver a synchronous program in a complex, fast-paced environment. Each consulting experience has its own unique context, and our expertise lies in the ability to compensate and adjust to meet the demands of the particular situation. At times, this can feel like being in a pressure cooker, but by the end of the season we can always reflect back and realize how much we have enjoyed the challenge.

For example, in almost every presentation to a group of coaches, there is always that one coach who sits at the back of the room, with arms crossed, and seems disinterested. In any other social situation, this would be considered rude. The challenge for the sport psychology consultant is to impact this individual and make a connection with him or her. The goal is to change the coach's negativity by reaching him or her through an example or an experience that he or she can relate to and that also has relevancy to sport psychology. As the consultant, having a clear mission provides direction, motivation, feedback, meaning, and a sense of purpose. It is this foundation that fosters the ability to maintain perspective and passion as you work through the difficult times.

Know Thy Consulting Self

To become a more effective sport psychology consultant, you must know yourself. What are your strengths? What do you need to improve? What do you enjoy about consulting? How well do you manage your time and energy? What can you do and what can't you do? The answers to these questions provide the framework for continuing self-improvement for the sport psychology consultant. One of the greatest compliments the lead author ever received from a professional athlete was when the athlete thanked him for introducing him to himself. Like the athlete, it is critical to know who you are so your identity doesn't get totally distorted in the consultant role. Also, this knowledge of who you are and why you engage in this work will help you deal with the rejection that is an inevitable part of consulting (i.e., your suggestions are not followed or you are not chosen for the role). We often reflect upon a story that the lead author likes to share in relation to this idea:

> I remember when I first began working in applied sport psych; I visited one of my mentors, Dr. Bruce Ogilvie. When I told him about my first opportunity with a professional baseball team, he told me something profound. He warned, "You are going to be fired! Rejection is part of the consulting process." I remember feeling a sense of disbelief at his words. "That won't happen to me," I thought.

But he was absolutely correct—the reality of this work is that you will experience rejection, on both a grand scale (e.g., management terminating your services, or failing to be hired in the first place), as well as on a smaller scale (e.g., players avoiding you). This rejection from the players is an endemic part of sport psychology consulting, as not all of them are ready for what you have to offer, nor do some even see a need for it. It took us a while to adjust to this. It doesn't mean we are not trying to get everyone involved, but sometimes the consultant has to be patient and wait for the teachable moment. This requires patience, confidence, and acknowledgment of your consulting self so that you can maintain perspective and clarity as you cope with the distractions and frustrations that go with the job.

Knowing yourself will also be critical in determining what situations and/or sports you want to work with. For example, in some sports sexuality issues are prevalent, and if one is homophobic it will likely be an uncomfortable environment and not be a good fit. Furthermore, certain sports may not be appropriate choices for you. The lead author was hesitant to work with boxers based on his philosophical values, but recognized that there was a point to be learned about concentration within this sport. He figured what better group of athletes to learn about concentration from, because if the boxer loses concentration he or she receives immediate feedback, usually in the form of a debilitating jab or uppercut. In addition, the culture of a sport is an important component in determining if we want to work in that situation. For example, the golf-country club culture is totally different from the rugby culture, and while the two may share many similarities, the skill set required of a sport psychology consultant working within those environments can be very different (Halliwell, Orlick, Ravizza, & Rotella, 2003).

We strongly believe that, as a consultant, you have to "bring yourself to the dance." Knowing and being yourself is one of your greatest assets because you are being authentic, and athletes/coaches have keen intuition to determine if someone is not being authentic.

Realities and Expectations of Peak Experience in the Consulting Process

In our work with athletes, we always have them reflect on their best performances. Even though this superior level of performance doesn't happen often, there is a lot we can learn from it. When athletes are "in the zone," or at peak performance levels, they consistently report that they are totally immersed, confident in their preparation, focused in the present, possess a relaxed concentration, and are thinking clearly. As sport psychology consultants we, too, can get into this "zone," but just like any other performance, this experience is fairly rare. You cannot always be in the zone, and it is unrealistic to set too high a standard for yourself or your team. We personally think we are in the zone about 20% of the time; for the rest of the time we are compensating and adjusting. In our work with athletes we want them to set the conditions for being in the zone by being prepared, maintaining a present focus, thinking clearly, and having that relaxed concentration. As consultants you have to do similar things, but recognize that there are going to be those days when you are not in the zone. For example, jet lag, illness, back pain, or issues in one's personal life all interfere with the present focus needed to approach peak experiences. We must actively get better at having what we call a "good lousy day."

As we always tell athletes, you have to learn to be "comfortable being uncomfortable." As consultants, there will be times that you will feel awkard. Just like athletes, you must learn to deal with the setbacks and rejections and persevere through the adversity. Some of these distractions will be the number of players who want to be involved in the program, as well as the amount of support you will receive from the coaches, administrators and/or physios/athletic trainers. Sometimes people are threatened by outsiders and they may attempt to sabotage what you are trying to do. This is where you must work to gain support at all levels, although many times this is not possible and you must be prepared to deal with it effectively and work within that context (Ravizza, 1988). This is similar to what we say to athletes when we tell them to focus on what they can control. You must have methods to go to when adversity presents itself. For those consulting days when you are in the zone, go with the experience and thank the "gods of sport consulting." Most days, however, will be more ordinary and will require a lot of hard work. From our years of experience, we have identified four skills that provide the consultant with a strategy, or "something to go to," when adversity happens. These are (1) preparation, (2) routines, (3) focus, and (4) performance evaluation. The development of these skills provides a contingency plan to deal with adversity, because adversity will occur. Be prepared to embrace it and use it to your advantage, instead of losing your focus because everything isn't going well. The mastery of these four areas will enhance your ability to mange your consulting day more effectively.

Preparation: Prepare to Prepare

One of the primary things a consultant has control over in the quest for peak consulting experiences is preparation. It is vital to immerse yourself in the preparation. You have to know the context in which you will be working. This includes knowledge of the sport, the group dynamics of the team, the politics of the team and/or organization, and the specific demands of the sport. You must be prepared to adjust your program to the unique context of the situation and sport (e.g., open vs. closed sports, team vs. individual sports, contact vs. non-contact sports). For example, working with a women's basketball team has both subtle and blatant differences from working with a men's basketball team. You must know the history of the team, the coach's philosophy, previous sport psychology consultants who may have worked with the team, and the unique context in which you will deliver the program. There are many ways to obtain this information, but it is essential to do your homework in each of these areas. All of this is in addition to the basic consulting and counseling skills. Good, solid preparation enables you as the consultant to build your confidence and deliver an effective program.

This preparation also allows you to design and implement your performance enhancement program to meet the demands of that unique situation. Developing short-, medium-, and long-range goals and objectives is important. As coaches and players know, a contingency plan is necessary for when the original plan doesn't work. As a consultant, you have to be flexible. We can likely all recall the times we have had a well-established plan, which then promptly changed when we began our day with the team. We must quickly adjust our plans to deal with the unforeseen circumstances of a team sport environment. This is why working with a team is dramatically different from teaching an academic class or working on an individual basis with athletes, because there are so many factors over which you have no control (e.g., access to the team, sufficient time to deliver your program, the amount of support by the coaching staff). Most times, once we have been working with a team and have a clear understanding of the history, coach, and team dynamics, we can go in ready for whatever may present itself. Not surprisingly, these have been some of our most productive days.

Similar to the athlete, we have to have a game plan, but we also need to be flexible in order to meet the demands of that day. This is very important in our consulting performance because our aptitude for dealing with adversity serves as an example for the athletes. Our actions count, and they are definitely watching. If you, as the consultant, are going to expect the athlete to deal effectively with obstacles, then you must be prepared to model this behavior yourself. How you handle interruptions, audio-visual or technical malfunctions during the presentation, athletes or coaches who are not paying attention, and other unexpected difficulties will be observed by all. Your credibility can be seriously compromised if you are unable to handle yourself when a problematic situation occurs—and it will.

When you are gaining entry with a team/coaching staff there will be a point at which you will have to perform, so prepare for this. You must earn their respect and trust or you will not be able to work productively. With one major American university's football team, the first author had to give a preliminary presentation to the 11 assistant coaches, who then evaluated whether to have him continue with the remainder of the team. After gaining their approval, he had to present to 25 key players. When he did this, the head coach positioned his seat so he could observe him and watch the players' non-verbal reactions to the presentation. You are going to be evaluated at all levels, so be ready for it, and realize that if you expect to gain their trust you are going to have to earn it!

The Use of Routines

Sport is driven by routines. There are game day routines, pre- and post-game routines, and pre- and post-performance or practice routines. Athletes are accustomed to getting ready to perform and to learn from their performances. The same holds true for sport psychology consultants. For some, getting dressed is an important transition to symbolically shift from the personal life to the consulting role. The drive or walk to the consulting area is when we begin our routine. We review our plan, get centered and balanced, and immerse ourselves in a present focus perspective so that when we meet the team we are ready. We then take a few moments to check-in, monitor ourselves, make any needed adjustments,

and "Get Big" when we walk into the pressure of the situation. Throughout the lead author's consulting experiences he has also always debriefed during the car or plane ride home to process the lessons learned from that experience. Just as we ask the athletes to learn each day, we have to learn things to keep getting better at what we do. And when we no longer want to get better, or feel as if there is no longer anything new for us to learn, it is time to retire.

Another important part of the post-consultation routine for us is checking in with other professionals in this field. At times, we have had the opportunity to collaborate with fellow sport psychology consultants, and these experiences have provided us with wonderful insights because we are in the environment together and, inevitably, see the same situation from slightly different perspectives. We would strongly encourage any consultant to collaborate with someone if and when the opportunity presents itself. The capability to debrief after consulting sessions with a colleague who is familiar with the pressures and expectations of the work can help you to fully appreciate the similarities and differences of your perceptions, and can go a long way toward helping to improve your own personal consulting skill set (Balague, Dee, & Ravizza, 2005; Ravizza, 1995).

Present Focus

Just as it is essential for an athlete to be totally immersed in the present moment to perform to his or her potential, so too the consultant must be in the present. We cannot emphasize this enough. At times this present focus just happens, but when adversity occurs, a present focus is critical if one is to compensate and adjust effectively. We always tell athletes to do everything they can to perform at their best, but not to be surprised by adversity when it occurs. This resiliency occurs in the "here and now." For consultants, an analogous example would be when you start your day with a presentation for the coaches and it doesn't go well, and you have 10 minutes to get ready for a presentation to the team. You must let go of the presentation to the coaches before you move on to the next thing. This may sound simple, but it is more difficult that it may first appear. Not surprisingly, this is also what a lot of our work with athletes is about—keeping them focused on performing, in the present moment, and as positive as they can be.

This process or skill of maintaining present focus is about self-control. The first and most important step in maintaining a present focus is taking responsibility for your performance. As a consultant you don't have control of what goes on around you, you only have control of how you choose to respond to it. Many factors associated with consulting in an athletic setting—such as players, coaches, access, and management—are out of your range of control. In order to maintain your present focus, it is important to remember that what you do have is control over yourself. You must be in control of yourself in order to maintain your present focus. The extent to which you are in control of your thoughts and feelings is directly related to your success with the team. Just as we tell athletes that they do not have control of the end results, we as consultants don't have control over whether we are going to be selected to work with a team. We do, however, have control over giving ourselves the best opportunity for success. That is all you are going to have control of, and this type of focus on the process will help you perform and deliver your program in a more effective manner. Remember, players and coaches will be observing how you handle adversity.

Another prerequisite to present focus is awareness (Ravizza & Hanson, 1995). You have to recognize what is going on in your environment. We relate performance to the experience of driving a car (Ravizza, 2005). We have to recognize the traffic or signal lights we confront during our journey. When the light is green, one is aware of it and just moves forward without additional thought. When the light is yellow, one must check the traffic and make a decision whether to continue forward, or make an adjustment. When the light is red, one must stop until ready to move forward again. This signal light analogy has two functions in relation to consulting performance. The first is to help recognize potentially stressful situations. For example, when your presentation time is shortened, or when certain key players may not be able to attend a meeting, the consultant must be able to recognize this new situation and make the necessary adjustments. The second function is to help recognize how you experience the pressure—what happens in your body, with your thoughts, and behaviors. For example, do you respond to pressure with an elevation in heart rate, an alteration in your attentional control, and/or a decline in patience? As consultants, if we know our stressors and how we experience them, we can be better prepared to deal with them. In comfortable situations, we simply perform our role to the best of our ability. When we are not comfortable, we must recognize it early and do something before we begin to spiral out of control. As consultants, when you begin to spiral out of control you must take responsibility for your performance and continually monitor yourself in the environment to recognize the need to make adjustments. This will better enable you to remain on task and get the job done in an effective manner.

Through our years of experience, we have developed a simple process that allows us to make continuous adjustments in the midst of the consulting experience by following a routine we commonly refer to as "The R's." As already described above, the preliminary requirement of "The R's" are individuals' willingness to take responsibility for their actions. Recognizing where you are in a situation and accepting that you have the power to adapt and adjust to the fluctuations within that situation are critical prerequisites for this model to be effective. As shown in Figure 1, "The R's" model of self-control in performance is a cyclical process of continual adjustments. The following is a brief explanation of each step in the process, and some practical examples of how this model works.

Recognize—Signal Lights

After people have accepted responsibility for their actions and reactions in any given situation, they are able to recognize what is going on around them. The previous section on developing and improving awareness describes this initial step. Before you are able to make any adjustments to your reactions in a given situation, you must first be aware of what those reactions are. If everything is going well and you recognize that the "lights are green," you can proceed directly to "Refocus" because no further adjustments are necessary; simply refocus on the task at hand. If, however, you must make adjustments, then you must proceed to the next step in the cycle—"Release."

Figure 1. The R's Model for Self Control in Performance

RESPONSIBILITY

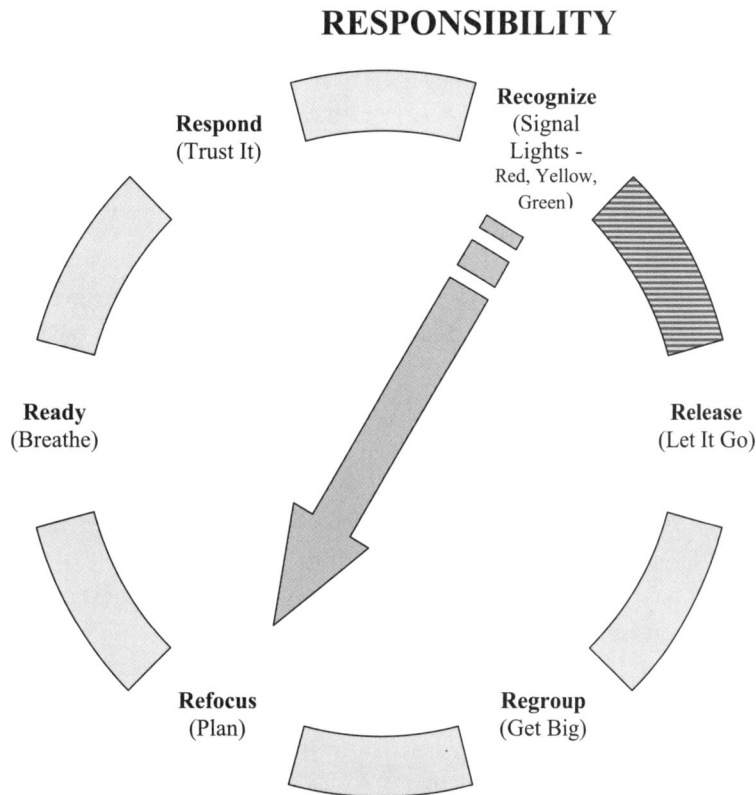

Respond
(Trust It)

Recognize
(Signal Lights -
Red, Yellow,
Green)

Ready
(Breathe)

Release
(Let It Go)

Refocus
(Plan)

Regroup
(Get Big)

Release—Let It Go

One must establish techniques to let things go. For example, we use breathing techniques, progressive relaxation methods, and individual coping strategies to let go of thoughts and feelings that might interfere with performance. If someone is being a pain in the neck, after you have finished the interaction, tighten your shoulders and then release them. This way you consciously tighten the muscle, gather up all the residual tension that might be remaining, and then let it all go in one action. It helps to rid you of that individual's negativity before the next interaction. If you are distracted by the previous interaction, you may miss key insights in your subsequent meeting and lose your present focus. This is the same issue on which we work with athletes, because if they make a mistake or get called for a penalty, they can't afford to dwell on it or they will lose the proper focus.

Regroup—Get Big

After you let it go, regain your composure, stand tall, get centered, and get ready to perform. A technique that we find useful is to monitor the way we walk from one interaction to the next. We learned this from working with golfers when we have them monitor the way they walk from one shot to the next. When they struggle, they begin to lean forward and walk faster. Not surprisingly, this energy is going to affect their next shot. Another approach is to locate a focal point, which is a productive tool to help regain your composure. By focusing on that external object, it helps to shift your focus from an internal perspective to a more external perspective.

Refocus—Get Back to Your Plan

When you are in control of yourself, things slow down; you can focus more clearly, and subsequently determine a plan of action for the next task at hand. If your mind is racing, and you are not focused, how can you think effectively to make a commitment to what you are trying to do and execute the required skill or provide the needed information?

Ready—Breathe Deep

Now that you are in control and can think more clearly, you are ready to perform. A productive way to do this is to take a slow, steady, breath. We believe this breath is extremely critical to an athlete's or consultant's performance because it is such a basic but effective technique. However, it is not easy to remember to breathe calmly when adversity strikes. The breath pulls you to the present and brings oxygen to the brain so you can think clearly. The breath also allows you to release if you focus on the exhalation, and activate if you focus on the inhalation. We have found this to be a very productive way to "check in" and determine if we are ready for the next situation.

Respond—Trust Yourself

The final step of this cycle is to trust your preparation, your experience, and your intuition. As a consultant you have prepared a lifetime for this. There are so many times you just have to be centered and balanced, and know that you are prepared. Trust yourself and just do what you do.

Performance Evaluation

A final and critical issue we review with athletes, which is equally important for a consultant to consider, is performance evaluation. In athletics, failure is part of the process—there will always be a winner and a loser. It is the nature of sport. As sport psychology consultants, we help athletes learn and adjust from their failures. This is analogous to the "black box recorder" when an airplane crashes. The recorder is located after the crash so that the information can be analyzed and procedures can be implemented to eliminate the problem. As consultants, we all make mistakes, but the key is to learn from them. This is where a support group can help you process your experience and provide a perspective that is productive and often affirming. Our willingness to be honest and learn from each other is what allows our field to remain vital and continue to help athletes and coaches achieve their full potential through sport.

Long-term Strategies for Taking Care of Yourself

Just as we inform athletes that they have a support group to help them in their quest for excellence, that they must take care of themselves physically, emo-

tionally, and spiritually, and that they have to make a commitment to learning and getting better, so we as their consultants must do the same. As a consultant, establish a support group with people you can share ideas with, ask questions, and gain perspective. A support group should have people who are accepting, yet able to offer critical feedback, and provide information that can support you. As we always tell athletes, when we have a problem, we know what we want to hear before we ever decide who we are going to call. Athletes have a support system that consists of coaches, athletic trainers, massage therapists, sport psychology consultants, personal trainers, and friends. As consultants, we need others with whom we can share ideas, successes, and failures. As caregivers and educators, it is imperative to make time for our own personal needs. If you do not care for yourself, you will eventually burn out. For example, during the intense involvement of working with athletes and coaches at an Olympic Games, it is easy to get totally involved in the experience. It is critical in an environment such as this to take some time for yourself during and after this involvement. When traveling with a team, we know to take some time for ourselves to get away from the players and coaches. This helps us to be more reflective, recharge ourselves, and is vital in ensuring we don't lose perspective, which helps to regain that critical balance.

Keep Learning

The quest for excellence is an ongoing journey. We have to keep growing and developing. This is why attending conferences, reading books and journals, sharing ideas with coaches and players, keeping a consulting journal, and exchanging ideas with colleagues in the field is so important. We have found sport psychology consulting to be like an onion: There are layers and layers to it. Just when you think you have complete understanding, some event or situation arises that shifts your perspective. We find this to be exciting and stimulating...and isn't this exactly what the athlete goes through in his or her quest for excellence?

Summary

It has been the purpose of this chapter to demonstrate how the sport psychology skills and issues that we teach athletes can be used by sport psychology consultants. One of your greatest teaching tools is to role model the skills and issues that you present. After all, working as a sport psychology consultant is just as much of a performance as being an athlete is, just on a different playing field. We can build our credibility and effectiveness by incorporating the skills that we encourage athletes to use to enhance our own performance.

References

Balague, G., Dee, M., & Ravizza, K. (2005). Team consulting as a team. In *Proceedings of the Annual Conference of the Association for the Advancement of Applied Sport Psychology* (p. 34). Vancouver, BC, Canada.

Halliwell, W., Orlick, T., Ravizza, K., & Rotella, R. (2003). *Consultant's guide to excellence*. Excel Press: Chelsea, QC, Canada.

Ravizza, K. (1988). Gaining entry with athletic personnel for season-long consulting. *The Sport Psychologist, 2,* 243-254.

Ravizza, K. (1995). A mental training approach to performance enhancement. In K. P. Henschen & W. F. Straub (Eds.). *Sport psychology: An analysis of athlete behavior* (3rd ed.), (pp. 35-44). Longmeadow, MA: Mouvement Publications.

Ravizza, K., & Hanson, T. (1995). *Heads up baseball: Playing the game one pitch at a time*. Indianapolis, IN: Master's Press.

Section III
Psychology of Exercise

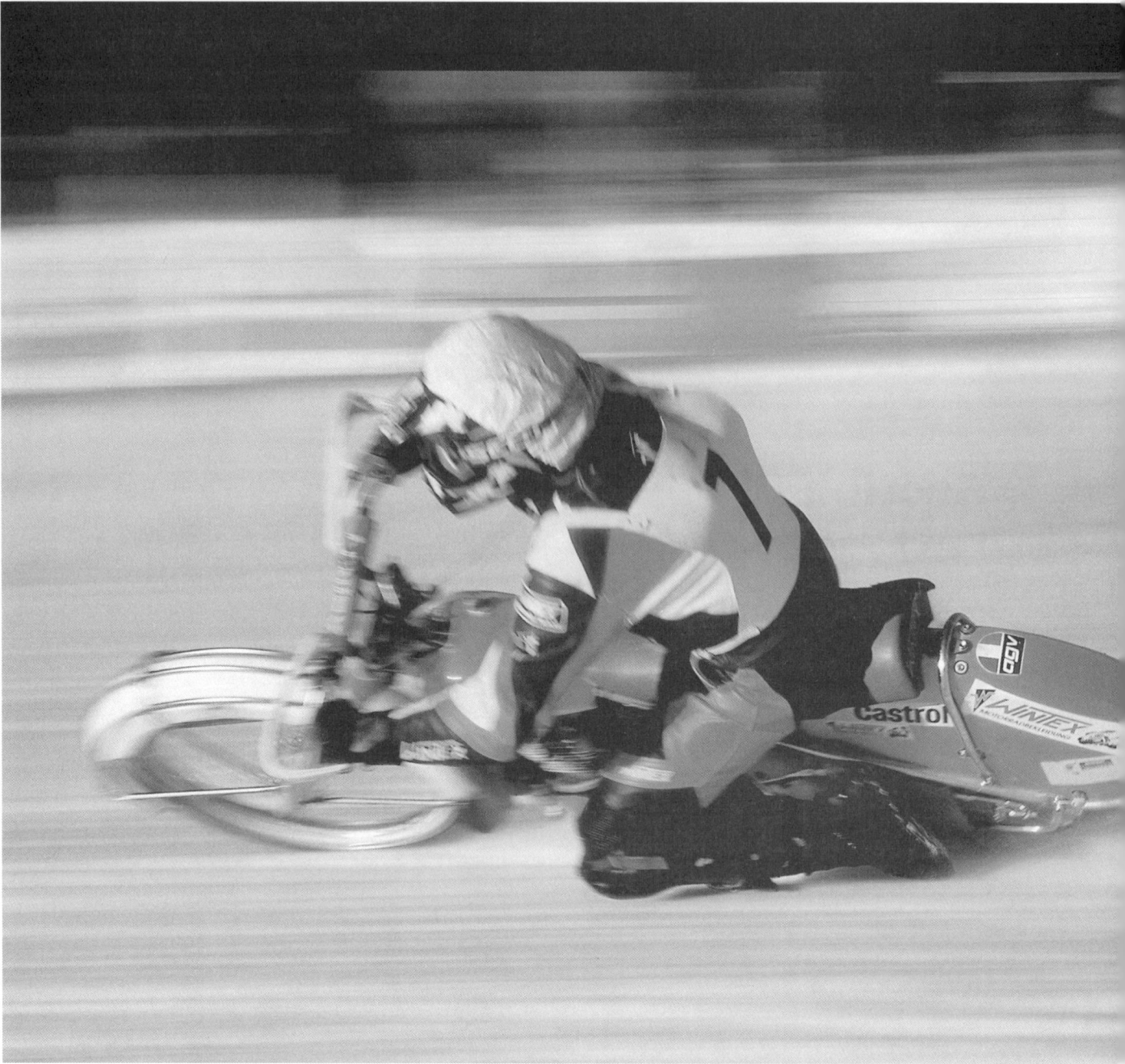

6

Applied Exercise Psychology: Promoting Activity and Evaluating Outcomes

NANETTE MUTRIE

Physical inactivity has become a central topic in public health and is now attracting concern from national and international agencies (Lankenau et al., 2004). In 2004, The World Health Organization (WHO) endorsed a global strategy on diet, physical activity, and health, indicating that inactivity is not just a problem for developed countries (WHO, 2004). WHO recognized that physical activity levels worldwide were falling as a result of industrialization, urbanization, and economic development. The global strategy was developed from a May 2002 mandate from member nations. The main principles of the WHO global strategy are summarized in Figure 1.

Many governments have adopted policies aimed at increasing the percentage of the population who are active enough to gain the well-documented health benefits. For example, the Scottish government created "Let's make Scotland more active" (http://www.scotland.gov.uk/library5/culture/lmsa-00.asp), which is a strategy that aims to have 50% of the Scottish population meet the minimum recommendations for activity by the year 2022 (Scottish Executive, 2002). The western world's obesity epidemic highlights a need to know how to increase activity levels. This has brought the topic of physical activity (as one part of the issue of obesity) to the attention of health professionals and politicians. A

- Appropriate regular physical activity is a major component in preventing the growing global burden of chronic disease.

- At least 60% of the global population fails to achieve the minimum recommendation of 30 minutes, moderate intensity physical activity daily.

- The risk of getting a cardiovascular disease increases by 1.5 times in people who do not follow minimum physical activity recommendations.

- Inactivity greatly contributes to medical costs—by an estimated $75 billion in the USA in 2000 alone.

- Increasing physical activity is a societal, not just an individual problem, and demands a population-based, multi-sectoral, multi-disciplinary, and culturally relevant approach.

Figure 1. Main principles of the WHO global strategy on diet physical activity and health (2004).

sedentary lifestyle is now the norm for the majority of the populations in developed countries. For example, the activity level of two thirds of the European population is not sufficient to meet current recommendations. However, a high proportion of individuals believe in the efficacy of physical activity for obtaining and promoting good health; over 90% of the populations in each of 15 European countries believed that physical activity had numerous health benefits, and there was little variation in this belief by age or socio-economic status (Kearney et al., 1999). Understanding how to effectively increase physical activity[1] levels in the population is one of the most pressing issues in the field of exercise science and medicine; without dramatic change to the percentage of people who are regularly active, the now well-documented health benefits of regular activity for individuals, communities, and populations cannot be realized. The gap between positive attitudes to physical activity and actual behavior represents a challenge for exercise psychology. How exercise specialists, health promoters, government or national agencies can most effectively intervene is a problem waiting to be solved (Mutrie & Woods, 2003), and exercise psychologists have a vital role to play in finding the solution.

Frameworks for policy development in the area of physical activity call for multidisciplinary strategies that could provide successful increases in physical activity (Shephard et al., 2004). The study of the determinants (such as gender, socio-economic status, attitude, and motivation) and consequences (such as improved physical and mental health) of physical activity and interventions within the developing field of exercise psychology has therefore increased dramatically over the last decade (Biddle & Mutrie, 2001) and the title change of the ISSP's official journal from *International Journal of Sport Psychology* to *International Journal of Sport and Exercise Psychology* reflects this trend. In this chapter, I aim to review what is known about how to increase physical activity, to re-assert the role of psychology in this process, to provide examples of how applications of exercise psychology have been used to promote activity and evaluate outcomes, and to suggest future directions for applied exercise psychology.

The Role of Psychology in Physical Activity Behavior Change

Several reviews of interventions aimed at promoting physical activity have now been conducted (Hillsdon Foster, Naidoo, & Crombie, 2003; Hillsdon, Thorogood, & Foster, C. , 2005; Kahn et al., 2002). In addition, Kahn et al. (2002) also produced an evi-

[1] I use *physical activity* (PA) as a general term that refers to any movement of the body that results in energy expenditure above that of resting level. Exercise is often (incorrectly) used interchangeably with PA, but exercise refers to a subset of PA in which the activity is structured, often supervised, and undertaken with the aim of maintaining or improving physical fitness or health. In considering how to increase the activity levels of a population, all modes of activity [including that performed at work, at home, and in leisure] must be taken into account, and so the term *physical activity* is more appropriate than the term *exercise*.

dence-based set of recommendations (Fielding et al., 2002). Their systematic review was commissioned by the US Task Force on Community Preventive Services as an element in the Guide to Community Preventive Services. Information about the Guide to Community Services and its importance for Public Health can be found at http://www.thecommunityguide.org/. The methods used to construct this systematic review are described in Briss et al., (2000) and involved extensive and rigorous procedures, including the appointment of a review team; the development of a conceptual framework for the review; the systematic searching, retrieval, and review of relevant evidence; and a summary of the strength of the body of evidence through the use of standard techniques. The body of evidence was then designated as strong, sufficient, or insufficient. These techniques are similar to those used by Cochrane reviews (http://www.cochrane.org/).

An even more recent review comes from the Health Development Agency in the UK (Hillsdon et al., 2003). This "review of reviews" summarizes the evidence from 16 systematic reviews and meta-analyses of interventions that promote physical activity for adults. Using these two recent reviews as a starting point, I have selected four themes that summarize what successful interventions should be based on, show the importance of exercise psychology, and provide guidance on developments that should be addressed within the exercise psychology community.

Theme 1: The Use of Behavior Change Models
The evidence suggests that interventions will be more successful if they are based on a model of behavior change, and this should also allow better understanding of why interventions may or may not work. For example, Kahn et al.'s (2002) review showed that interventions using a cognitive and behavioral framework produced a median net increase of 35.4% in time spent in physical activity (interquartile range of 16.7% to 83.3%). However, practitioners and researchers are left with a problem: which model to use? There is no model of behavior change that is universally accepted as the most appropriate for studying physical activity and exercise behavior (Mutrie & Woods, 2003). Perhaps the most frequently used models are the Theory of Planned Behaviour (Ajzen, 1985) and the Transtheoretical Model of Behaviour

Change as applied to exercise (Marcus et al., 1994), which show the strong link exercise psychology has with health psychology. Each of these models has support and criticism (Mutrie & Woods, 2003) and both can provide the framework that the reviews tell us will lead to more successful interventions. However, there is plenty of scope for developing specific models that have direct application to physical activity as well as models that take into account the wide range of determinants that are known to influence physical activity behavior. There is also a need to refine the measurement tools that are available for these models as they relate to physical activity before we might be able to say which model is best.

Initial work with these models focused on description of how they worked in physical activity and exercise, but now we need to focus on explanations of what aspects of these models create behavior change. For example, in a recent study we aimed to identify key processes (from the Transtheoretical Model) associated with movement between the stages of exercise behavior change using a longitudinal design (Lowther, Mutrie, & Scott, in press; Lowther, Mutrie, & Scott, 2002). Generally, for progress through the stages of exercise behavior change over the course of 12 months, the process of self-liberation appeared to be particularly important at each stage. In addition, the process of stimulus control appeared important when progressing from contemplation to preparation, and progression from action into maintenance was associated with increased use of social liberation and helping relationships. This type of information is only now emerging in the literature and we need more of this kind of knowledge in order to design and deliver interventions.

While reviews have shown that interventions based on these behavior change models are effective, there is clearly a need to take a wider perspective. Behavior change happens within a particular socio-cultural context and models need to expand to include the wider determinants of activity, such as the "walkability" of the environment people live in (Owen, Humpel, Leslie, Bauman, & Sallis, 2004) or the socio-economic circumstances in which they find themselves. Developing such comprehensive models is another challenge for exercise psychology. One model that offers much promise in this regard is the socio-ecological model proposed by Sallis &

Owen (2002). This model suggests that there are many environments that influence physical activity behavior, ranging from local policies, organizational structures, the built environment, and both interpersonal and individual issues.

This leads me to comment on the finding from reviews that not much is known about how changes to the built environment might influence physical activity. In the meantime the idea that "if you build it they will come" is pervasive for both physical recreation and sport facilities. This way of thinking suggests that simply having bike lanes or sports facilities nearby will automatically increase physical activity. There is ample evidence that the provision of facilities by themselves will not encourage a large percentage of people to be more active. For example, most towns have always had pavements but the rates of walking have declined. People choose not to use the stairs even when they are easily found. Bike lanes by themselves will not necessarily encourage more people to cycle; even in Denmark where there is a very positive cycling environment with bike lanes separated from traffic, health promoters and city planners had to use a variety of promotional prompts to increase the percentage of the population who choose to cycle. Understanding how the environment interacts with individuals remains another challenge for exercise psychology. A new organization, the International Physical Activity and the Environment Network (IPEN), has been formed to increase knowledge and awareness of how the environment influences physical activity. More information about IPEN can be found at http://www. ipenproject.org/.

The field of environmental psychology is devoted to the topic of understanding people's perceptions of their environment. An association with exercise psychology would aid in the development of this field (Owen, Humpel, Leslie, Bauman, & Sallis, 2004). The use of stair prompts is one simple example of how this can be achieved. Points of choice prompts are usually visual cues (such as posters) that are strategically placed in a position where people can be influenced as they make a decision between being active or passive (such as stair or escalator use). Kahn et al.'s (2002) review showed that baseline rates of stair use were low (usually less than 12% of the potential population chose the stairs without the

prompt). However, the median increase in stair use, following a prompt, was 53.9% for the five studies included in the review, and the range of effect sizes was a net increase of 5.5% to 128.6%. In a study we conducted in Glasgow on this topic (Blamey, Mutrie, & Aitchison, 1995), we aimed to discover if Scottish commuters would respond to motivational signs encouraging them to "Stay Healthy, Save Time, Use the Stairs." The signs were placed in a Glasgow city center underground station where stairs (30 steps) and escalators were adjacent.

The study spanned a 16-week period and a total of 22,275 observations were made on Mondays, Wednesdays, and Fridays between 8.30 and 10 a.m. during eight of those weeks. The eight observation weeks were split into four stages: a one-week baseline, a three-week period when the sign was present, a two-week period immediately after the sign was removed, and two one-week follow-ups (during the fourth and twelfth weeks after intervention). Observers recorded the number of adults using the escalators and stairs and categorized them by sex. Those carrying luggage or with pushchairs were excluded. A comparison was made between the baseline week stair use and each of the seven subsequent observation weeks. This process was repeated for the total sample as well as for males and females separately.

Stair use during the one-week baseline period was around 8%. This increased to the order of 15-17% during the three weeks that the sign was present. Figure 2 shows the overall percentage improvement from baseline compared to each of the subsequent seven weeks. Stair use significantly increased after the signs were in place and continued to increase during the three intervention weeks. A sudden decrease in stair use occurred after the sign was removed. At the 12-week follow-up, stair use remained significantly higher than at baseline. There is, however, an obvious downward trend suggesting a possible eventual return to baseline levels. It was found that females were more likely to use escalators than males at all times. These results are illustrated in Figure 2.

Interviews were also conducted as part of the Blamey et al. (1995) study. These were conducted during the time taken to go up the escalator or walk up the stairs—about 45 seconds. Stair users reported saving time and health as the main motivating factors, while escalator users cited laziness and the time

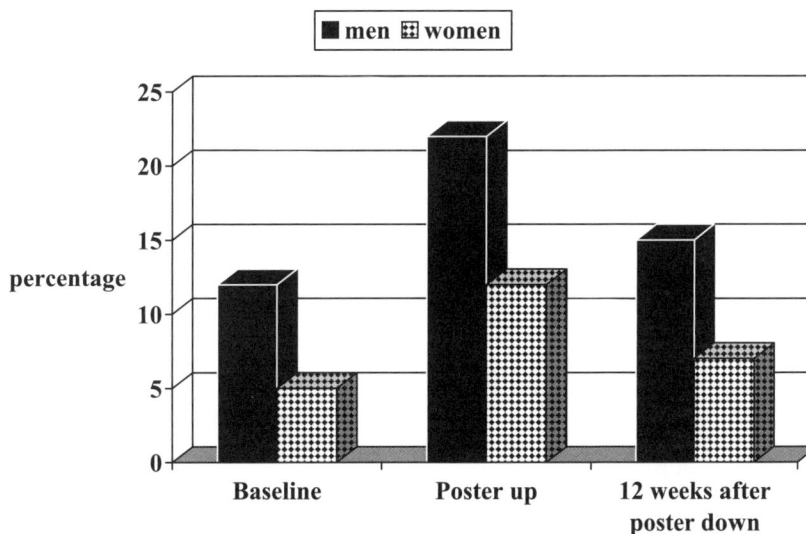

Figure 2. Percentage of commuters using the stairs before and after poster prompt (Blamey et al., 1995).

and effort required by stair climbing as the main barriers. In general, males reported higher levels of physical activity and lower perception of the effort required to climb stairs than females. Adults over 50 years of age gave a higher rating of the perception of effort required to climb the stairs.

Work by Kerr and colleagues have added to this literature by exploring where to locate the message (Kerr et al., 2001b). They concluded that banners with messages on the stair risers (i.e., between each step) may be twice as effective as point-of-choice posters that are located at a position where the person makes a decision between going up the stairs or the elevators (Kerr et al., 2001a). Such prompts can be used creatively and could become an integral part of stair design. Imagine the possibility that every building with an escalator or lift would also carry a motivational prompt to choose the stairs instead!

The reviews show that we have no evidence (yet) of how policies or legislation actually influence population levels of activity and this is another area for exercise psychologists to play a role in partnership with others. If interventions require changing the environment, policy, and legislation, along with individual behavior, then this brings with it increasing levels of complexity for evaluation. If we consider, for evidence of cause and effect, that randomized controlled trials are the design we should aim for, then we are immediately faced with some difficult

issues. Randomization can be difficult at the level of the individual and becomes increasingly fraught with political and pragmatic problems when dealing with geographic areas, communities, policy actions, and legislation. There is a long list of challenges that await researchers who might want to evaluate how "natural experiments" influence health and, in particular, physical activity. Such natural experiments might consist of investment in new playgrounds, the closure of local sport facilities, traffic calming or congestion schemes. Decisions about such interventions are made for many different reasons but may have an important impact on physical activity, although we have not, as of yet, found a way to evaluate it—perhaps because forward planning and new thinking are required to overcome the methodological challenges (Ogilvie, Mitchell, Mutrie, Petticrow, Platt, in press). For these purposes, a range of new and more comprehensive evaluation strategies need to be developed. Such strategies need to be driven by the theory of the interventions; they need to work in relation to ecological models of health and they also need to consider indicators that are relevant at the level of communities, populations, and settings rather than simply the individual. These strategies are challenging and psychologists need to be part of the evaluation teams that will put these strategies into practice. To be part of such evaluation teams psychologist may well have to learn a range of new evaluation skills (Blamey & Mutrie, 2004).

One example of a new standard for designing and implementing interventions can be found by considering the framework suggested the Medical Research Council (MRC) in the UK (Campbell et al., 2000). This framework suggests that for complex interventions (i.e., an intervention with many parts to it), several stages of design and development are required. Initial stages involve exploration of the literature, perhaps in the form of a systematic review, to ensure that the best theoretical intervention is chosen. Intermediate stages involve determining how elements of the intervention might influence behavior and testing the feasibility of the intervention in a realistic setting. Final stages of this framework include a definitive trial, which will usually involve randomization and control conditions to robustly determine the effect of the intervention, and then further study to determine if the intervention has the same effects in less controlled conditions. This framework is depicted in Figure 3. In summary,

for the theme relating to the use of behavior change models for promoting activity, exercise psychologists must develop specific models relating to physical activity and must work in partnership with other professionals to encourage such behavior change. Simultaneously, we must appreciate that an increase in a population's level of physical activity is not a problem that psychologists alone can solve. Finally, we have to learn new evaluation skills to help provide robust evidence regarding how to achieve physical activity behavior change. There is a clear need for partnership working in this area.

Theme 2: The Role of an Exercise Specialist
The second theme that emerges from the review of what works in physical activity promotion refers to the extra benefit of including referral to an exercise specialist. Such a person might provide support for long-term change but must also use behavior change principles. Physical activity counseling is a new application of exercise psychology. Such a process

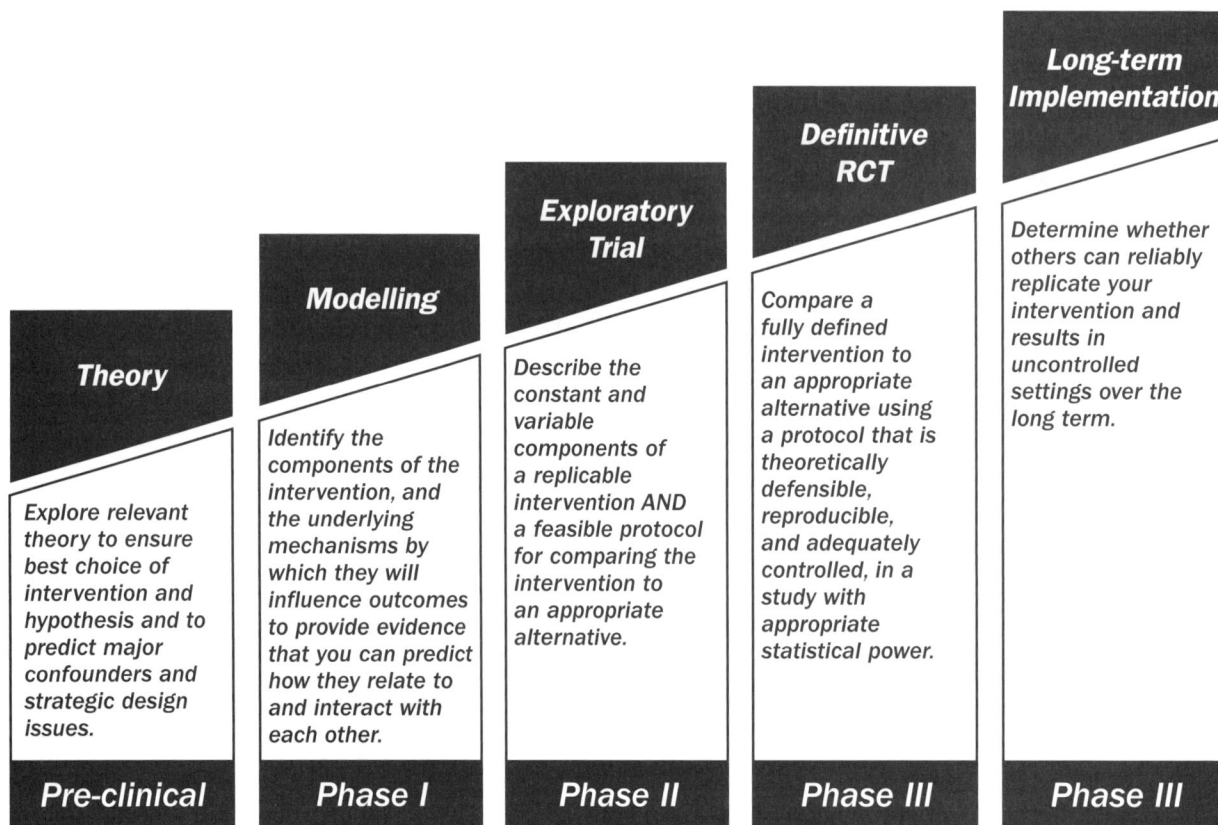

Theory

Explore relevant theory to ensure best choice of intervention and hypothesis and to predict major confounders and strategic design issues.

Pre-clinical

Modelling

Identify the components of the intervention, and the underlying mechanisms by which they will influence outcomes to provide evidence that you can predict how they relate to and interact with each other.

Phase I

Exploratory Trial

Describe the constant and variable components of a replicable intervention AND a feasible protocol for comparing the intervention to an appropriate alternative.

Phase II

Definitive RCT

Compare a fully defined intervention to an appropriate alternative using a protocol that is theoretically defensible, reproducible, and adequately controlled, in a study with appropriate statistical power.

Phase III

Long-term Implementation

Determine whether others can reliably replicate your intervention and results in uncontrolled settings over the long term.

Phase III

Figure 3. The MRC framework for designing and implementing complex interventions (Campbell et al., 2000).

includes knowledge of exercise prescription and contraindications and has usually focused on those with knowledge of exercise physiology. Knowledge of motivations and barriers to behavior change, along with counseling skills, are also needed. We developed a set of guidelines (see Figure 4) for such procedures (Loughlan & Mutrie, 1995) and they have been shown to be effective in increasing activity for community participants (Lowther et al., 2002) and clinical populations (Kirk, Mutrie, MacIntyre, & Fisher, 2004). This provides another role for exercise psychologists in providing appropriate training for a variety of health professionals who need to provide effective physical activity counseling. Such professionals might include doctors, nurses, physiotherapists, health promotion specialists, personal trainers, fitness professionals, mental health workers, community workers, and home health visitors. If all of these professionals could effectively deliver counseling to promote increased activity, we might begin to realize the increase in activity across the population that most countries require.

Theme 3: Promoting Walking

Perhaps the majority of sport and exercise psychologists started their careers in relation to sport , for example by providing mental skills training, and enjoy sport performance themselves. It is therefore hard for people who love sport to understand that sport will not solve the problem of inactivity when we consider the population as a whole. The segments of the population most in need of increasing activity levels are the least likely to have ever enjoyed sport and the notion of going to the gym is alien to them. Sport is truly a minority activity for most adults, and the "active living" message, which is now adopted worldwide (Pate et al., 1995), is the key to getting such people more active. In most developed countries there is a clear and steep gradient in sports participation from youth to older adults, and there is usually a social class gradient with the more affluent participating more than others. In addition, there is usually a gender divide showing more men than women participating. In contrast, walking has been found to be the mode of activity that is most popular.

Step 1   Determine Physical Activity History

Discuss the reasons that the person has for wanting to increase activity. Take note of when the person was last active, the kinds of activities they might like now, and a measure of recent physical activity, e.g. 7-day recall.

Step 2   Discuss Decision Balance

Ask the person to consider the pros and cons of increasing activity for themselves. If there are more cons than pros, ask them to consider how to minimize some of the cons.

Step 3   Ensure social support

Determine with the person what kind of support they might need and who can provide it.

Step 4   Negotiate Goals

Help the person set realistic and time-phased goals for gradually increasing activity up to a level they have determined, e.g. in 4 weeks time I would like to be walking for 30 minutes more on at least 3 days of the week. Write these goals down.

Step 5   Discuss Relapse Prevention

If there is time, or if the counseling session is with someone who is already active, a discussion regarding how to prevent relapse from regular activity should take place.

Step 6   Provide Information on Local Opportunities

All information on relevant local activities, such as walking paths, swimming pools, and classes should be on hand to supplement discussion as required.

Figure 4. Main steps in a physical activity counseling session (Loughlan & Mutrie, 1995).

In a population study of residents in the West of Scotland, we found that walking was the single most popular mode of activity with almost half of the respondents reporting at least one two-mile walk (3.2 kilometres) in the past month. We also showed that for those capable of walking at least one quarter of a mile, there was no decrease in walking across three age cohorts ranging from young people to those aged over 55 years, while there was a decrease across age cohorts for other activities.

In addition, walking seems to be the mode of activity most amenable to change through intervention; it is also capable of overcoming many barriers to activity, such as time or expense; and has been described as the nearest activity to perfect exercise (Morris & Hardman, 1997). Walking could also be a very important mode of activity in relation to health, as epidemiological studies have found a reduced risk of mortality among men who walked 20 or more kilometres per week (Lee & Paffenberger, 2000). There is a strong case for the promotion of walking as an expanded area of study in its own right, and exercise psychologists should focus on it in an attempt to develop our understanding of how to increase the percentage of the population who regularly walk.

Although reviews support the use of walking as the most likely mode of activity to appeal to the inactive segment of the population, we are still in the early days of knowing exactly how to promote these findings. We have recently used both written materials and pedometers to encourage walking, with mixed levels of success. The first study used written materials to determine if a self-help intervention, delivered via interactive materials (the "Walk in to Work Out" pack), could increase active commuting behavior (walking and cycling) (Mutrie et al., 2002). The participants were 295 employees who had been identified as thinking about, or actually doing, some irregular walking or cycling to work. The intervention group received the "Walk in to Work Out" pack, which contained written interactive materials based on the Transtheoretical Model of Behaviour Change, local information about distances and routes, and safety information. The control group received the pack six months later. Focus groups were also conducted after six months. The results showed that the intervention group was almost twice as likely to increase walking to work as the control group at six months (odds ratio of 1.93, 95% Confidence Interval of 1.06 to 3.52). The intervention was not successful at increasing cycling. These results are illustrated in Figure 5 and show that it is possible to change the

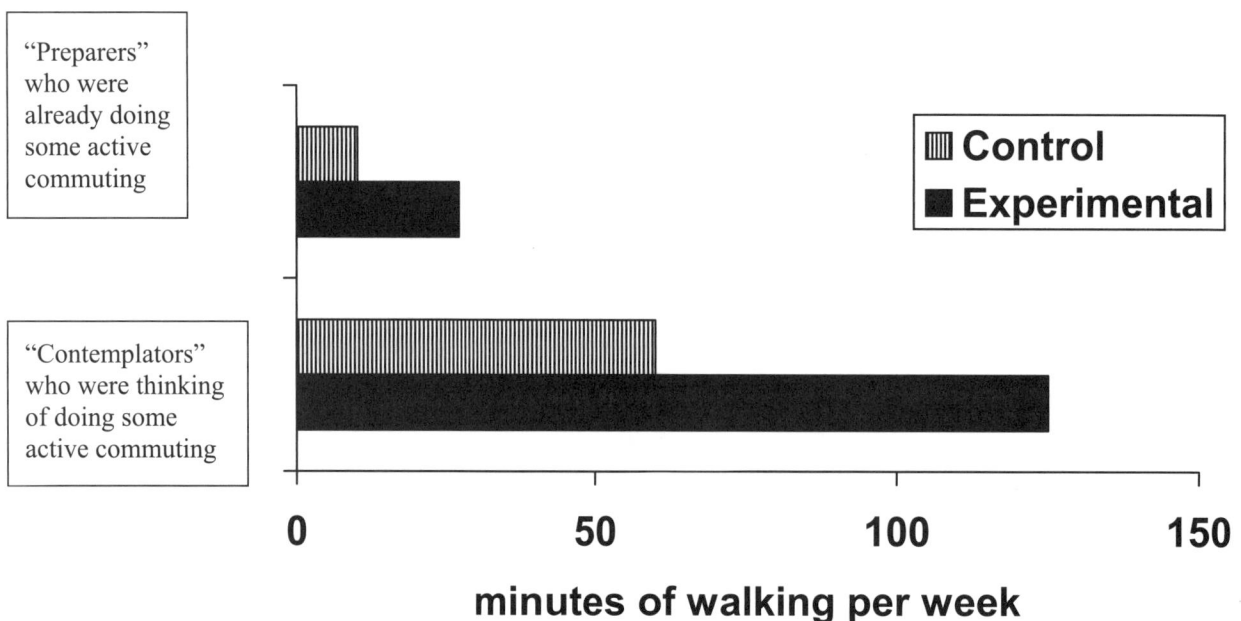

Figure 5. Results from a randomized controlled trial in which the experimental group received materials aimed at helping them to "walk in to work out" (Mutrie et al., 2002).

way that people travel to work, and in doing so, more physical activity is created. This kind of approach may have added benefits in reducing pollution and congestion from motor vehicles. The pedometer study (Mutrie et al., 2004) had less favorable long-term effects. Pedometers are small mechanical devices, usually with an electronic display, that count walking steps when they are worn on the wearer's waistband. They are currently extremely popular and can be found for purchase in many sports and leisure outlets. They may even be given away free in breakfast cereals or, surprisingly, from fast food companies. In our study, we wanted to examine the motivational effect of a pedometer for increasing walking. Fifty participants were randomly assigned to a 4-week walking program following a goal-setting program based on pedometer step-counts (intervention group) or a similar walking program based on minutes (control group). Step-counts were obtained at baseline and at weeks 4, 16, and 52 for all participants. Questionnaires based on the TTM in full were also completed at these time-points. Both groups significantly increased their step-counts from baseline to week 4. Both groups significantly decreased step-counts over time, and at week 52, step-counts

returned to baseline. These findings are illustrated in Figure 6. From these results it appears that pedometers have no advantage over goals set in minutes and that even those who are motivated to increase their walking find it difficult to sustain initial increases in the long term. Pedometers are currently very popular but we clearly need to know more about how to use them to increase walking over the long term. Walking behavior offers a multitude of possibilities for future research by exercise psychologists, and Owen and colleagues have recently set out a framework for this research agenda (Owen, Humpel, Leslie, Bauman, & Sallis, 2004).

Theme 4: The Need for Further Research

All reviews of physical activity promotion comment on the lack of evidence for promoting physical activity to black and ethnic minority groups. We may have been guilty of researching those populations that are easy to reach, although this may be defensible given the short history of exercise psychology. It is now time to focus on the hard to reach—to learn about the different needs of population segments such as children, older adults, black and ethnic minori-

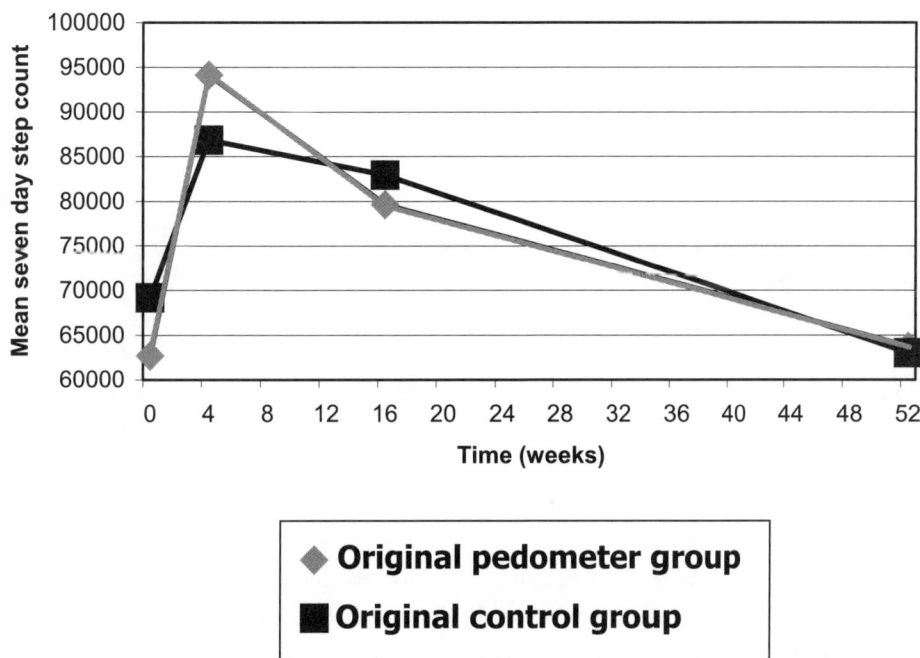

Figure 6. Weekly step counts over time for those who originally used a pedometer and those who did not (Baker et al., under review).

ties, and clinical populations. In addition, evidence of long-term behavior change is missing. There is plenty of scope for further research to determine what works for whom and for how long.

Outcomes Issues

There is an overemphasis in the public health literature on the physical rather than mental health outcomes from physical activity. As exercise psychologists we can make another important contribution to this field by focusing on the mental health benefits of regular activity. One way to do this is to link to the growing literature on positive psychology.

Seligman (2002) suggested that the goal of positive psychology is to "learn how to build the qualities that help individuals and communities not just positive psychology often make reference to the capacity for sport experience to achieve some of endure and survive but also flourish" (p. 8). Seligman and others who write about the goals of positive psychology (but non-sport related physical activity) will help both individuals and communities survive and flourish. At an individual level, physical activity has the capacity to prevent mental illness, to foster positive emotions, and to buffer individuals against the stresses of life. Therefore, when physical activity is seen as the norm within a community, both health and social capital can increase (Mutrie & Faulkner, 2004). This link to positive psychology develops the principle that the body is important to how we think, feel, and behave. The principles of psychosomatic medicine have clearly established the idea that how we think and feel will affect the functioning of the body. However, the reverse is also true. There is also a somato-psychic principle which is very much in line with the principles of positive psychology (Harris, 1973). The somatopsychic principle is neatly displayed in the well-known phrase "mens sana in corpore sano," which means "a healthy mind in a healthy body."

Gaining physical strength or capacity allows us to feel more confident in our ability to do everyday tasks, perhaps provides us with a more positive perception of our physical selves, and thus can influence our self-esteem. Seligman (2002) further argues that building strengths should be at the forefront of treating mental illness. Building physical capacity has a somatopsychic impact on those people who are suf-

fering from poor mental health. The most compelling evidence comes from studies in the area of clinical depression. For example, two recent meta-analyses reported effects sizes of 0.72 (Craft & Landers, 1998) and 1.1 (Lawlor & Hopker, 2001) for exercise as compared to no treatment for depression, and both meta-analyses showed effects for exercise that are similar to those found from other psychotherapeutic interventions. One recent study has also shown that exercise equalled the effect found from a standard anti-depressant drug after 16 weeks (Blumenthal et al., 1999), and after six months there were some indications that those who had continued to exercise had additional benefits in comparison with those taking the drug (Babyak et al., 2000).

For people with severe and enduring mental health problems, improvement in quality of life tends to enhance the individual's ability to cope with and manage their disorder. Preliminary evidence suggests that regular physical activity can improve positive aspects of mental health (such as psychological quality of life and emotional well-being) in people with mental disorders. Positive psychological effects from physical activity in clinical populations have been reported, even among those individuals who experience no objective diagnostic improvement (Faulkner, 2005). The evidence shows a positive link between psychological well-being and regular physical activity, and this epitomizes the principles of positive psychology (Biddle, Fox, & Boutcher, 2000).

Conclusions and Implications for the Promotion of Health

Exercise psychologists have an important role in the task of increasing the percentage of people who are physically active. Particular contributions include the development of appropriate theoretical frameworks for interventions, training professionals in appropriate counseling skills, and focusing on walking as a key mode of activity for promotion. Such contributions must involve partnership working with other psychologists (such as health and environmental psychologists) and other professionals; it may also involve new evaluation techniques and research approaches. There are many gaps in our current knowledge, such as finding an effective way to reach the "hard to reach" segments of our populations, making long-term evaluations, and learning to comprehensively evaluate the wider determinants of a physically active life. Finally, there is a role for exercise psychologists to reassert the somatopsychic rationale for physical activity and emphasise the importance of mental health benefits from regular activity. The emerging field of positive psychology offers a framework for this approach.

Issues for Debate and Discussion

The above conclusions suggest to me at least two immediate questions for debate and discussion. First, are we, as sport and exercise psychologists, providing the same level of training in exercise psychology as we do in sport psychology? Almost all accreditation processes that exist around the world focus on assuring quality in the delivery of support for sport performers. I challenge you when reading this chapter to check out any national accreditation schemes or plans that you have in your own country and encourage the inclusion of exercise psychology training if it is not already there. Some examples do exist, such as the British Association of Sport and Exercise Sciences (BASES) supervised experience process, pursued in either exercise or sport psychology. More details can be found on the BASES web site (http://www.bases.org.uk/).

Second, is exercise the correct title? Would physical activity psychology show the wider concern for all types of activity? Would this change align us more with health psychology than sport psychology and would this be a good or bad thing? Questions within a book chapter cannot, of course, be answered adequately. However, I hope that you can answer them at least for yourself, and at best, debate them at future meetings of the International Society for Sport Psychology.

References

Ajzen, I. (1985). From intentions to actions: A theory of planned behavior. In J. Kuhl & J. Beckmann (Eds.), *Action control: From cognition to behavior* (pp. 11-39). New York: Springer-Verlag.

Babyak, M., Blumenthal, J. A., Herman, S., Khatri, P., Doraiswamy, M., Moore, K., et al. (2000). Exercise treatment for major depression: Maintenance of therapeutic benefit at 10 months. *Psychosomatic Medicine, 62*(5), 633-638.

Baker, G., Mutrie, N., & Lowry, R. (under review). The effectiveness of pedometers as motivational tools in both the short- and the long-term.

Biddle, S. J. H., Fox, K. R., & Boutcher, S. H. (2000). *Physical activity and psychological well-being.* London: Routledge.

Biddle, S. J. H., & Mutrie, N. (2001). *Psychology of physical activity: Determinants, well-being, and interventions.* London: Routledge.

Blamey, A., & Mutrie, N. (2004). Changing the individual to promote health-enhancing physical activity: The difficulties of producing evidence and translating it into practice. *Journal of Sports Sciences, 22*(8), 741-754.

Blamey, A., Mutrie, N., & Aitchison, T. (1995). Promoting active living: Increasing stair walking by motivational stimulus cues. *British Medical Journal, 311,* 289-290.

Blumenthal, J. A., Babyak, M. A., Moore, K. A., Craighead, W. E., Herman, S., Khatri, P., et al. (1999). Effects of exercise training on older patients with major depression. *Archives of Internal Medicine, 159*(19), 2349-2356.

Briss, P. A., Zaza, S., Pappaioanou, M., Fielding, J., Wright-De Aguero, L., Truman, B. I., et al. (2000). Developing an evidence-based guide to community preventive services—methods. *American Journal of Preventive Medicine, 18*(1), 35-43.

Campbell, M., Fitzpatrick, R., Haines, A., Kinmonth, A. L., Sandercock, P., Spiegelhalter, D., et al. (2000). Framework for design and evaluation of complex interventions to improve health. *British Medical Journal, 321*(7262), 694-696.

Craft, L. L., & Landers, D. M. (1998). The effect of exercise on clinical depression and depression resulting from mental illness: A meta-analysis. *Journal of Sport & Exercise Psychology, 20,* 339-357.

Faulkner, G. E. J. (2005). Exercise as an adjunct treatment for schizophrenia. In G. E. J. Faulkner & A. H. Taylor (Eds.), *Exercise, health and mental health. Emerging relationships* (pp. 27-47). London: Routledge.

Fielding, J. E., Mullen, P. D., Brownson, R. C., Fullilove, M. T., Guerra, F. A., Hinman, A. R., et al. (2002). Recommendations to increase physical activity in communities. *American Journal of Preventive Medicine, 22*(4), 67-72.

Harris, D. V. (1973). *Involvement in sport: A somatopsychic rationale for physical activity.* Philadelphia: Lea & Febiger.

Hillsdon, M., Foster, C., Naidoo, B., & Crombie, H. (2003). *A review of the evidence on the effectiveness of public health interventions for increasing physical activity amongst adults: A review of reviews.* London: Health Development Agency.

Hillsdon, M., Thorogood, M., & Foster, C. (2005). *Interventions for physical activity* (Cochrane review): Oxford: Update Software.

Kahn, E. B., Ramsey, L. T., Brownson, R. C., Heath, G. W., Howze, E. H., Powell, K. E., et al. (2002). The effectiveness of interventions to increase physical activity—a systematic review. *American Journal of Preventive Medicine, 22*(4), 73-108.

Kearney, J. M., Graaf, C. d., Damkjaer, S., & Engstrom, L. M. (1999). Stages of change towards physical activity in a nationally representative sample in the European Union. *Public Health Nutrition, 2*(1a), 115-124.

Kerr, J., Eves, F., & Carroll, D. (2001a). Encouraging stair use: Banners are better than posters. *American Journal of Public Health, 91,* 1192-1193.

Kerr, J., Eves, F., & Carroll, D. (2001b). The influence of poster prompts on stair use: The effects of setting, poster size and content. *British Journal of Health Psychology, 6,* 397-405.

Kirk, A. F., Mutrie, N., MacIntyre, P. D., & Fisher, M. B. (2004). Promoting and maintaining physical activity in people with type 2 diabetes. *American Journal of Preventive Medicine, 27*(4), 289-296.

Lankenau, B., Solari, A., & Pratt, M. (2004). International physical activity policy development: A commentary. *Public Health Reports, 119*(3), 352-355.

Lawlor, D. A., & Hopker, S. W. (2001). The effectiveness of exercise as an intervention in the management of depression: Systematic review and meta-regression analysis of randomised controlled trials. *BMJ, 322,* 1-8.

Lee, I.-M., & Paffenberger, R. S. (2000). Associations of light, moderate, and vigorous intensity physical activity with longevity. The Harvard alumni health study. *American Journal of Epidemiology, 151*(3), 293-299.

Loughlan, C., & Mutrie, N. (1995). Conducting an exercise consultation: Guidelines for health professionals. *Journal of the Institute of Health Education, 33*(3), 78-82.

Lowther, M., Mutrie, N., & Scott, E. M. (in press). Identifying key processes of exercise behaviour change associated with movement through the stages of exercise behaviour change. *British Journal of Health Psychology.*

Lowther, M., Mutrie, N., & Scott, M. (2002). Promoting physical activity in a socially and economically deprived community: A 12 month randomized control trial of fitness assessment and exercise consultation. *Journal of Sports Sciences, 20,* 577-588.

Marcus, B. H., Eaton, C. A., Rossi, J. S., & Harlow, L. L. (1994). Self-efficacy, decision-making and stages of change: An integrative model of physical exercise. *Journal of Applied Social Psychology, (24),* 489-508.

Morris, J. N., & Hardman, A. E. (1997). Walking to health. *Sports Medicine, 23*(5), 306-333.

Mutrie, N., Carney, C., Blamey, A., Crawford, F., Aitchison, T., & Whitelaw, A. (2002). "Walk in to work out": A randomised controlled trial of a self help intervention to promote active commuting. *Journal of Epidemiology and Community Health, 56*(6), 407-412.

Mutrie, N., & Faulkner, G. E. J. (2004). Physical activity: Positive psychology in motion. In P. A. Linley & S. Joseph (Eds.), *Positive psychology in practice* (pp. 146-164). New Jersey: Wiley.

Mutrie, N., & Woods, C. (2003). How can we get people to be more active? A problem waiting to be solved. In J. McKenna & C. Riddoch (Eds.), *Perpsectives on health and exercise* (pp. 131-152). Basingstoke: Palgrave McMillan.

Mutrie, N., Wright, A., Wilson, R., & Gunnyeon, K. (2004). Do pedometers motivate people to walk more? *Journal of Sports Sciences, 22*(3), 254.

Ogilvie, D., Mitchell, R., Mutrie, N., Petticrew, M., & Platt, S. (in press). Evaluating health effects of transport interventions: Methodological case study. *American Journal of Preventive Medicine.*

Owen, N., Humpel, N., Leslie, E., Bauman, A., & Sallis, J. F. (2004). Understanding environmental influences on walking—review and research agenda. *American Journal of Preventive Medicine, 27*(1), 67-76.

Pate, R. R., Pratt, M., Blair, S. N., Haskel, W. L., Macera, C. A., Bouchard, C., et al. (1995). Physical activity and public health: A recommendation from the Centers for Disease Control and Prevention and the American College of Sports Medicine. Journal of the *American Medical Association, 273,* 402-407.

Sallis, J., & Owen, N. (2002). Ecological models of health behavior. In K. Glanz, F. Lewis & B. Rimer (Eds.), *Health behavior and health education* (3rd ed., pp. 462-484). San Francisco: Jossey-Bass.

Scottish Executive. (2002). *Let's make Scotland more active.* Edinburgh: Scottish Executive

Seligman, M. E. P. (2002). Positive psychology, positive prevention and positive therapy. In C. Snyder & S. Lopez (Eds.), *Handbook of positive psychology* (pp. 3-9). New York: Oxford University Press.

Shephard, R. J., Lankenau, B., Pratt, M., Neiman, A., Puska, P., Benaziza, H., et al. (2004). Physical activity policy development: A synopsis of the WHO/CDC consultation, September 29 through October 21 2002, Atlanta, Georgia. *Public Health Reports, 119*(3), 346-351.

World Health Organization. (2004). *Global strategy on diet, physical activity and health.* Retrieved September 29, 2006, from http://www.who.int/dietphysicalactivity/publications/facts/obesity/en/

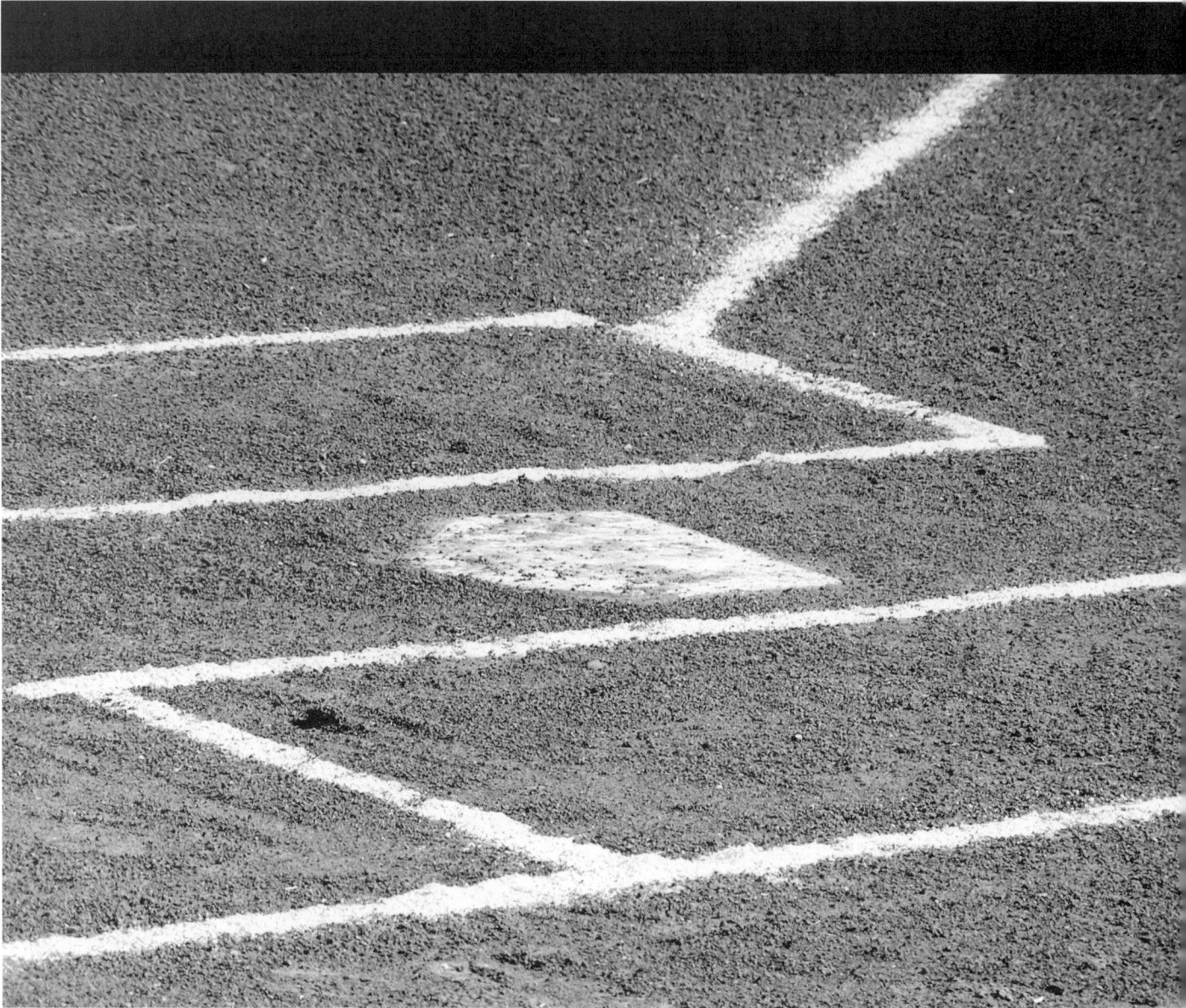

Courtesy of stock.xchng

7

Exercise Relative to Other Treatments for Reduction of Anxiety/Depression: Overcoming the Principle of Least Effort

DANIEL M. LANDERS AND BRANDON ALDERMAN

The relationship between exercise and reduction of anxiety and depressive symptoms was examined scientifically in the early part of the 20th century. Case studies and correlational studies were first used to examine these relationships (Franz & Hamilton, 1905; Vaux, 1926). Today there are several experimental studies with participants who have normal levels of anxiety (Bahrke & Morgan, 1978; deGeus, Lorenz, van Doornen, Visser, & Orlebeke, 1990; DeVries, Wisell, Bilbulian, & Moritani, 1981; Driscoll, 1976; Steptoe, Edwards, Moses, & Mathews,

1989) and depression (Blumenthal et al., 1989, 1991; Galye, Spitler, Karper, Jaeger, & Rice, 1988; McNeil, LeBlanc, & Joyce, 1991; Moses, Steptoe, Mathews, & Edwards, 1989; Roth, Bachter, & Fillingim, 1990). These experimental studies have used study participants who have either normal levels of anxiety and depression or score above average on an anxiety or depression-screening instrument (Stich, 1998).

Randomized clinical trials (RCT) with clinically depressed and anxious study participants have also been conducted. These studies have used clinical patients diagnosed with panic attack (Broocks, Bandelow, & Pekrun, 1998), unipolar major and minor depression (Babyak et al., 2000; Blumenthal et al., 1999; Dunn, Trivedi, Kampert, Clark, & Chambliss, 2005; Singh, Clemens, & Fiatarone, 1997; Singh, Clemens, & Singh, 2001), and depression resulting from another mental disorder (see Craft & Landers, 1998). These RCT studies have consistently demonstrated the efficacy of exercise in reducing anxiety and depression in certain types of clinical patients. At this time, no RCT studies were found in which a majority of the study participants had any of the following DSM-IV anxiety and depressive disorders: dysthemic disorder, bipolar disorder (I & II), cyclothymic disorder, posttraumatic stress disorder, acute stress disorder, generalized anxiety disorder, anxiety disorder due to a general medical condition, and substance-induced anxiety disorder. Experimental research is needed to examine exercise effects on these anxiety and depressive disorders.

In addition to experimental and RCT studies, there are numerous quasi-experimental and correlational studies examining exercise effects on anxiety, depression, and positive mood. Along with experimental studies, these non-experimental studies have been included in several narrative reviews and at least 13 English-language, meta-analytic reviews (Arent, Landers, & Etnier, 2000; Calfas & Taylor, 1994; Carlson, 1991; Craft & Landers; 1998; Kugler, Seelbach, & Kruskemper, 1994; Landers & Petruzzello, 1994; Lawlor & Hopkor, 2001; Long & van Stavel, 1995; McDonald & Hodgdon, 1991; North, McCullagh & Tran, 1990; Petruzzello, Landers, Hatfield, Kubitz, & Salazar, 1991; Schlicht, 1994; Stich, 1998). With the exception of the Schlicht meta-analysis, which used a different inclusion criterion than other meta-analyses (Landers & Arent, 2001), these reviews show that exercise, as an intervention, consistently improves positive mood and reduces anxiety and depression scores. These effects are consistently observed for men/women; young/old people; in clinical/normal populations; with human/animal subjects; in the United States/European countries; in different research laboratories; in correlational/cross-sectional studies as well as experimental studies; with different types of exercise (e.g., aerobic or anaerobic, acute or chronic); and with different operational measures of anxiety, depression, and mood state. Meta-analyses

reveal that the overall magnitude of these exercise effects in non-clinical populations is generally "small to moderate" (ES_{range} = .15 to .56), but "large effects" (ES_{range} = .72 to .94) are commonly observed in clinically anxious or depressed people.

The Nature of the Relationship: Is It Causal?

The consistency and magnitude of exercise effects on improved mood state have led Mutrie (2000) to suggest that the relationship may be described as "causal in lowering depression scores in clinical patents." To better understand how conclusions can be weighted in science, Hill's (1965) guidelines/criteria for determining causation are present in Table 1. In determining strength of association, each study is examined and an effect size is calculated by dividing the mean difference (e.g., experimental/treatment group minus no treatment/control group, or pretest minus posttest values) by the pooled variability (i.e., pooled standard deviation or standard error) that exists in that study. Conceptually, an effect size is a measure of the meaningfulness of the relationship and these effect sizes can range from zero to infinity with small effect sizes ranging from .20 to .40, moderate ranging from .41 to .70, and large ranging from .71 on up (Cohen, 1992). Meta-analyses are most often the source of effects sizes because they combine the results from multiple studies and therefore these effect sizes are based on more subjects and are more stable and representative than effect sizes derived from individual studies. Large numbers of subjects are needed to offset the risk of making Type I errors (i.e., saying something is significantly different when it isn't) and Type II errors (saying something is not different when it actually is different).

Type I errors are minimized by insuring that the mean difference between groups would not occur by chance any more than five times in 100 replications; Type II errors, by having sufficient numbers of participants in each of the groups to minimize the variability. With this in mind, Sackett (1989) has assessed the quality of studies (Levels 1 to 5) and given each level a letter grade (A through C). According to him, the best research evidence (Level 1) comes from large randomized trials with clear-cut results. These are experimental studies where subjects have

Table 1. Hill's (1965) Guidelines/Criteria for Causation

Strength of Association – an average effect size from several studies.

Consistency – effect seen in different places, by different people, at different times, and in different circumstances.

Specificity – limited to a single cause for a single effect, but if other criteria are met, lack of specificity is not a fatal flaw.

Temporal Sequence – does physical activity precede changes in mental health?

Dose Response Gradient – change in the dependent variable is dependent on increased dose/ duration of exposure (e.g., exercise).

Biological Plausibility – results are in harmony with understanding of the response of cells, tissues, organs, and organisms to stimuli.

Coherence – possible mechanisms should not conflict with our understanding of the natural history and biology of mental illness.

Experimental Evidence – existence of experimental studies with very large (Grade A) or relatively small (Grade B) study samples that support the predicted relationship.

been randomly assigned to experimental and control groups. These studies have a low risk of error and therefore receive a grade of A. Level 2 evidence is derived from small randomized trials with uncertain results. In this case, the study receives a grade of B because there is a moderate to high risk of error. The only difference between Levels 1 and 2 is that Level 1 research has a very large sample size. This large sample size minimizes the risk of making a Type II error. One advantage of meta-analyses is that Level 1 (Grade A) evidence can be produced by combining the results of several Level 2 (Grade B) studies. This has occurred only because the sample size has been greatly increased. Even if the sample size was vastly increased in Grade C studies (Levels 3, 4, and 5), this would not produce Level 1 or 2 evidence because these are not controlled experimental studies and therefore there is an increased likelihood of Type I errors.

Another criterion for causation is the consistency of the findings (Table 1). It is important to have large reviews of the literature (either quantitative or narrative reviews) that can potentially show the same or similar results for men/women, young/old people, in clinical/normal populations, with human/animal subjects, in the United States/European countries, in different research laboratories, in Grade C studies/Grade A&B studies, with different types of exercise (e.g., aerobic or anaerobic, acute or chronic),

and with different operational measures for selected mental health variables. Specificity is another guideline for causation, but it is rarely achieved when dealing with human behavior. For instance, there are many ways to treat panic attack patients besides exercise (e.g., drugs, psychotherapy). Hill has noted the difficulty in meeting this criterion and has said that failure to meet this criterion is not a fatal flaw as long as the other criteria for causation are met.

Temporal sequence, as a criterion for causation, can be established by examining epidemiological and experimental studies. Epidemiological studies that follow cohorts over time allow for the determination of whether activity precedes reductions in mental health variables. These Grade C studies are limited, however, in the control of all extraneous variables. Experimental studies are designed to control for extraneous variables and thus are vital for determining causation. In experimental studies, where subjects are randomly assigned to treatment (e.g., exercise training) or control (no exercise training) groups prior to an intervention period (e.g., exercise training program), it can also be determined if exercise precedes changes observed in psychological outcomes. Dose-response studies (preferably experimental) that have examined at least two or more levels of exercise intensity and duration are also useful in determining how much exercise is needed to produce desired changes in the psychological variable of interest. This information is very important in developing exercise prescriptions for individuals with mental health problems.

Evidence for biological plausibility and coherence can be found in human and animal studies that have examined exercise in relation to physiological mechanisms believed to be important for creating better mood states. Many of these studies have used an animal model to be able to directly measure biochemical or structural changes in the brain after the animal has been sacrificed. Animal studies offer the investigators control of variables that are often uncontrollable in human research, but there is always the concern about the validity of the models used to examine depression and anxiety in animals generalizing to human mental health issues (Dishman, 1997). Although biological plausibility must be satisfied for a relationship to be causative, psychological explanations can also be considered.

Mutrie concluded that there was support for all causal criteria (except specificity), whereas Arent, Rogers, and Landers (2001) found support for only some criteria (strength of association, consistency, temporal sequence, and biological plausibility), limited support for experimental evidence and coherence, and weak experimental support for dose-response gradient. Recent human experiments now show dose-response effects of exercise for both anxiety reduction (Arent, Landers, Matt, & Etnier, 2005; Bartholomew & Linder, 1998; Ekkekakis, Hall, & Petruzzello, 2004; He, 1998) and for depression (Dunn et al., 2005). The dose-response criterion for causation has now been met and shows that moderate levels of exercise (40% to 75% of VO_2 or HR_{max}) reduce levels of anxiety and depression. Finally, coherence is also met because the results for exercise as an antidepressant and anxiolytic does not conflict with our understanding of the natural history and biology of mental illness.

Although there is now ample experimental evidence for dose-response gradient and coherence, it is still debatable if there are enough RCT studies to support a causal relationship that chronic exercise programs reduce depression and anxiety in clinically depressed people (Blumenthal et al., 1999; Babyak et al., 2000; Dunn et al., 2005; Singh et al., 1997, 2001) or people who experience panic attack (Broocks et al., 1998). The U.S. Surgeon General's Report on

Mental Health (1999) specifies that the level of evidence required for psychotherapy to be well established is at least two published experiments with group designs that have demonstrated efficacy. The experimental evidence for exercise as a treatment intervention clearly exceeds this criterion for both anxiety and depression. It also appears that exercise as an intervention meets this criterion for RCT trials with patients who have minor or major unipolar clinical depression. Two of the RCT studies have examined depression during follow-up (Babyak et al., 2000; Singh et al., 2001), but no studies examining anxiety disorders during a follow-up period were found.

Whether there are enough RCT studies to justify support for a causative relationship for the effects of exercise on specific anxiety and depressive disorders remains to be seen. Overall, some would regard what is presented here as sufficient evidence to conclude that exercise can be considered causal as it relates to reductions in depression and anxiety. Others may not believe that there is enough evidence to justify a conclusion of causation. They would probably point to the possibility of methodological problems in RCTs, and the insufficient number of RCT studies, which have examined patients with anxiety disorders during a follow-up period. To receive more attention from general practice physicians, psychologists, and psychiatrists, more RCT studies with suitable methodological controls (e.g., adequate randomization and complete blinding in outcome assessment) are needed before widespread clinical acceptance will be achieved (Lawlor & Hopker, 2001).

How Does Exercise Compare to Other Interventions?

While evidence continues to mount in favor of exercise as an intervention for anxiety and depression, it is worthwhile to compare exercise to other psychological and pharmacological treatments that are commonly used to treat those with anxiety or depressive disorders. Obviously, if it cannot be shown that exercise is as good as or better than drugs or psychotherapy, there would be no reason for health care professionals to recommend it to their patients. Research information is now available to compare exercise to various types of psychological therapies

Table 2. Meta-Analyses Comparing Exercise With Other Treatments for Depression and Anxiety

Comparison	Depression	Anxiety
Psychotherapy vs. No Treatment =	.30 to 1.22	.85
Cognitive Therapy vs. No Treatment =	.96 to 1.73	.70
Behavioral Therapy vs. No Treatment =	1.02	.91
Cognitive-Behavioral Therapy vs. No Treatment =	.85	1.79
Tri- & Tetra-Cyclic Drugs vs. No Treatment =	.51 to .75	.52
SSRI Drugs vs. No Treatment =	.52 to 1.12	.94
Exercise vs. No Treatment Controls =	.88 (k=18)	.94 (k=11)
Exercise vs. Psychotherapy =	.14 (k=8)	.10 (k=6)
Exercise vs. Recreational Activities =	.73 (k=4)	.65 (k=3)
Exercise vs. Relaxation/Meditation =	.41 (k=3)	.11 (k=3)
Exercise vs. Structured Social Interactions =	.03 (k=5)	-----------

Note. Meta-analyses upon which these overall effect sizes are based are Allen, Hunter, and Donohue (1989, as cited in Stich, 1998, p.59); Gaffan, Tsaousis, and Kemp-Wheeler (1995); Nordhus and Pallesen (2003); Quality Assurance Project (1983, 1985); Robinson, Berman, and Neimeyer (1990); Schroeder and Dush (1987); Steinbrueck, Maxwell, and Howard (1983); Stich (1998); van Balkom et al. (1993); Westen and Morrison (2001).

(e.g., cognitive therapy, behavior therapy, cognitive-behavioral therapy) and drug treatments (e.g., tricyclic antidepressants, selective serotonin-reuptake inhibitors [SSRIs], tranquilizers). The effect sizes reported in several studies are summarized in Tables 2 and 3. In each of these tables, the number of studies (symbolized by k) used in calculating effect sizes is listed for the exercise comparisons. The number of studies for treatments other than exercise ranged from 8 to 200. Effect sizes were derived from meta-analytic findings of several authors (see Stich, 1998 for a review of these studies).

As can be seen for clinical depression (Table 2), exercise produces better anti-depressive effects than waitlist or no treatment control groups or groups engaging in recreational activities or relaxation/meditation. Exercise is not better or significantly worse than interventions involving psychotherapy or structured social interaction. When compared to no treatment control groups, exercise produces effect size results that are in the same range as psychotherapy, cognitive therapy, behavioral therapy, cognitive-behavioral therapy, and various kinds of drugs. Similar results are evident for anxiety reduction (Table 2). Exercise is a better anxiolytic than no treatment control groups and groups engaging in relaxation/meditation or unstructured recreational activities. Exercise

is at least as good as psychotherapy in reducing anxiety. The magnitude of the exercise effect is also in the same range as drug interventions for reducing anxiety. Although tranquilizers are no longer drugs of choice for reducing symptoms of anxiety and depression, DeVries et al. (1981) found that following acute exercise, resting muscle action potentials (i.e., more muscle calming) were lower than following the use of the minor tranquilizer meprobanate.

Exercise Combined with Other Treatments

It appears that exercise is effective in reducing anxiety and depression, but would the effects of exercise be even greater if it were combined with either psychotherapy or with drugs? Effect sizes from studies that have combined treatment interventions for depression and anxiety are presented in Table 3. Positive effect sizes indicate that the effect of the intervention on the left is larger and thus more meaningful than the intervention on the right, whereas a negative effect size indicates that the effect of the intervention on the right is larger and more meaningful than the intervention on the left. This table reveals that although exercise is not significantly different from therapy when examined singly, exercise

Table 3. Effect Sizes for Combined Treatments

Reduction in Depression	
Exercise vs. Therapy =	.14 (k=8)
Exercise vs. Exercise + Therapy =	-.49 (k=1)
Exercise + Therapy vs. Therapy =	+.92 (k=3)
Exercise + Drugs vs. Exercise =	-----------
Antidepressant Drugs + Behavior Therapy vs. No Treatment =	+.95 (k=86)
Reduction in Anxiety	
Exercise vs. Therapy =	.10 (k=6)
Exercise vs. Exercise + Therapy =	-1.18 (k=1)
Exercise + Therapy vs. Therapy =	+.60 k=2)
Exercise + Drugs vs. Exercise =	+1.12 (k=1)
Drugs + Behavioral Therapy vs. No Treatment =	+.47 (k=86)
Therapy + Drugs vs. Placebo Control =	+1.09 (k=8)
Therapy + Drugs vs. Exposure =	+.26 (k=5)

Note. Meta-analyses upon which these overall effect sizes are based are Blumenthal et al. (1999); Clum, Clum, and Surls (1993); Stich (1998); van Balkom et al. (1993).

does enhance the antidepressant and anxiolytic effect of therapy when they are used in combination. The benefit of combining exercise with drugs is not as clear. Blumenthal et al. (1999) found that a combination of exercise and medication (Zoloft) was not as good as exercise alone or medication alone in reducing depression scores. The combination of exercise and drugs, however, showed greater anxiolytic effects than exercise alone.

The Time Course of Exercise Relative to Drugs

It is also of interest to know the time course of the exercise effects. Two studies have examined this, but only for the relationship between exercise and drugs. In randomized clinical trial studies, researchers (Blumenthal et al., 1999; Broocks et al., 1998) found that when compared to exercise, drugs produced quicker anxiolytic and antidepressive effects (@4 weeks), but by 8 weeks and at the end of the chronic exercise training program (10-16 weeks), exercise and antidepressant medications produced comparable effects.

Exercise Compliance and the Principle of Least Effort

What about the willingness of people to use exercise as a treatment intervention? Whereas drugs and therapy are essentially passive treatments, exercise is more active and involves considerable physical effort. According to Zipf (1949), individual and collective behavior is governed by the *principle of least effort.* In organizing our work, we typically minimize the distance between objects, we reduce the size and weight of objects, and we minimize the frequency of performing repetitive tasks by redesigning a single tool to do more jobs. All of these behaviors are undertaken to minimize effort over time. If this principle is true, we might expect that more people would opt for drugs or psychotherapy because they involve considerably less physical effort.

There is some limited evidence in studies comparing drugs to exercise that this may be the case. Broocks et al. (1998) showed that the overall dropout rate was 31% for the exercise group and 27% for the placebo group. There were no dropouts in the medication group. Only one participant in the exercise group dropped out after the first training session because she did not think that exercise was the right treatment for her. Other dropouts from the exercise group occurred at weeks 6-8 of the intervention period because participants did not feel that their symptoms were improving. Blumenthal et al. (1999) did not find a significant difference in dropout rates among exercise, medication, and combined exercise/medication groups, but the dropout rate in the exercise group and combined groups (26.4% & 20.0%) were higher than for the medication group (14.6%). Both studies suggest that it may be harder to get clinically depressed or anxious patients to adhere to an exercise program than it is for them to adhere to a drug treatment. Although the principle of least effort may account for differences in initial compliance with an exercise regimen, it is clear that the vast majority of patients are willing to endure the rigors of an effortful exercise-intervention program.

Post-Intervention Follow-Up Effectiveness of Exercise

There is some evidence for the persistence of exercise effects beyond the intervention period. There are two clinical trial studies examining patients 6 months (Babyak et al., 2000) and 26 months (Singh et al., 2001) after the intervention. Babyak et al. reported that, at follow-up, formerly institutionalized people who exercised had lower rates of depression (30%) than those who had received medication (52%) or combined exercise/drugs (55%). Participants in the exercise group were also more likely than those in the medication group to be partially or fully recovered. Only 8% of people in the exercise group had relapsed compared with 38% in the medication group and 31% in the combined group. Sixty-four percent of people in the exercise group and 66% of the people in the combined group continued to exercise, whereas 48% of people in the drug group initiated an exercise program. Only 7% of people in the exercise group, 40% in the combination group, and 26% in the drug group were still using medication. At least in this study, exercise appears to have a better long-range outcome than antidepressant medication.

Singh et al. (2001) showed that elderly people assigned to an exercise group had significantly less depression than the control group at 26-months following a 20-week resistance-training intervention.

The relative improvements in depression scores for the exercise group were 1.5 to 2.5 times greater than for control participants, and both psychological and somatic subscales of the Beck Depression Inventory were improved with exercise. One-third of the outpatients who were still exercising at 26 months following the intervention "showed that active exercisers demonstrated a trend toward greater long-term response than either exercisers who had stopped lifting weights or controls" (p. M501).

Health Risks and Benefits of Exercise Relative to Other Treatments

How does exercise compare to other interventions when it comes to possible adverse side effects (health risks) or health benefits other than reductions in anxiety and depression? Compared to other psychological and drug treatments, the health risks/side effects of exercise are minimal (e.g., time, sore muscles/cramps, perspiration/fatigue, and effort expenditure) and the health benefits are considerable (e.g., less depression/anxiety; longer life; less body fat; and reduced risk of cardiovascular disease, high blood pressure, dementia/Alzheimer's disease, colon, breast, and prostate cancers, falling, arthritis, NID-diabetes) (Corbin & Pangrazi, 1996; Fratiglioni, Paillard-Borg, & Wimblad, 2004; Holmes, Chen, Feskanich, Kroenke, & Colditz, 2005; Giovannucci, Liu, Leitzmann, Stampfer, & Willett, 2005). Drugs and psychotherapy produce few health benefits beyond reducing depression and anxiety and there are costs associated with therapy (e.g., considerable cost and time) and cost and adverse side effects associated with drugs (e.g., ~$300 per week, lethargy/confusion, sleep disturbances, weight gain, bleeding, flushing/sweating, muscle spasms, heart and lung problems in newborns, sexual dysfunction, seizures, heart arrhythmias, and suicidal thoughts)(Chambers et al., 2006; Hu et al., 2004; Mayers & Baldwin, 2005; Rappaport, Prince, & Bostic, 2005; Ruetsch, Viala, Bardon, Martin, & Vacheron, 2006; Serebruany, 2006).

Compared to exercise, some drugs (tri-cyclic antidepressants, monoamine-oxidase inhibitors) can cause weight gain, and this can increase depression. In fact, this is one of the major reasons for non-adherence to drug treatments among depressed individuals not selected by weight (Deshmukh & Franco, 2003). There is, however, some evidence that some SSRIs may induce weight loss in the acute phase of treatment, and they may also be useful as an adjunct to cognitive-behavioral therapy for treating weight loss in obese individuals with and without mood problems (Ricca et al., 1996). In the elderly population, pharmacotherapy as a treatment for depression has also been shown to increase the risk of falling and hip fractures (Ray, Griffen, Scheffner, Baugh, & Melton, 1987; Thapa, Gideon, Cost, Milam, & Ray, 1998).

Although the purpose of prescribing antidepressant and anxiolytic drugs is to raise levels of serotonin and norepinephrine, it is difficult to measure brain levels of serotonin (5-HT) and norepinephrine (NE), and they are rarely examined in clinical practice. After elimination of other possible problems (e.g., thyroid dysfunction or anemia) that could cause lethargy or tension, prescriptions for antidepressant or anxiolytic drugs are usually based on individuals' self-report of symptoms. Without knowing one's initial level of serotonin or norepinephrine or its levels after drug administration, it is difficult for physicians to know if serotonin and norepinephrine are in the normal range of human values (100-450 pg/ml for NE & 101-283 ng/ml for 5-HT). It has already been pointed out that sub-normal levels of NE and 5-HT increase the risk of depression, anxiety, insomnia, anger, and obesity. What has not been pointed out is that abnormally high levels of NE increase the risk of high blood pressure, which is linked to cardiovascular disease, whereas abnormally high levels of 5-HT increase the risk of carcinoid heart disease, compulsive behavior, and obsessive tidiness. Without primary care physicians knowing plasma levels, and particularly brain levels of serotonin and norepinephrine, there is potential risk of significant side effects with the use of antidepressant and anxiolytic drugs.

Summary

Overall, these results show that exercise is effective as an alternative treatment for anxiety and depression, and it enhances positive mood. It produces consistent anxiolytic and antidepressant effects that are of the same magnitude as effects derived from drugs or many of the more common psychological interventions. Exercise combined with, or as an adjunct to, psychotherapy produces even better anxiolytic or antidepressant results, but it is unclear at this time whether exercise is more effective for reducing depression when combined with drugs. Compared to exercise, drugs appear to be more effective and desirable to patients early in an intervention period, but by the middle to the end of the intervention period, exercise is as effective as drugs. During follow-up, however, there is only one study (Babyak et al, 2000) and thus, limited evidence that exercise is better than drugs (less depression and relapse rates and better adherence). In addition, compared to other treatments, exercise has minimal adverse side effects and has many physical and mental health benefits.

Even though more experimental evidence is needed, particularly in regard to RCT studies with anxiety and depressive disorders other than major and minor depression and panic attack, it is concluded that the research evidence available at this time warrants the recommendation that exercise be used by general practice physicians and mental health professionals as an alternative or as an adjunct to drugs or various forms for psychotherapy. For people with mild to moderate depression, this research evidence has recently led investigators to encourage primary care providers to recommend exercise as either adjunct therapy (Craft & Perna, 2004), or as an alternative to drug therapy (Hardie, 2005).

Currently in both the United Kingdom and in Australia, people who are diagnosed with an anxiety or depressive disorder can receive money from government health care providers to allow them to offset the cost of health/fitness club membership. This has come about through the realization by health care providers in these countries that the research evidence for the anxiolytic and anti-depressive effects of exercise is substantial and that exercise should be encouraged with financial support. Problems still remain, however, because primary care providers have often not been educated in the efficacy of exercise as an intervention, so they do not recommend it as often as other treatments. In fact, in the United Kingdom, 78% of physicians who prescribed antidepressive medication in the past three years had done so because they believed that suitable alternatives were not available (Hardie, 2005). The guidelines of the Mental Health Foundation in the United Kingdom now state that antidepressant drugs should be avoided as a first-line treatment for mild depression, and that primary care physicians should more often recommend exercise as a first-line treatment. With numerous research studies demonstrating that exercise is an effective treatment option, the Mental Health Foundation is now embarking on a year long campaign to educate general practitioners on the use of exercise as a first-line treatment intervention for mild depression. Based of the findings presented in Table 3, it would also be of benefit to use exercise as an adjunctive therapy for more major forms of anxiety or depressive disorders, particularly when combined with some type of psychotherapy.

References

Arent, S. M., Landers, D. M., & Etnier, J. L. (2000). The effects of exercise on mood in older adults: A meta-analytic review. *Journal of Aging and Physical Activity, 8,* 407-430.

Arent, S. M., Rogers, T. J., & Landers, D. M. (2001). Mental health and physical activity. *Sportwissenschaft, 31,* 239-254.

Arent, S. M., Landers, D. M., Matt, K. S., & Etnier, J. L. (2005). Dose–response and mechanistic issues in the resistance training and affect relationship. *Journal of Sport and Exercise Psychology, 27,* 92-110.

Babyak, M., Blumenthal, J. A., Herman, S., Khatri, P., Doraiswamy, M., Moore, K., et al. (2000). Exercise treatment for major depression: Maintenance of therapeutic benefit at 10 months. *Psychosomatic Medicine, 62,* 633-638.

Bahrke, M. S., & Morgan, W. P. (1978). Anxiety reduction following exercise and meditation. *Cognitive Therapy and Research, 2,* 323-333.

Bartholomew, J. B., & Linder, D. E. (1998). State anxiety following resistance exercise: The role of gender and exercise intensity. *Journal of Behavioral Medicine, 21,* 205-219.

Blumenthal, J. A., Emery, C. F., Madden, D. J., George, L. K., Coleman, R. E., Riddle, M. W., et al. (1989). Cardiovascular and behavioral effects of aerobic exercise training in healthy older men and women. Journal of *Gerontology: Medical Sciences, 44,* M147-M157.

Blumenthal, J. A., Emery, C. F., Madden, D. J., Schniebolk, S., Walsh-Riddle, M., George, L. K., et al. (1991). Long-term effects of exercise on psychological functioning in older men and women. *Journal of Gerontology: Psychological Sciences, 46,* P352-P361.

Blumenthal, J. A., Babyak, M. A., Moore, K. A., Craighead, W. E., Herman, S., Khatri, P., et al. (1999). Effects of exercise training on older patents with major depression. *Archives of Internal Medicine, 159,* 2349-2356.

Broocks, A., Bandelow, B., & Pekrun, G. (1998). Comparison of aerobic exercise, chomipramine, and placebo in the treatment of panic disorder. *American Journal of Psychiatry, 155,* 603-609.

Calfas, K. J., & Tylor, W. C. (1994). Effects of physical activity on psychological variables in adolescents. *Pediatric Exercise Science, 6,* 406-423.

Carlson, D. L. (1991). *The effect of exercise on depression: A review and meta-analysis.* Unpublished doctoral dissertation, Wisconsin School of Professional Psychology, Milwaukee.

Chambers, C. D., Hernandez-Diaz, S., Van Marter, L. J., Weber, M. M., Louik, C., Jones, K. L., et al. (2006). Selective serotonin-reuptake inhibitors and risk of persistent pulmonary hypertension of the newborn. *New England Journal of Medicine, 354,* 636-638.

Clum, G. A., Clum, G. A., & Surls, R. (1993). A meta-analysis of treatments for panic disorder. *Journal of Consulting and Clinical Psychology, 61,* 317-326.

Cohen, J. (1992). A power primer. *Psychological Bulletin, 112,* 155-159.

Corbin, C. W., & Pangrazi, R. (Eds.). (1996, July). What you need to know about the Surgeon General's Report on Physical Activity and Health. *Physical Activity and Fitness Research Digest, 2*(6), 1-8.

Craft, L. L., & Landers, D. M. (1998). The effect of exercise on clinical depression and depression resulting from mental illness. *Journal of Sport and Exercise Psychology, 20,* 339-357.

Craft, L. L., & Perna, F. M. (2004). The benefits of exercise for the clinically depressed. Primary Care Companion to the *Journal of Clinical Psychiatry, 6,* 104-111.

De Geus, E. J. C., Lorenz, J. P., van Doornen, L. J. P., de Visser, D. C., & Orlebeke, J. F. (1990). Existing and training induced differences in aerobic fitness: Their relationship to physiological response patterns during different types of stress. *Psychophysiology, 27,* 457-478.

Deshmukh, H., & Franco, K. (2003). Managing weight gain as a side effect of antidepressant therapy. *Cleveland Clinic Journal of Medicine, 70,* 614-618.

DeVries, H. A., Wisell, R. A., Bilbulian, R., & Moritani, T. (1981). Tranquilizer effect of exercise. *American Journal of Physical Medicine, 60,* 57-60.

Driscoll, R. (1976). Anxiety reduction using physical exertion and positive images. *The Psychological Record, 26,* 87-94.

Dunn, A. L., Trivedi, M. H., Kampert, J. B., Clark, C. G., & Chambliss, H. O. (2005). Exercise treatment for depression: Efficacy and dose response. *American Journal of Preventive Medicine, 28,* 1-8.

Ekkekakis, P., Hall, E. E., & Petruzzello, S. J. (2004). Practical markers of the transition from aerobic to anaerobic metabolism during exercise: Rationale and a case for affect-based exercise prescription. *Preventative Medicine, 38,* 149-159.

Franz, S. I., & Hamilton, G. V. (1905). The effects of exercise upon retardation in conditions of depression. *American Journal of Insanity, 62,* 239-256.

Fratiglioni, I., Paillard-Borg, S., & Wimblad, B. (2004). An active and socially integrated lifestyle in late life might protect against dementia. *Lancet Neurology, 3,* 343-353.

Gaffan, E. A., Tsaousis, I., & Kemp-Wheeler, S. M. (1995). Researcher allegiance and meta-analysis: The case of cognitive therapy for depression. *Journal of Consulting and Clinical Psychology, 63,* 966-980.

Galye, R. C., Spitler, D. L., Karper, W. B., Jaeger, R. M., & Rice, S. N. (1988). Psychological changes in exercising COPD patients. *International Journal of Rehabilitation Research, 11,* 335-342.

Giovannucci, E. L., Liu, Y., Leitzmann, M. F., Stampfer, M. J., & Willett, W. C. (2005). A prospective study of physical activity and incident and fatal prostate cancer. *Archives of Internal Medicine, 165,* 1005-1010.

Hardie, A. (2005). Exercise "best cure" for depression. Retrieved from http://news.scotsman.com/index.cfm?id=331212005

He, C. X. (1998). *Exercise intensity, duration, and fitness effects on mood and electroencephalographic activity.* Unpublished doctoral dissertation, Arizona State University, Tempe.

Hill, A. T. (1965). The environment and disease: Association or causation? *Proceedings of the Royal Society of Medicine, 58,* 295-300.

Holmes, M. D., Chen, W. Y., Feskanich, D., Kroenke, C. H., & Colditz, G. A. (2005). Physical activity and survival after breast cancer diagnosis. *Journal of the American Medical Association, 293,* 2479-2486.

Hu, X. H., Bull, S. A., Hunkeler, E. M., Ming, E., Lee, J. Y., Fireman, B., et al. (2004). Incidence and duration of side effects and those related as bothersome with selective serotonin-reuptake inhibitor treatment for depression: Patient report versus physician estimate. *Journal of Clinical Psychiatry, 65,* 959-965.

Kugler, J., Seelbach, H., & Kruskemper, G. M. (1994). Effects of rehabilitation exercise programmes on anxiety and depression in coronary patients: A meta-analysis. *British Journal of Clinical Psychology, 33,* 401-410.

Landers, D. M., & Arent, S. M. (2001). Physical activity and mental health. In R. N. Singer, H. A. Hausenblas, & C. M. Janelle (Eds.), *Handbook of sport psychology* (2nd ed., pp. 740-765). New York: Wiley.

Landers, D. M., & Petruzzello, S. J. (1994). Physical activity, fitness, and anxiety. In C. Bouchard, R. J. Shephard, & T. Stevens (Eds.), Physical activity, fitness, and health (pp. 868-882). Champaign, IL: Human Kinetics.

Lawlor, D. A., & Hopker, S. W. (2001). The effectiveness of exercise as an intervention in the management of depression: Systematic review and meta-regression analysis of randomized controlled trials. *British Medical Journal, 322,* 768-777.

Long, B. C., & van Stavel, R. (1995). Effects of exercise training on anxiety: A meta-analysis. *Journal of Applied Sport Psychology, 7,* 167-189.

Mayers, A. G., & Baldwin, D. S. (2005). Antidepressants and their effect on sleep. *Human Psychopharmacology, 20,* 533-559.

McDonald, D. G., & Hodgdon, J. A. (1991). *The psychological effects of aerobic fitness training: Research and theory.* New York: Springer-Verlag.

McNeil, K., LeBlanc, E., & Joyce, M. (1991). The effect of exercise on depressive symptoms in the moderately depressed elderly. *Psychology of Aging, 3,* 487-488.

Moses, J., Steptoe, A., Mathews, A., & Edwards, S. (1989). The effects of exercise training on mood and perceived coping ability in anxious adults from the general population. *Journal of Psychosomatic Research, 33,* 47-61.

Mutrie, N. (2000). The relationship between physical activity and clinically defined depression. In S. J. H. Biddle, K. R. Fox, & S. H. Boutcher (Eds.), *Physical activity and psychological well-being* (pp. 46-62). London: Taylor & Francis.

Nordhus, I. H., & Pallesen, S. (2003). Psychological treatment of late-life anxiety: An empirical review. *Journal of Consulting and Clinical Psychiatry, 71,* 643-651.

North, T. C., McCullagh, P., & Tran, Z. V. (1990). Effect of exer-

cise on depression. *Exercise and Sport Science Reviews, 18,* 379-415.

Petruzzello, S. J., Landers, D. M., Hatfield, B. D., Kubitz, K. A., & Salazar, W. (1991). A meta-analysis on the anxiety-reducing effects of acute and chronic exercise. *Sports Medicine, 11,* 143-192.

Quality Assurance Project (1983). A treatment outline for depressive disorders. *Australian and New Zealand Journal of Psychiatry, 17,* 129-146.

Quality Assurance Project (1985). Treatment outlines for the management of anxiety states. Australian and New Zealand *Journal of Psychiatry, 19,* 138-151.

Rappaport, N., Prince, J. B., & Bostic, J. Q. (2005). Lost in the black box: Juvenile depression, suicide, and the FDA's black box. *Journal of Pediatrics, 147,* 719-720.

Ray, W. A., Griffen, M. R., Scheffner, W., Baugh, N. K., & Melton, L. J. (1987). Psychotropic drug use and the risk of hip fracture. *New England Journal of Medicine, 316,* 313-319.

Ricca, V., Mannucci, E., Di Bernard, M., Rizzello, S. M., Cabras, P. L., & Rotella, C. M. (1996). Sertaline enhances the effects of cognitive-behavioral treatment on weight reduction of obese patients. *Journal of Endocrinology Investigation, 19,* 727-733.

Robinson, L. A., Berman, J. S., & Neimeyer, R. A. (1990). Psychotherapy for the treatment of depression: A comprehensive review of controlled outcome research. *Psychological Bulletin, 108,* 30-49.

Roth, D. L., Bachter, S. D., & Fillingim, R. B. (1990). Acute emotional and cardiovascular effects of stressful mental work during aerobic exercise. *Psychophysiology, 27,* 694-701.

Ruetsch, O., Viala, A., Bardon, H., Martin, P., & Vacheron, M. N. (2006). Psychotropic drugs induced weight gain: A review of the literature concerning epidemiological data, mechanisms and management. *Encephale, 31,* 507-516.

Schlicht, W. (1994). Does physical exercise reduce anxious emotions? A meta-analysis. *Anxiety, Stress, and Coping, 6,* 275-288.

Schroeder, H. E., & Dush, D. M. (1987). Relinquishing the placebo: Alternatives for psychotherapy outcome research. *American Psychologist, 42,* 1129-1130.

Serebruany, V. L. (2006). Selective serotonin reuptake inhibitors and increased bleeding risk: Are we missing something? *American Journal of Medicine, 119,* 113-116.

Singh, N. A., Clemens, K. M., & Fiatarone, M. A. (1997). A randomized controlled trial of progressive resistance training in depressed elders. *Journal of Gerontology: Medical Sciences, 52A,* M27-M35.

Singh, N. A., Clemens, K. M., & Fiatarone-Singh, M. A. (2001). The efficacy of exercise as a long-term antidepressant in elderly subjects: A randomized controlled trial. *Journal of Gerontology: Medical Sciences, 56A,* M497-M504.

Steinbrueck, S. M., Maxwell, S. E., & Howard, G. S. (1983). A meta-analysis of psychotherapy and drug therapy in the treatment of unipolar depression with adults. *Journal of Consulting and Clinical Psychology, 51,* 856-863.

Steptoe, A., Edwards, S., Moses, J., & Mathews, A. (1989). The effects of exercise training on mood and perceived coping ability in anxious adults from the general population. *Journal of Psychosomatic Research, 33,* 537-547.

Stich, F. A. (1998). *A meta-analysis of physical exercise as a treatment for symptoms of anxiety and depression.*

Unpublished doctoral dissertation, University of Wisconsin-Madison.

Thapa, P., Gideon, P., Cost, T., Milam, A., & Ray, W. (1998). Antidepressants and the risk of falls among nursing home residents. *New England Journal of Medicine, 339,* 875-882.

U.S. Department of Health and Human Services (1999). *Mental health: A report of the Surgeon General—executive summary.* Rockville, MD: Author.

Van Balkom, A. J., Bakker, A., Spinhoven, P., Blaauw, B. M., Smeenk, S., & Ruesink, B. (1997). A meta-analysis of the treatment of panic disorder with or without agoraphobia: A comparison of psychopharmacological, cognitive-behavioral, and combination treatment. *Journal of Mental Disease, 105,* 510-516.

Vaux, C. L. (1926). A discussion of physical exercise and recreation. *Occupational Therapy and Rehabilitation, 6,* 320-333.

Westen, D., & Morrison, K. (2001). A multidimensional meta-analysis of treatments for depression, panic, and generalized anxiety disorder: An empirical examination of the status of empirically supported therapies. *Journal of Consulting and Clinical Psychiatry, 69,* 875-899.

Zipf, G. K. (1949). *Human behavior and the principle of least effort: An introduction to human ecology.* Cambridge, MA: Addison-Wesley.

Section IV
Cognitive Psychology and Psychophysiology

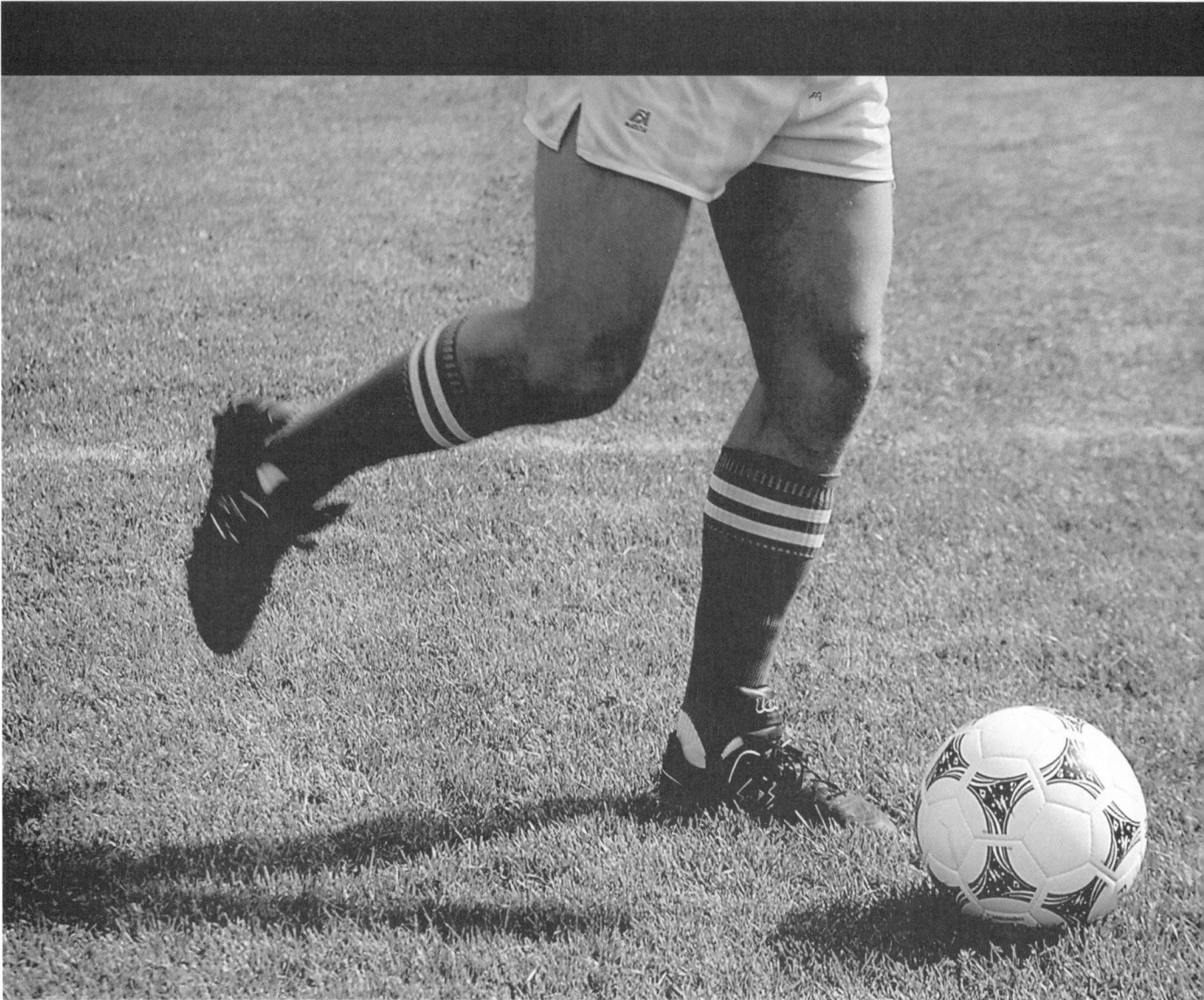

8

A Psychological Approach to the Organization of Voluntary Movements

FRANZ MECHSNER

Introduction

How is it possible that we move according to our intentions, in an abundantly flexible way? Thereby we creatively invent novel movements and can often immediately execute them in a way that is perfectly adapted to the functional goal we have. I will argue that the key to understanding movement organization and control lies in the flexible, creative, and thereby perfectly adapted function of our psychological system. According to this view, humans perform voluntary movements by way of constructing the adequate perceptual-conceptual movement representations.

Since the mid-eighties, the debate in movement science has been dominated by the controversy between the motor program approach and the synergetic action approach. According to the motor program approach, patterns of muscular activation are precisely pre-structured before a movement starts, whereas according to the synergetic approach, muscular patterns self-organize in response to the tuning of specific control parameters. In both traditions, however, organizing the correct pattern of muscular activation is considered the primary problem. In recent years, several scholars have re-emphasized the importance of anticipated perceptual effects and the crucial role of mental representations in action control (in the tradition of James and Bernstein, among others). In this spirit, new approaches to human voluntary movements have emerged with the proposal that the crucial step in movement control is the construction of appropriate psychological representations. These representations may include goal states as well as dynamical components. It is assumed that these representations primarily govern the flexible and adaptive tuning of motor commands and muscular activity patterns.

In other words, it is suggested that human voluntary movements are planned, performed, and stored in memory as perceptible events, known as *gestalts* (German word for perceptual configuration, as emphasized by the German gestalt psychologists in the early 20th century), with a strong role of anticipatory representations. Motor commands are never addressed and organized as such in any stage of the process. Instead, they are automatically and implicitly tuned in direct correspondence to perceptual-cognitive, or psychological, activity.

Strange as that turn of view (saying that the psychological apparatus is the primary system for motor control) might appear at first sight, it does nothing but analogize movement to other human activities such as perception and cognition. It is possible to understand perception and cognition without explicitly considering their material basis (namely neuronal activity), and it is posed here that it is equally plausible to comprehend voluntary movements without explicitly considering their material basis (namely neuronal and musculo-skeletal activity).

I will argue that *efferences* (i.e., neuronal motor pathways) should not be ascribed a special status in the nervous system—as compared to neurons in the brain that bring about, say, perception. It has traditionally been claimed that movement planning and executing involves a particular step that explicitly maps the anticipated perceptible movement effects to the adequate pattern of efferent commands. How this step might be brought about has remained a mystery. Not only do the necessary computations seem utterly intricate, if not *a priori* impossible due to the ever-changing properties of the neuronal-muscular-skeletal system. It is also completely enigmatic how information in a psychological format that plausibly emerges from collective properties of neuronal networks could be explicitly related to physical motor commands.

I consider these problems actually insurmountable. However, there is a way out—namely to change view and conceive the contribution of neuronal-muscular pathways in movement performance *in strict analogy* to the role of purely neuronal pathways in mediating purely perceptual-cognitive processes. In principle, that seems quite possible. A purely neuronal pathway internal to the brain conveys activity from neurons to other neurons. A pathway transforming neuronal activity into muscular activity and back into (sensory) neuronal activity again does exactly the same, in effect. The crucial step is then to appreciate that the roles of purely neuronal, brain-internal pathways and the roles of neuronal-muscular-neuronal pathways might be *identical* insofar as both kinds of pathways contribute to the *material* (and never explicitly addressed) activity of the physiological network that collectively mediates *psychological* processes. If so, motor behavior is controlled in the same way as perception and cognition and thus can basically be understood as perceptual and cognitive (i.e., genuinely psychological) activity.

A Perceptual-Cognitive Approach to Voluntary Movement Control

The psychological (perceptual-cognitive) approach to human voluntary movement control implies two main claims: First, all of the amazing capabilities of our cognitive system, including perfect improvisation, are directly available for motor control at all levels. Second, motor commands are never addressed and organized as such in any stage of the process. Instead, they are automatically and implicitly tuned in direct correspondence to perceptual-cognitive activity. For a comparison, to steer a car along a curved road it is certainly most important that the electrical signals to the wheels be tuned appropriately. However, those signals are never addressed and organized as such. Control is more about the mapping of steering wheel movements to situational task constraints and the corrections that are necessary due to imperfect mapping.

In the following, I will discuss some pieces of experimental evidence in favor of a psychological approach. There are also two strong theoretical reasons why the hypothesis of a psychological approach is worth exploring. First, if the controlling system is purely and directly psychological in nature, movement control might directly take advantage of the whole of perceptual-cognitive capabilities. That would be possible only in a very limited way if motor control implied a complicated system of mapping perceptual-cognitive movement design to a detailed pattern of motor commands. Second, it might well turn out that it is actually impossible to determine the appropriate motor command pattern from the myriads of relevant variables that are effective in a given situation. The first argument may appear a little obscure at this place in the discussion, but I hope that it will become clearer in the course of the chapter. The relevance of the second argument is immediately obvious. As far as I know, Bernstein (1967) was the first to argue that motor commands that are appropriate to the intention and situation could not be reliably determined and organized as such by the system, for principal reasons. If Bernstein was right in that regard, one actually has no other option than to discard any efference-oriented approach, and instead look seriously for alternative mechanisms of human motor control.

I am rather convinced that efference-oriented approaches would definitely not work. I will not go into detail in this regard and will mainly ask whether a purely perceptual-cognitive approach is thinkable at all as an alternative framework and whether there is experimental and theoretical evidence in favor of it. I will conclude that a purely perceptual-cognitive movement control principle is plausible. Moreover, it seems to have very attractive characteristics in light of everyday and experimental evidence.

Perceptual-cognitive approaches to human voluntary movements have not been particularly embraced by the scientific community in the past. Regardless, I am neither the only one nor the first to propose such an approach. I rely on related ideas by Bernstein (1967), Hoffmann (1993, 2003), Ivry, Diedrichsen, and colleagues (Ivry, Diedrichsen, Spencer, Hazeltine, & Semjen, 2004), James (1890), Lotze (1852), Metzger (1972), Prinz, Hommel, and colleagues (Prinz, 1990, 1997; Hommel, 1998; Hommel, Muesseler, Aschersleben, & Prinz, 2001), Schack (2002), and others. It is fair to say, however, that certainly not all of these authors would agree to the notion of a purely psychological approach as proposed here.

A Psychological Approach to Bimanual Coordination

In bimanual movements there are spontaneous coordination tendencies, in particular the so-called symmetry tendency. In my view these tendencies are best understood by way of a perceptual-cognitive approach. My argument will proceed in three steps.

First, spontaneous coordination phenomena between persons, as well as between persons and moving objects, seem to provide evidence for an important role of perceptual-cognitive control principles. Second, in some bimanual coordination paradigms, spontaneous coordination seems to be completely under perceptual-cognitive control (apart from minor details that are not perceptible to begin with). Third, a generalization of this supposition seems plausible. Spontaneous coordination in periodic movements might generally be brought about by way of perceptual-cognitive control mechanisms.

Spontaneous Person-Person and Person-Object Coordination Is Governed by Perceptual Factors

Perceptual factors can shape spontaneous coordination and even define transition tendencies. For instance, two people looking at each other tend to synchronize oscillatory movements of the limbs as well as hand-held pendulums, and to switch in symmetry at higher velocities (Schmidt, Bienvenu, Fitzpatrick, & Amazeen, 1998; Schmidt, Carello, & Turvey, 1990; Schmidt & O'Brian, 1997). Similar phase transitions also occur in rhythmic coordination of one single limb with an oscillating visual cue (Wimmers, Beek, & van Wieringen, 1992). It is plausible that the transitions are analogous or equivalent to the well-known action slips in human performance (see Norman, 1981), thus pointing to the perceptual-cognitive nature of voluntary movement coordination. In conclusion, several authors have considered the possibility that spontaneous coordination phenomena are generally *abstract* (Saltzman, 1995) or *informational* (Kelso, 1994) in nature.

It has to be emphasized that perception and action seem not to be arbitrarily associated in the form of stimulus-response chains, but seem to make sense as a unified whole, according to perceptual grouping principles, such as rhythmic coherence and symmetry. Transitions into the perceptually defined preferred mode are spontaneous, with the adequate muscular activation patterns automatically and effortlessly tuned in service to the perceptually defined movement tendency. In addition, the induced perceptually defined movement patterns are novel at the relevant dimension. Recall that pattern transitions of this type become obvious especially in very quick movements, which nicely illustrates the proposed direct quality of perceptual-cognitive control.

To conclude, direct perceptual-cognitive (psychological) control appears possible. The evidence is rather suggestive. If the system has the capacity to apply a perceptual-cognitive control principle at all, it would not be surprising to learn that this capacity is generally applied in human movement control. In the following, I will discuss some other phenomena in spontaneous interlimb coordination, in particular the symmetry tendency that has widely been explained in terms of preferred patterns of efferent commands and muscular activity.

The Symmetry Bias in Bimanual Finger Wiggling
The symmetry tendency in the classical bimanual finger-wiggling paradigm as introduced by Cohen (1971) and Kelso (1981, 1984) is one of the most investigated motor phenomena. A person places his or her arms parallel on a table and stretches out both index fingers. Two kinds of periodical movements are instructed: The symmetrical pattern involves moving both fingertips synchronously toward the sagittal midline and synchronously away from it (Figure 1A). The parallel pattern is defined as one fingertip moving away from the sagittal midline synchronously with the other fingertip moving toward the midline, and vice versa (Figure 1B). The symmetrical pattern can be performed virtually up to the highest possible wiggling frequencies of the fingers. In stark contrast, the parallel pattern is stable only at moderate speed, but deteriorates at higher speed, with spontaneous transitions to the symmetrical pattern occurring at higher speed. Such spontaneous coordination phenomena have attracted considerable research interest. The characteristic and impressive stability phenomena in connection have, above all, inspired the dynamical systems approach to action and cognition (Haken, Kelso, & Bunz, 1985; Kelso, 1995).

It has often been emphasized that symmetric movements of homologous limbs involve synchronous contractions of homologous muscles (Cohen, 1971; Kelso, 1984). Thus, the symmetry tendency might mirror an underlying tendency toward co-activation of homologous muscles. For a possible interpretation, bilateral cross-talk in homologous efferent neuronal pathways might lead to a co-activation and assimilation tendency in those pathways (Cattaert, Semjen, & Summers, 1999; Swinnen, 2002).

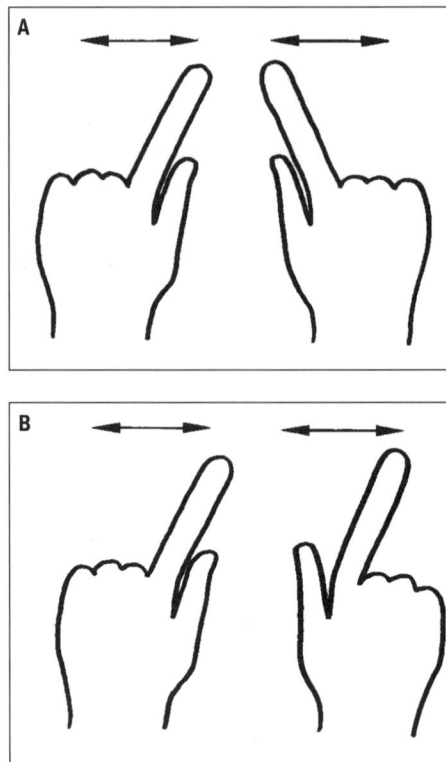

Figure 1. Finger oscillation patterns in the experiment by Kelso (1984). A: symmetrical movements, B: parallel movements. Reprinted with permission.

**The Symmetry Bias Seems to Be
Defined in Terms of a Perceptual Pattern**
Mechsner, Kerzel, Knoblich, and Prinz (2001) suggested that the symmetry tendency in a version of the bimanual finger-wiggling task does not mirror a co-activation tendency of homologous muscles, but rather, it demonstrates perceptual mirrorsymmetry independent of the muscles and, thus, motor commands involved. They asked participants to perform adductive-abductive bimanual index finger oscillations in the transverse plane. The hands were placed parallel in mirrorsymmetry to the sagittal midline and individually positioned either palm down or palm up. Two of the four possible palm combinations were congruous, that is with both palms up or both palms down, and two of them were incongruous, with one palm up and the other palm down (Figure 2).

Participants were instructed to perform mirrorsymmetrical and parallel movements at increasing metronome speed. Participants were instructed that

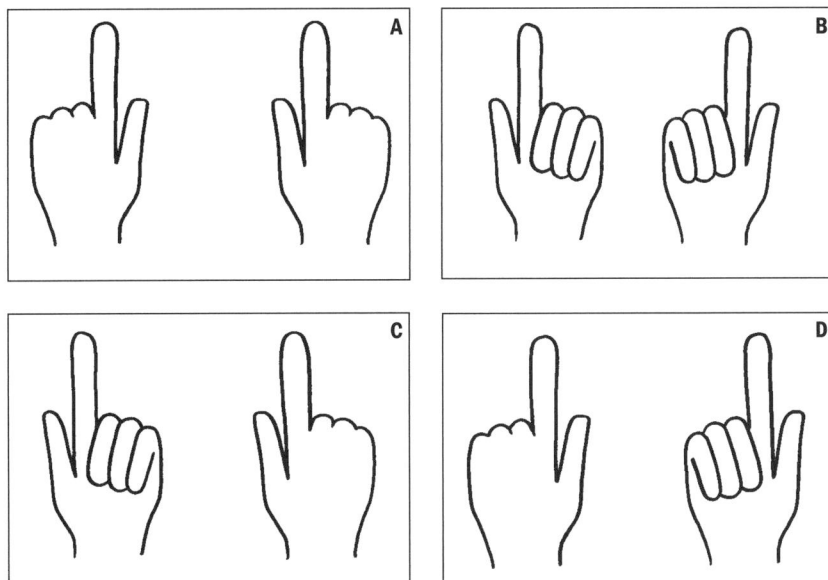

Figure 2. Palm positions in the experiment by Mechsner et al. (2001). Congruous positions with (A) both palms down or (B) both palms up. Incongruous positions (C, D) with one palm up and the other palm down.

if they felt a tendency to slip out of the instructed pattern they should not resist too much, but should adopt the more comfortable pattern. The crucial condition was defined by the incongruous palm settings. If there was a dominant tendency toward co-activation of homologous muscles, then the parallel pattern should be more stable than the symmetrical pattern. In contrast, if there was a dominant tendency toward spatial perceptual mirrorsymmetry, then the symmetrical pattern should be more stable than the parallel pattern.

As for the results, instructed symmetrical movements were quite successfully performed to the highest movement frequencies, independent of palm position. In contrast, parallel movements were correctly performed only at low metronome speed. At increased speed, the parallel pattern dissolved considerably. Transitions to the symmetrical movement pattern frequently occurred (Figure 3). Virtually the same result was revealed if the participants' view of the hands was occluded (Mechsner, 2005a; see also Mechsner & Knoblich, 2004).

In conclusion, Mechsner et al. (2001; Mechsner, 2005a) hypothesized that the symmetry tendency in periodic bimanual finger adduction and abduction is toward perceptual mirrorsymmetry, be the mediating perceptual medium vision or proprioception. At least with occluded vision, the mediating perceptual modality is plausibly kinesthetic proprioception, which may play a prominent role in the first case.

From these results one might conclude that per-

ceptual-cognitive control, including an automatic and flexible tuning of muscular activity, fully explains the symmetry tendency in the finger oscillation paradigm. Swinnen (2002) pointed to the particular strength of the symmetry tendency in intrapersonal coordination as compared with interpersonal and person-object coordination. He argued that this particular strength points to the special and important role of the homologous muscle principle in intrapersonal coordination. The reported experiment by Mechsner et al. (2001), however, revealed that the symmetry tendency was virtually equally strong in the congruous and incongruous palm positions, thus without regard to the homology or nonhomology of the involved muscles. An alternative, perceptual explanation for the particular strength of the intrapersonal symmetry bias might be that proprioception is of particular importance here, in contrast to interpersonal coordination. In other words, bimanual coordination seems solely and exclusively defined in terms of perceptual factors here, whereas muscles and motor commands do not matter because they are automatically and flexibly tuned in service to the perceptually defined event.

A Psychological Approach to
Spontaneous Coordination

Is the hypothesis plausible that bimanual coordination is generally perceptual-cognitive in nature? To note, even if homology of involved muscles would be an important factor in bimanual coordination,

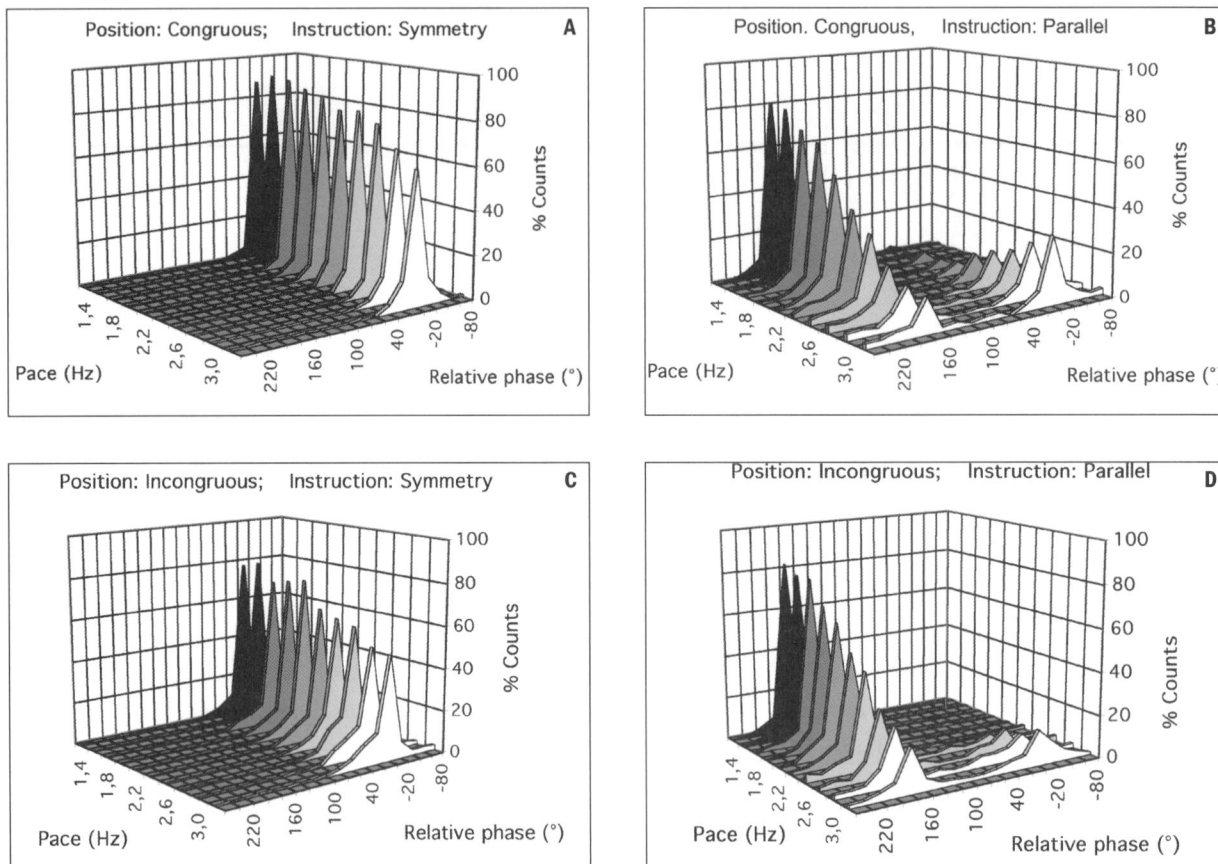

Figure 3. Histogram plots of relative phase counts, as a function of metronome frequencies, (Mechsner et al., 2001). With congruous palm positions, instructed symmetry, i.e., 0° relative phase (A) is reliably performed up to the highest frequencies, whereas instructed parallel movements, i.e., 180° relative phase (B) are reliably performed only at low frequencies. At high frequencies, transitions into symmetry are obvious. The same stability characteristics hold with incongruous palm positions (C, D).

that would not speak against this idea, as homology is clearly confounded with perceptual factors. Material support for the proposed hypothesis may be found in experimental results on bimanual coordination in split-brain patients. Franz, Eliassen, Ivry, and Gazzaniga (1996) had callosotomy patients and control participants draw two three-sided boxes synchronously, one with each hand. Controls performed with ease when the to-be-drawn boxes were oriented in a symmetrical fashion, but had considerable problems when drawing boxes in non-symmetrical orientations. In stark contrast, callosotomy patients performed the symmetrical and the non-symmetrical task equally well, without difficulties. The authors concluded that interference in this task occurred at a cortical level of movement organization. Eliassen, Baynes, and Gazzaniga (1999) provided further evidence suggesting that the critical spatial interactions reflect communication between parietal cortical re-

gions, a well-known locus for spatial cognition.

There are results in the literature, however, that at first sight might be—and have been—taken as evidence that a perceptual-cognitive control principle is certainly not universally valid in spontaneous coordination. Riek, Carson, and Byblow (1992) studied finger flexion and extension in a much similar way as Mechsner et al. (2001) studied bimanual finger adduction and abduction, but obtained strikingly different results. Participants performed bimanual index finger oscillations in the transverse plane, with their hands either prone or supine (Figure 4). Movements of the index fingers were restricted to flexion and extension. All participants received symmetrical as well as parallel movement instructions under all four combinations of right and left hand positions. With increasing frequencies, involuntary transitions occurred only when flexion in one hand went together with extension in the other hand, in the instructed

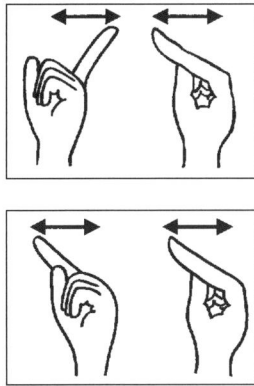

Figure 4. Finger movement patterns under incongruous hand positions (Riek et al., 1992). A: symmetrical oscillations; B: parallel oscillations.

movement pattern. Thus, after the transition, flexion was always synchronous with flexion and extension with extension. Further variations of hand positions would provide convincing evidence that the revealed flexion-flexion bias seems to be maintained fully independent of the absolute and relative position of the hands.

Riek et al. (1992) concluded that there was a strong tendency toward co-activation of homologous muscles. To possibly explain that result, Carson (2004) underlined that there are notable differences between flexors and extensors. The finger flexors are stronger than the extensors, requiring a smaller proportion of motor units to be activated in order to produce a given level of force. Flexors receive a greater share of monosynaptic inputs from the motor cortex in nonhuman, and probably also human, primates. Activation of flexors enhances the excitability of contralateral flexors. Carson named further neuro-musculo-skeletal factors that might contribute to the observed flexion-flexion bias. To explain the contrasting results by Mechsner et al. (2001), Carson hypothesized that there are no similarly significant differences between the adductors and abductors of the fingers. The presence versus absence of those differences might explain why the coupling tendencies in bimanual index flexion and extension are so substantially at variance with the tendencies in adduction and abduction.

Material Factors Organize under Perceptual-Cognitive Guidance

What does the result by Riek et al. (1992) mean in connection with the present considerations? Is it thinkable that the observed flexion-flexion bias is perceptual-cognitive in nature? Carson (2004) claimed

that this is certainly not so. His argument goes along the following lines. First, he considered it plausible that neuro-musculo-skeletal factors are the basis of the flexion-flexion bias. Second, neuro-musculo-skeletal factors are clearly different from perceptual factors. Carson concluded that the flexion-flexion bias is not perceptually defined. Thus, Mechsner et al. (2001) overstated their case with their hypothesis that spontaneous coordination might, in general, be perceptual-cognitive in nature. Carson instead proposed that spontaneous coordination is governed by a coalition of perceptual, neuro-musculo-skeletal, and other factors.

Obviously, it would be ridiculous to deny an important role of physical, and in particular, neuro-musculo-skeletal factors in movement coordination (although the relevant factors are not a priori obvious but need to be determined in every paradigm). A perceptual-cognitive approach, however, does not in the least imply such a denial. Quite to the contrary, one has to appreciate that perceptual and cognitive factors can only guide and control the form of well-adapted action if they are well-adapted to physical factors. Thus, in our connection, the relevant question is not to ask whether physical factors are relevant for coordination at all. Clearly they are. The crucial point in our connection is the following: Do the relevant physical factors blindly mix beyond perceptual-cognitive control (as is the case in unforeseen and unplanned falling)? Or does the controlling system actually control their influence according to perceptual-cognitive principles and criteria, by way of addressing their perceptual correlates and consequences? I argue that the second view is rather plausible in the bimanual finger flexion and extension paradigm and, in consequence, that a perceptual-cognitive approach might well be adequate here.

Recently, Oullier, DeGuzman, Jantzen, and Kelso (2003) conducted an experiment with pairs of persons who performed periodic unimanual flexion and extension movements of the index fingers. The two participants grasped a horizontal bar from above or below and looked at each other. The results of that experiment revealed a tendency to interpersonally synchronize flexion with flexion and extension with extension, independent of whether the individual hands grasped the bar from above or below. Because the observed flexion-flexion bias holds between persons, it is clearly perceptual-cognitive in nature. That outcome strongly points to the possibility that the flexion-flexion bias might be perceptual-cognitive in nature in intra-personal bimanual coordination also.

What kind of perceptual factors might possibly be relevant in bringing about the flexion-flexion coupling bias? For a start, consider an observation by Carson (1996). In unimanual periodic index finger flexion and extension following a metronome pace, there was a clear tendency to perform flexion, rather than extension, on the beat. Moreover, if extension on the beat was instructed, there was a strong bias to switch to flexion on the beat with increasing metronome frequencies, but not vice versa. Why is this? Why are periodic finger movements coupled to periodic metronome beats? And what is the crucial difference between flexion and extension that leads to the revealed bias to perform flexion on the beat?

A hypothetical explanation might go like this. In accordance with the findings of Ivry and colleagues (Ivry, Spencer, Zelaznik, & Diedrichsen, 2002; Ivry et al., 2004; Kennerly, Diedrichsen, Hazeltine, Semjen, & Ivry, 2002), one might hypothesize that participants tend to conceive one flexion-extension cycle as a unified event, with flexion as the perceptually most salient or accentuated subevent. The stronger salience of flexion as compared with extension corresponds to the stronger salience of the beat as compared with the pause. The series of flexions is coupled to the series of beats because it creates a uni-

fied, perceptually defined rhythmic event (for comparable lines of thought see Ivry et al., 2002; Ivry et al., 2004). If so, a possible perceptual explanation of the flexion-flexion bias is obvious: Flexion in one hand might be preferably coupled to flexion, and not to extension, in the other hand because in that manner, the sequences of the perceptually most salient subevents go together in both event streams.

Mechsner (2005b) tested the relative salience hypothesis in the following experiment. Participants were requested to flex and extend their left index finger in the transverse plane, with the hand either prone or supine. At the same time, the right forearm was to oscillate in the transverse plane, at the same pace. Thereby, the hand grasped an arrow, with a red head pointing outward or inward (see Figure 5). Participants were instructed to synchronize either finger flexion or extension with an arm movement in or opposite to the direction of the arrow head. Under the assumption that a movement in the direction of the arrow head is more salient than a movement in the opposite direction, I expected that participants would preferably synchronize finger flexion with arrow movements in the direction of the head rather than with movements in the opposite direction. As the experiment revealed, that is exactly what happened. Independent of the left hand position (prone or supine) and the arrow direction (outward or inward) there was a strong tendency to synchronize finger flexion with a contralateral arm movement

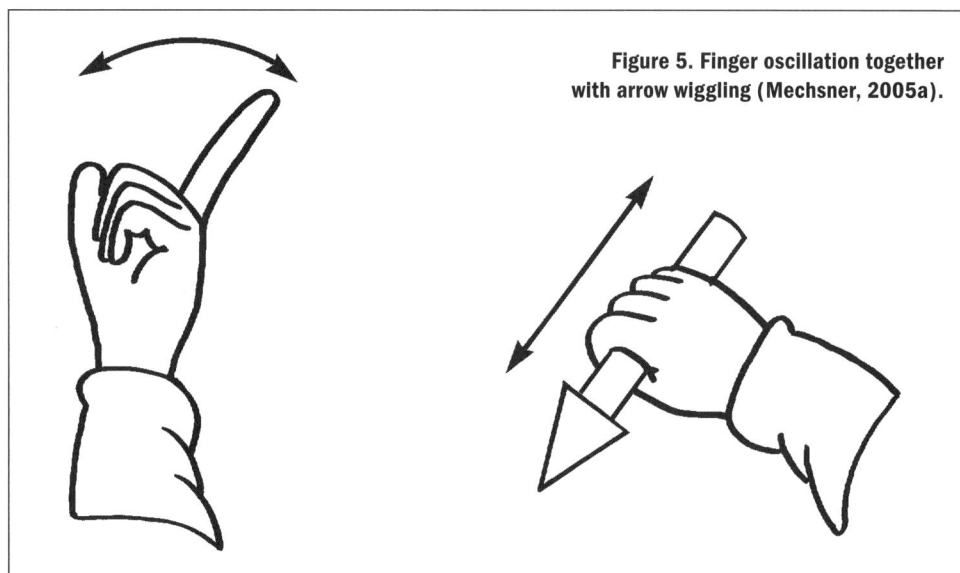

Figure 5. Finger oscillation together with arrow wiggling (Mechsner, 2005a).

in the direction of the arrow. (That tendency was clearly revealed in addition to a tendency toward mirrorsymmetry that was also obvious.)

I conclude that the relative salience hypothesis is rather plausible, at the least, as a partial-perceptual-cognitive explanation of the flexion-flexion bias. Recent results by Kelso, Fink, DeLaplain, and Carson (2001) nicely fit into the proposed explanatory scheme. Participants performed periodic unimanual flexion and extension movements of the index finger to the pace of a metronome, with either flexion or extension going toward a physical stop. In short, individuals were drawn to patterns of coordination in which the beat and the touch coincided in time, regardless of whether flexion or extension movements were producing the touch. If one assumes that a finger movement touching the stop tends to be perceived as more salient than a movement that reverses in the air, that outcome fits well the proposed relative salience hypothesis.

In conclusion, I would like to emphasize that a perceptual-cognitive origin of the flexion-flexion bias is plausible. The relative salience hypothesis may or may not be part of the explanation; the important message here is that a co-activation of homologous muscles in the spontaneously adopted coordination mode does not in the least exclude the idea that the preferred pattern is defined in terms of perceptual-cognitive factors.

To emphasize again, the relevance of physical factors does not contradict a purely perceptual-cognitive approach to bimanual coordination as proposed here. The controlling system might actually control their influence by way of addressing their perceptual effects and consequences. If so, then the relevant perceptual-cognitive factors and criteria do not necessarily reveal the underlying relevant biomechanical constraints. For illustration, consider the above hypothesis that the flexion-flexion occurs because finger flexion is more salient than extension and salient events tend to be synchronized. That is a purely perceptual-cognitive explanation of the flexion-flexion bias that might be fully sufficient for a first interpretation. For this level of explanation, it plays no role, whereas neuro-muscular-skeletal factors might provide the material basis for that coordination tendency.

It is crucial to point out that a consideration of material factors addresses a level of movement coordination categorically different than that of the perceptual-cognitive level. The material and the perceptual-cognitive level are certainly dependent on each other, in that the psychological level emerges from the material one. However, they imply different viewpoints, and can thus not directly influence each other as such. In a related vein, Koehler (1947, p. 162) pointed out: "In psychology we have often warned against the stimulus error, that is, against the danger of confusing our knowledge about the physical conditions of sensory experience with the experience as such." (For similar considerations, see Metzger, 1972).

Similar considerations may hold for the influence of pre-wired higher reflexes, such as the tonic neck reflex or the crossed extensor reflex. If people move according to the movement patterns facilitated by such reflexes, one may rightly say that this was because of the motoric facilitation. In the view proposed here, however, the movements do not blindly follow a motoric bias. The motoric facilitation may well result in sensory consequences, which are actually controlled by way of a perceptual-cognitive control scheme. For instance, the facilitated movement might feel particularly easy and comfortable and thus be preferred to a certain degree.

In that connection, it would not come as a surprise for a perceptual-cognitive approach that the system settles into movement patterns that fulfill physically defined optimality criteria, such as minimum energy expenditure. Plausibly, perceptual-cognitive preferences are evolved as means to cope with the physical reality. Already, everyday experience tells us that it feels good to move smoothly and effortlessly. Most interestingly—and well in line with the previous notion—is Feldenkrais's (1991) system of movement education that builds on the assumption that simply paying attention to one's movements often leads to improved performance.

To sum up, in a perceptual-cognitive approach to spontaneous coordination phenomena, the importance of physical, and in particular, neuro-musculoskeletal factors, would never be denied. According to that approach, however, the physical effects are controlled by way of perceptual-cognitive factors and criteria. Whether this is actually the case remains to be explored.

Beyond the Symmetry Tendency: The Role of
Perceptual-Conceptual Grouping Factors

Swinnen (2002) has proposed that isodirectionality and symmetry are important grouping principles governing spontaneous coordination tendencies. Beyond this proposal, it is plausible to expect that manifold perceptual factors and principles may play a role in coordination tendencies, as may be inferred from the many grouping principles proposed by researchers of the Gestaltist tradition (Koehler, 1947). That assumption holds in spite of the admitted problem that grouping principles of that kind are often suggested intuitively and ad hoc in the light of certain phenomena, although their theoretical status, as well as the area of their applicability, are usually unclear, and their predictive value is often rather limited.

Symmetry itself is confounded with many possible grouping factors. For instance, the probably perceptual symmetry tendency revealed by Mechsner et al. (2001) in the finger-wiggling model is not simply toward mirrorsymmetry. Mechsner (2005a) replicated the experiment with the participant's arms placed orthogonal to each other (Figure 6), again with the hands placed palm up and palm down. Two oscillation modes were possible and instructed: First, in the mid-down mode, the finger of the sagittally placed arm moved toward the sagittal midline when the finger of the vertically placed arm moved toward the body. Second, in the mid-up mode, the finger of the sagittally placed arm moved toward the midline when the finger of the vertically placed arm went away from the body. Most surprising, the results revealed that the mid-down mode was much more stable than the mid-up mode, with a strong transition tendency into mid-down, if mid-up was instructed. One may interpret this as a symmetry tendency that is defined in arm coordinates. Further confounds are obvious, however, and need to be investigated.

It might well be that the symmetry tendency has been overemphasized by scientists. In the usual experiments on coordination tendencies, the limbs are moved without objects to be manipulated and without meaning. In that condition, more low-level perceptual grouping principles might be dominant, which might be the reason that a symmetry tendency is usually obvious. But what if meaning and movement goals come into play? In that condition, high-level principles of a semantic nature might dominate movement conceptualization. Franz, Zelaznik, Swinnen, and Walter (2001) investigated half-circle drawing by both hands. They revealed that a bimanual pattern is much more stable if both hands work together in drawing a circle, than if a less meaningful, though equally symmetrical, figure is the result. Many bimanual gestures are not symmetrical on all dimensions, but are nevertheless spontaneously

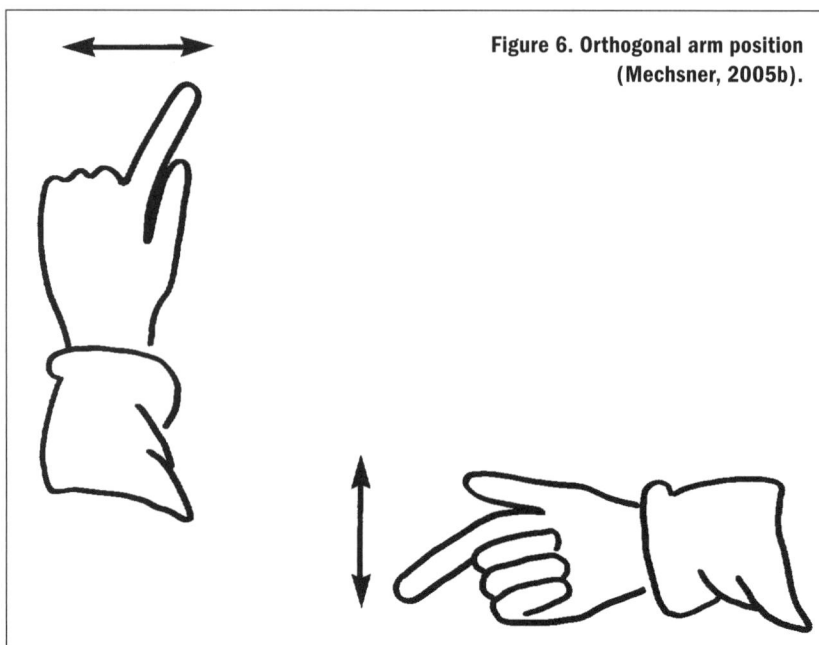

Figure 6. Orthogonal arm position (Mechsner, 2005b).

executed in the adequate situation. Bimanual actions are generally not symmetrical. In motoric approaches to bimanual coordination, a bodily defined symmetry tendency should, as a rule, be predicted to disturb and make more difficult such movements. Might it be, however, that the conceptualization of an action fully determines its difficulty and the loci of interference? In the following, I consider some arguments and experimental results that suggest that the answer is yes.

Economical Coding and Focused Control

If one assumes that the perceptual-cognitive system is actually solely responsible for organizing and guiding movement performance, the following question immediately arises: How does the system organize movements effectively under its seemingly strong capacity limitations (Miller, 1956)? If the controlling system, in order to perform a complex movement, had to specify sub-movements of all the involved joints or the contractions of all the involved muscles or the like, then that would probably put too much of a burden on cognitive resources. Obviously, a kind of sparse, or economic, coding is needed that nevertheless guides the flexible and automatic tuning of the required motor structures. As we will see in the following, there is good evidence for such an economic coding principle. It can be considered a focused coding principle. The perceptual-conceptual Gestalt of a movement in its environment as an integrated whole seems actually to be what matters for coordination costs, and the Gestalt is specified in a most strategic, economic way.

From earlier experiments, it seems that the controlling system does not actually have to specify the complete set of joint angle changes or muscular contractions in order for the body to move. In reaching movements, general movement parameters such as direction and amplitude have been investigated. Rosenbaum (1980, 1983) had participants perform goal-directed reaching movements of a short or long amplitude, with the right or the left hand, toward or away from the body. Thus, there were 2x2x2 = 8 reaction alternatives altogether. The crucial experimental manipulation was to pre-inform, or precue, the participant as to a selected parameter or parameter combination before the imperative signal appeared, which would then give information about the remaining parameters. It turned out that reaction time (RT) systematically decreased depending on the number of the precued parameters. Rosenbaum concluded that action preparation mainly means specification of perceptible motor parameters. RT mainly reflected the time needed for the remaining specifications after the imperative signal was given, plus an execution time that was rather similar in the different conditions.

If one assumes that the perceptual-cognitive system does the whole job of movement organization, it may appear quite obvious at first sight that an appropriately chosen complete set of bodily defined parameters has to be specified, so that the bodily form of the movement is fully determined by these parameters. The reported results of the prespecification experiments by Rosenbaum (1980, 1983) might be taken as evidence in favor of such a body parameterization approach, as I call this hypothesis here. Note that, in those experiments, participants could perform the reaching movements only after hand, direction, and amplitude had been specified; thus, these three movement dimensions might be assumed to form a complete set of parameters in the case of reaching. Further support for the body parameterization hypothesis may be found in results on bimanual interference by Heuer and colleagues (Heuer, 1993; Heuer, Kleinsorge, Spijkers, & Steglich, 2001; Heuer, Spijkers, Kleinsorge, van der Loo, & Steglich, 1998; Spijkers, Heuer, Kleinsorge, & van der Loo, 1997; Spijkers, Heuer, Steglich, & Kleinsorge, 2000). Those authors showed that bimanual movements of anatomically nonhomologous fingers of different amplitudes or directions are initiated more slowly than movements of anatomically homologous fingers of the same amplitudes or directions. Instruction of unequal amplitudes or directions resulted in bimanual assimilation, such as lengthening of the shorter amplitude and shortening of the longer amplitude. The symmetry advantage (or the asymmetry disadvantage), as well as bimanual assimilation, almost fully disappeared if the respective parameter values were sufficiently precued before presentation of the imperative go-signal. To note, the reported reaction time and assimilation effects were also present in unimanual movements following a bimanual parameter specification (Heuer et al., 2001). The authors concluded that the observed transient interference arises in connection with flexible planning of the investigated bodily defined movement parameters, that is, finger, amplitude, and direction. If movements are started before, say, the amplitude specification has reached steady state, the movement automatically seems to follow the amplitude that has been specified at that time. In sum, there is clear evidence that movement parameters can flexibly and successfully be planned on a perceptual-cognitive level. Execution virtually perfectly follows the perceptual-cognitive plan, be it already finished or still unfolding, with a possible small deviation due to some remaining static cross-talk.

In the light of the foregoing experiments and considerations, it might seem plausible to assume at first sight that specification of a complete set of bodily defined parameters is not only possible, but also a necessary step in movement preparation. Surprisingly, there is evidence telling a different story. Goodman and Kelso (1980) had participants perform movements of the same kind as in the experiment by Rosenbaum (1980). They did not prespecify the parameters, however, but precued the remaining possible targets. For instance, instead of precuing the right hand by symbolic information, they marked all the possible end positions to the right as possible movement targets. In this variation of Rosenbaum's task, reaction time was solely dependent on the number of remaining reaction alternatives, not on the number of unspecified parameters. Zelaznik and Hahn (1985) combined duration, hand, and finger as movement parameters. Similar to Goodman and Kelso (1980), however, they precued not one or more of these parameters, but directly the remaining possible targets. In this condition, the number of unspecified parameters had no effect on reaction time, which was solely dependent on the number of the remaining reaction alternatives.

Though, at first sight, specification of a complete set of bodily defined movement parameters seems a quite natural or even inevitable step in a perceptual-cognitive control scheme, such a step may actually be unnecessary in movement preparation. A specification of movement parameters can certainly be done, if required by the task, but such a step can easily be replaced by a specification of other movement characteristics, which are not necessarily to be defined in body coordinates. If one insists on as-suming that these characteristics are translated into bodily defined parameters (such as direction and amplitude) in a second step, one has to explain why parameter specification seems not to cause any costs dependent on the number of the still to-be-specified parameters. As will become obvious from the following experiments, not only are any such costs absent, but the overall costs can also be lowered if specification of bodily defined parameters is circumvented.

Recently, Diedrichsen and colleagues (Diedrichsen, Hazeltine, Kennerly, & Ivry, 2001; Diedrichsen, Ivry, Hazeltine, Kennerly, & Cohen, 2003) showed that higher RT costs, usually observed in asymmetrical movements, as compared with symmetrical movements, fully disappear if one does not instruct bodily defined movement parameters (such as amplitudes or directions), but instead presents the targets directly. Moreover, overall RT was dramatically reduced with externally specified targets, as compared with the condition in which the movement was instructed with regard to the body. Weigelt, Rieger, Mechsner, and Prinz (in press) explored that issue further. They revealed that the advantage for external targets is independent of whether those targets are cued directly; Weigelt et al. also found this to be true when targets are cued symbolically by way of arbitrarily associated symbols, such as letters or geometric forms. Thus, Diedrichsen et al.'s conclusion seems to hold independent of the information format: "When external goals are available, the two hands seem to be able to produce nonhomologous trajectories without difficulty." (Diedrichsen et al., 2001, p. 498).

In the experiments by Diedrichsen et al. (2001), as well as those by Weigelt et al. (in press), there was a considerable RT advantage if the targets were identical (with regard to color or to the labeling symbol), rather than if they were not identical. If one calls targets with identical features symmetrical with regard to the respective features, one may thus speak here of a symmetry advantage for external targets. Weigelt et al. revealed in an additional experiment that the advantage for bodily movement symmetry and the disadvantage for nonsymmetry recurred if all external targets were labeled by different letters or geometrical symbols (thus target equality was not possible). One may speculate that that outcome mirrors a general strategic principle in movement control: If the features of the instructed external target are not easy to perceive, participants look for other ways to make the perceptual structure of their movements—and thus control over them—easier.

Kunde and Weigelt (2005) showed that the advantage for external target symmetry holds not only for reaching movements, but also for bimanual object manipulation. Upon observing a barkeeper who put glasses from an inverted position on a table to an upright position on a shelf, always two at a time, they developed an experimental task. Two building bricks with a black end were presented to the participant in one of four possible starting positions (Figure 7). Participants had to place the bricks into either parallel or opposite orientations with regard to the black end by performing either mirrorsymmetrical or asymmetrical hand movements. The experimental question was whether there would be a RT advantage for symmetrical hand movements, for symmetrical start or end positions of the bricks, or for all of those cases. It turned out that fastest reactions occurred when the intended final brick orientations were symmetrical, independent both of the starting position of the bricks and whether or not the required bimanual hand movements were symmetric.

As it seems, bimanual interference and movement costs are mainly dependent on how the focus of control is defined. If there are easy-to-handle external targets, interference is defined in terms of those targets and not with regard to the body. If there is no external target, interference is defined in terms of bodily movement characteristics, that is, of internal targets. The previous experiments indicate that a complete parameterization of body movements, independent of the situation and of what the movement is for, does not take place. Instead, a sparse or economical coding principle for movements actually seems to hold: The difficulty of a given movement is not dependent on the bodily motion pattern as such; rather, it is dependent upon the way it is conceived on a psychological (i.e., perceptual and/or conceptual) level, together with the relevant characteristics of the external environment.

As already noted, the overall difficulty of both symmetrical and asymmetrical movements was dramatically reduced (as measured by RT) when external targets were instructed as compared to the condition in which bodily defined parameters were instructed. Mechsner et al. (2001) showed that even movements that are unrealizable when planned as a bodily defined motion pattern can be performed rather easily under a suitable perceptual conception that can be used for focused control. The production of nonharmonic frequency relationships (e.g. 5:6, 4:3) between periodic movements of the hands is virtually impossible for naive persons and is often hard or even intractable after long periods of practice (Summers, Ford, & Todd, 1993). In the experiment by Mechsner et al. (2001), right-handed participants circled two visible flags, by way of two cranks that were hidden under the table (Figure 8A). Owing to a gear system, isofrequency in the flags went together with a 4:3 frequency ratio in the hands. After a 15-20 min training, participants were instructed to circle the flags inward and to maintain the visual circling pattern either in mirrorsymmetry (Figure 8B) or antiphase (Figure 8C). In a trial of 30-s duration, they began at a velocity they considered slow and speeded up to a velocity they considered fast, but not beyond the point where visual control was lost. If they felt a tendency to slip from the instructed flag movement pattern to the other one, then they were to give in and perform the more comfortable pattern.

The main question of interest was whether the participants could perform the requested movement patterns at all. To keep the flags in isofrequency, participants had to circle the hands in a 4:3 frequency relationship. As has already been said, bimanual oscillations under this frequency relationship are virtually impossible to perform for naive persons, if instructed as such. In consequence, no body-oriented strategy is thinkable that might bring about isofrequency in the flags, not to mention symmetry and antiphase. Most interestingly, most participants performed symmetry in the flags rather well and were able to speed up. Antiphase was also managed at slow speed, but dissolved at higher speed, with a certain tendency to switch into symmetry (see Figure 9).

I consider those results a dramatic demonstration of the advantages of the economic coding or focused coding principle as proposed here. I hold that improvement of coordination as a result of practice mainly means figuring out and stabilizing a more and more suitable and economic way of representing the practiced movements, rather than establishing bodily defined movement patterns by way of repetition. Of

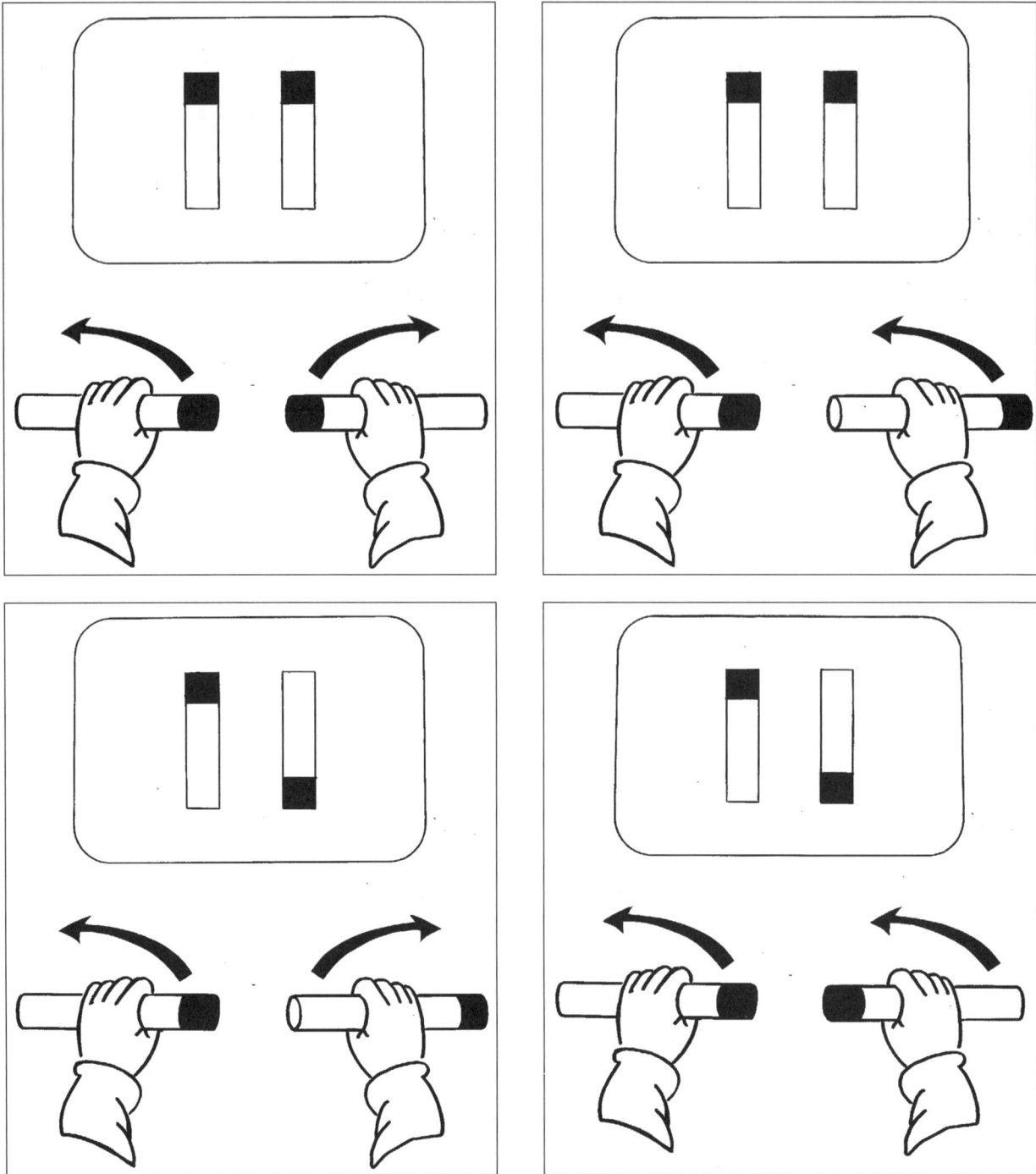

Figure 7. Bar-positioning experiment by Kunde, W., & Weigelt, M. (2005) Goal congruency in bimanual object manipulation. *Journal of Experimental Psychology: Human Perception and Performance, 31*(1), 145-156. Reprinted with permission. (A) Desired end position of bars: symmetrical; starting position of bars: symmetrical; required movement: symmetrical. (B) Desired end position of bars: symmetrical; starting position of bars: asymmetrical; required movement: asymmetrical. (C) Desired end position of bars: asymmetrical; starting position of bars: asymmetrical; required movement: symmetrical. (D) Desired end position of bars: asymmetrical; starting position of objects: symmetrical; required movement: asymmetrical.

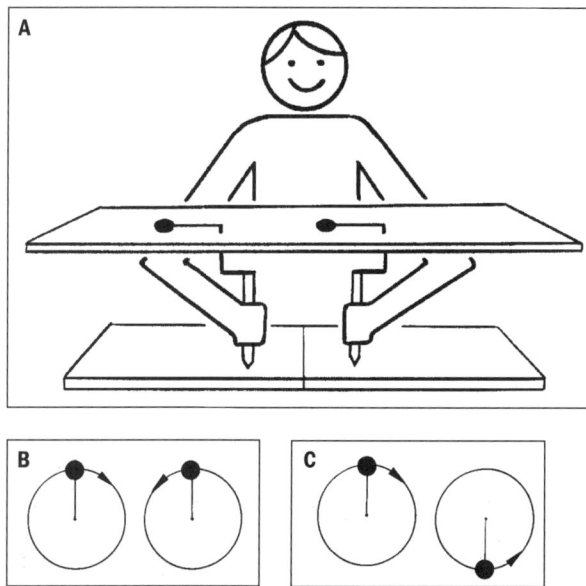

Figure 8. Apparatus and instructed movement patterns in the bimanual flag circling experiment by Mechsner et al. (2001). (A) Apparatus. (B) Symmetry. (C) Antiphase.

course, the perceptual representation of the movement has to be adequate. What is adequate has often to be figured out in the course of practice.

A suitable perceptual representation of movement characteristics and targets can be provided—at least in part—by a human guide or environmental cues. In consequence, one is relieved from mentally constructing it from scratch, which means that part of the usual task is circumvented. Thus, relying on external guidance may be an especially economic

way to make performance easy. Rosenbaum (2002) showed that participants were well able to perform otherwise impossible bimanual movements in a haptic pursuit task. Participants pushed their two middle fingers against buttons mounted under vertically oriented shafts that were displaced rapidly, continuously, and quasi-randomly in a horizontal plane either by one or two experimenters. One person is usually not able to actually move the hands independently. Participants did equally well, however, in the one- and two-experimenter conditions. That is most remarkable, in view of the fact that the shafts were moved essentially independently in the two-experimenter case. Those findings further support the more general idea that guidance provided by other persons or the environment may greatly support motor control. Obviously, a common functional medium for representing target-directed actions together with relevant characteristics of the environment is highly useful in this regard.

A Psychological Approach to Skilled Voluntary Movements

So far, we have considered movements that can be regarded as rather simple in a perceptual-cognitive control scheme (although they sometimes are complex in anatomical terms or in terms of patterns of muscular activation and motor commands). What about tasks that are seemingly more difficult, such as tying one's shoelace, skillfully executing a penalty

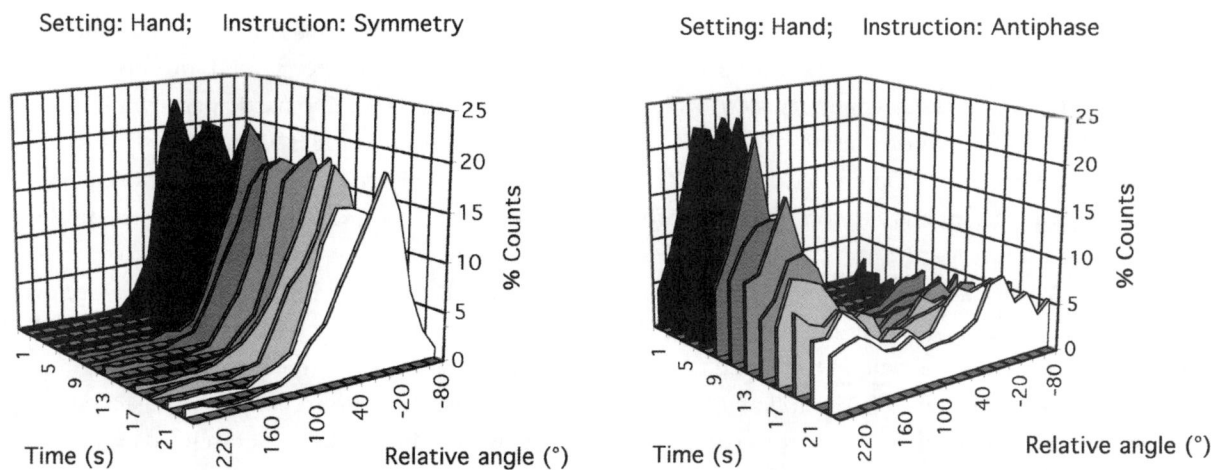

Figure 9. Histogram plots in analogy to Figure 3. The participants speeded up during a trial. A: Symmetry (0° relative angle) can be performed up to the highest frequencies. B: Antiphase movements (180° relative angle) can be performed only at low frequencies, with transitions into symmetry at high frequencies (from Mechsner et al., 2001).

in soccer, or performing a twisted somersault? In a series of investigations, which are unfortunately available only as a Habilitation thesis in German, Schack (2002) explored this issue on the basis that a perceptual-cognitive approach to skilled voluntary movements might be adequate. If so, one has to ask in the first place what kind of perceptual-cognitive representations make skilled performance possible.

Schack (2002) argued that any purposeful movement has to fulfill distinct functional demands that pose corresponding biomechanical problems to be solved by way of appropriate submovements. If movement control is actually purely perceptual-cognitive, these problems have to be solved by the perceptual-cognitive system. In consequence, the pattern of functionally essential motor problems and the corresponding submovements should be adequately represented in the long-term memory of skilled athletes. To explore that issue, Schack and Mechsner (2006) investigated the tennis serve in three groups of different expertise. Eleven high-level players performed in upper German leagues. Eleven low-level players performed in lower German leagues. Eleven nonplayers had virtually no experience with the game.

In a preparatory step, the task-adequate functional demands of the tennis serve were determined by way of biomechanical considerations and in discussions with experts. In that connection, a plausible set of functionally necessary phases and submovements was established. In a further step, a set of movement-related mental concepts at a medium level of categorization, so-called basic action concepts (BACs), was established by way of representation analyses. BACs turned out to be linked to the functional movement problems identified in the preparatory step, which are suitably solved by submovements.

First, in the pre-activation phase, the body and ball are put in position, and tension energy is provided in preparation for the strike. The following BACs were identified: (1) ball throw, (2) forward movement of the pelvis, (3) bending the knees, and (4) bending the elbow. Second, in the strike phase, energy is conveyed to the ball. The following BACs were identified: (5) frontal upper rotation, (6) racket acceleration, (7) whole body stretch motion, and (8) hitting point. Third, in the final swing phase the body is prevented from falling and the racket movement is decelerated after the strike. The following BACs

were identified: (9) wrist flap, (10) forward bending of the body, and (11) racket follow-through.

The functionally characterized BACs go along with perceptual characteristics, as a rule, and can be labeled by a linguistic mark. If they are mentally represented at all, then it makes sense to assume that they are represented in a corresponding way, namely, as concepts. In cognitive domains, research on expertise has revealed that high-level competence is characterized by well-integrated and organized mental networks of task-relevant knowledge. Correspondingly, if skilled athletes actually rely on perceptual-cognitive representations as their basic resource, then the existence of suitably integrated mental BAC networks in long-term memory is to be expected. In the following analysis, researchers asked whether there are mental BAC networks of that kind in which structure matches the functional demands of the task.

To test persons for relational structures in a given set of mental concepts, investigators have developed an experimental procedure called structural dimensional analysis (SDA) in the field of cognitive psychology (Lander & Lange, 1996). Schack (2002) adapted this method for investigating motor memory (structural dimensional analysis-motor = SDA-M). At the core of SDA-M is a multiple sorting task whose results are then submitted to a hierarchical cluster analysis. In the present experiment, the sorting task worked as follows. The respective participant was made familiar with the set of BACs by way of pictures with verbal BAC names as a printed heading. Then, one selected verbal BAC name was constantly presented on a computer screen, on top of a list of the remaining BACs. The participant was instructed to judge, for each of the BACs in the list, whether or not it was functionally close to the anchoring BAC on top. As a result, two sub-sets of BACs were produced and submitted to the same operation until the referee decided not to do any further splits. Because every BAC was used as an anchoring unit, this procedure resulted in 11 decision trees per participant.

The results of those subjective distance judgements were submitted to a hierarchical cluster analysis. Figure 10 shows the resulting dendrograms as averaged for the expert, low-level, and nonplayer groups. In a dendrogram, the path connecting two BACs gives a refined measure of the subjective

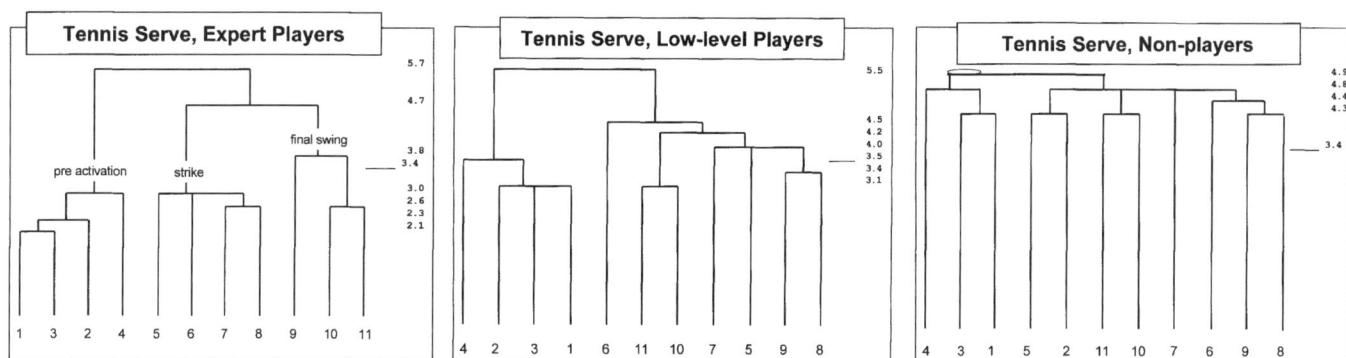

Figure 10. Results of a hierarchical cluster analysis of basic action concepts (BACs) in the tennis serve. Dendrograms are shown for (A) the expert group, (B) the low-level group and (C) for the non-player group (adapted from Schack & Mechsner, 2006). Numbers on the bottom denote the BACs (for the code, see text), the vertically aligned numbers the Euclidean distances. For each group, n = 11; p = .05; d_{crit} = 3.46.

Euclidian distance between those mental concepts, that is, how close together they belong. The tree structure of a dendrogram reflects the hierarchical grouping of the BACs. Clusters are significant (chosen level: p = .05) if the corresponding master node is placed below a critical level of dcrit = 3.51.

In experts, this hierarchical mental structure comes close to the functionally demanded structure of the tennis serve. The three functional phases, that is, pre-activation phase, strike phase, and final swing phase, are clearly visible in the dendrograms in the form of significantly separated subtrees. There was no significant difference between the mental BAC framework in experts and the functionally-demanded structure of the tennis serve. In low-level players and nonplayers, the results look much different. Here, the clustering of BACs mirrors less well the functionally demanded phases. In addition, the BACs are less clearly grouped, with no close neighborhoods, and the partial clusters are usually below the chosen significance level (p = .05). When considering the individual dendrograms, one realizes that the cognitive clusterings in experts are not significantly different among individuals, but they vary considerably among individuals in low-level players and nonplayers.

To note, hierarchical BAC networks in skilled movements show some resemblance to hierarchical cognitive control structures at a basic level, which

have been proposed by Rosenbaum, Kenny, and Derr (1983) for sequences of finger taps. Based on analyses of intertap intervals, these authors hypothesized that well-learned sequences are controlled by way of hierarchical perceptual-cognitive control structures, which bind together elemental sequences to those of higher orders.

Further experiments by Schack (2002) seem to support the notion that hierarchical BAC networks of experts correspond to a quite perfect and well-integrated procedural understanding of the entire movement scheme that is automatically activated whenever any part of it is mentally present. This means that the BAC network might not simply mirror a hierarchically organized mental sequence of intermediate movement goals. Beyond that, an implicit understanding of the whole movement might be revealed here, which allows control of the situation-adequate performance of every submovement in perfect flexible balance with the anticipated, actual, and finished performance of the other submovements in the respective situation. For instance, a small error in the performance of a submovement leads to a kind of performance of the following submovements, such that the error is intuitively corrected. Situational challenges may be perfectly and flexibly handled, in a well-adapted interplay of circumstantial intentions, perceptions, anticipations, and movements. If so, highly integrated BAC networks might form the representational counterpart of the often emphasized, but badly understood, automation in the course of practice—or what top athletes call their "feeling" for the movement. To note, BAC networks in long-term memory should not be considered rigid, program-like structures. If situation-adequate, one may skip customary movement phases and subphases, vary the scheme creatively, and so on.

Such intuitive action knowledge also seems important for everyday actions and might be largely based on proprioceptive competence (Smetacek & Mechsner, 2004). Cole (1995) has known and extensively investigated a person who had been functionally deafferented below the neck because of a peripheral neuropathy of the haptic and proprioceptive afferences. This person had learned to move rather well under visual feedback. The movements are often still clumsy, however, and are never really automated. Instead, any movement is extremely strenuous, seemingly because attentional demands are very high. The deficits observed in this case support the notion that the possibility of relying on proprioception and proprioceptive knowledge may be crucial for forming sufficiently economic and focused movement representations.

The Psychological System Might Be Responsible for Action Control

The foregoing considerations strongly suggest that movement organization is not about efferent commands, but is actually about goals and the functional (e.g., biomechanical) movement problems to be solved in that connection, with the motor commands automatically and flexibly tuned in service to the perceptual goals. In short, movement quality is dependent on how suitably the body-world system is conceived and represented, based on how well the relevant rules and interactions are implicitly, and sometimes explicitly, understood. A purely perceptual-cognitive control would imply that the whole organizational work is actually done in the psychological domain. If so, then moving means nothing else than figuring out and tuning suitable dynamic perceptual-conceptual representations of the body-world system, based on schemas of the relevant interactions in that system.

To throw a dart successfully, the system has to understand how characteristics of the body-world representation during throwing (including dynamic proprioceptive information) are tuned best, so that they can be developed into the body-world representation that includes the dart having hit the center of the target. And that's it. Because the dynamic interactions may slightly change from situation to situation, and the respective sensitivity may decline between situations, it is no surprise that even expert dart-throwers, who weigh and move the dart in their hands before each round, have to adapt by making a few practice throws. In that way, they update their intimate knowledge of how the whole system works, that is, their feeling for the movement.

If the controlling system had to address and determine motor commands during movements, myriads of detailed information on the situation would have to be integrated in order to actually determine the appropriate motor commands. Even given that this would be possible (which I strongly doubt) the apparatus and the to-be-executed calculations would in any case be extremely intricate. A psychological scheme seems to work much more economically, as was suggested in light of the experiments reported earlier. Though astonishing at first sight, this is not truly surprising, for it is well known that perception works in a most economic way by representing simple gestalts with only a few characteristic features and internal relationships instead of myriad details (Rock, 1995). Faces, for instance, are recognized and distinguished by way of very few characteristics, whereby the use of wholistic and figural characteristics depends on the situation and seems largely determined by perceptual-conceptual economics (Leder, Candrian, Huber, & Bruce, 2001). Another important and attractive feature of a purely perceptual-cognitive control scheme is that global characteristics can immediately be tuned. For instance, one automatically moves more gently in the company of gentle persons than of rude persons. It is hard to imagine how the system would be able to integrate gentleness information in order to calculate appropriate motor commands. It seems more plausible that the system is able to perceive the quality of gentleness in a person's movements and to immediately and directly perform accordingly.

Let us consider again the results from bimanual circling studies by Mechsner et al. (2001), because they shed some light on what it means to use a tool.

Povinelli (2000) claimed that using a tool demands more cognitive resources than moving the body in the same way without a tool. He argued that in the second case, only the bodily movement has to be organized, whereas in the first case the bodily movement plus the tool effect have to be organized. According to Povinelli, humans can cope better with the resource demands of body plus tool movements than can chimpanzees, because of their greater working memory capacity. Povinelli's theory is well in line with the body parameterization approach as described earlier. The results of Mechsner et al.'s bimanual circling experiment, however, clearly contradict that idea: Moving an appropriate tool (the flags can be considered tools) can actually be much less demanding than moving only the body in the same way, but without a tool. Similar considerations may be applied to language, where nonbodily effects, namely, speech sounds, are controlled. To produce speech, one has to perform very complicated movements of the vocal tract, which, in addition, change from situation to situation. One may plausibly assume that the patterns of motor commands are even more intricate and more variable. If a perceptual-cognitive control scheme holds, with the advantages of economic and focused coding considered earlier, then the bodily movement might actually not pose so much of a problem for the system, because the movements are performed in service to the sound and are organized so that the perception of the sound and the perception of bodily movements are integrated in a suitable way—similar to the performance of isofrequent flag movements by way of nonisofrequent hand movements.

So far, I have postponed a problem that is most fundamental for a psychological approach to human motor behavior, always lurking in the background. To move the body one has to activate the muscles in an appropriate way. How this is brought about has remained a riddle, so far.

Consider a very simple movement like flexing the arm around the elbow. To be exact, that movement is simple only in perceptual terms, but not in terms of motor commands. Direct perceptual-cognitive control would mean that only perceptual characteristics of the movement are controlled, but not the motor commands. Is it actually possible, however, to tune movements by directly tuning characteristic percep-

tual events? Frankly speaking, nobody knows. In a way, such a direct control scheme is hard to imagine. That might be the reason why movement scientists are so occupied with motor commands and with how the system might determine them appropriately. As has been argued in this chapter, however, there are several strong arguments in favor of a purely perceptual-cognitive control scheme. First, experimental evidence seems to show that it is possible and it works, in principle. Second, determining the appropriate patterns of motor commands or muscular contractions from intentions and situational constraints would be very difficult, if not impossible. Third, direct perceptual-cognitive control could work in a most economic way, while taking advantage of the economic principles of perceptual-conceptual organization. Fourth, the whole capabilities of the perceptual-cognitive system (including tuning representations that are not spatiotemporal in nature) could be directly used for movement control.

So let us try to go ahead with the idea that moving means directly tuning perceptions. Mysterious as such an idea may at first seem, it is actually rather obvious that the brain routinely and actively brings about intended perceptual changes in the phenomenal world without any reliance on motor commands, namely in the process of perceiving. Even if you do not move your eyes, you can still attend on purpose, particularly to green, or star-shaped, or long, or eatable objects in your visual field, or search and detect a hidden figure that means that you can willingly enhance the perceptual salience of environmental characteristics. Thus, perception is clearly an action here, even if you do not move at all. How is this action brought about? Plausibly, certain neuronal pathways have to become active so that the desired perceptual event can be brought about, but it is not plausible to assume that the system addresses and determines the activity of those pathways.

Is it conceivable that motoric action is brought about by way of the same kind of processes as is perceptual action? Muscular activity can, in principle, be replaced by activity of other devices that are controlled by neuronal brain activity. Birbaumer and colleagues (Kotchoubey, Schleichert, Lutzenberger, & Birbaumer, 1997; Kuebler et al., 1998) showed that persons can learn to control cursor movements on a screen by way of their EEG-activity. This ability is not dependent on remaining motor functions because even fully paralyzed persons (two of whom could not even breathe and were therefore artificially ventilated) were able to control the cursor, and even type letters by making use of such cursor movements (Birbaumer et al., 1999). The important message in our connection is that the brain, after some training whose mechanism is unclear, is able to settle into desired perceptual states. These states can be brought about by neuronal activity alone or in part by way of external devices that follow neuronal activity. In the first case only the network activity is changed; in the second case the external world is changed in addition, so that perceptual-conceptual changes in the phenomenal field can be produced.

If so, one may provocatively suggest that acting and perceiving are basically the same, in terms of brain processes. The brain is able to actively bring about changes in the phenomenal field. Sometimes the material pathways that bring about the phenomenal change include only neurons; then the process is called perception. Sometimes the material pathways that bring about the phenomenal change include not only neurons but also external devices such as muscles; then the process is called movement.

References

Bernstein, N. A. (1967). *The coordination and regulation of movement.* London: Pergamon Press.

Birbaumer, N., Ghanayim, N., Hinterberger, T., Iversen, I., Kotchoubey, B., Kuebler, A., et al. (1999). A spelling device for the paralysed. *Nature, 398,* 297-98.

Carson, R. G. (1996). Neuromuscular-skeletal constraints upon the dynamics of perception-action coupling. *Experimental Brain Research, 110,* 99-110.

Carson, R. G. (2004). Governing coordination. Why do muscles matter? In V. K. Jirsa & J. A. S. Kelso (Eds.), *Coordination dynamics: Issues and trends.* New York: Springer.

Cattaert, D., Semjen, A., & Summers, J. J. (1999). Simulating a neural cross-talk model for between-hand interference during bimanual circle drawing. *Biological Cybernetics, 81,* 343-358.

Cohen, L. (1971). Synchronous bimanual movements performed by homologous and non-homologous muscles. *Perceptual and Motor Skills, 32,* 639-644.

Cole, J. (1995). *Pride and a daily marathon.* Cambridge, MA: The MIT Press.

Diedrichsen, J., Hazeltine, E., Kennerly, S., & Ivry, R. B. (2001). Moving to directly cued locations abolishes spatial interference during bimanual actions. *Psychological Science, 12,* 493-498.

Diedrichsen, J., Ivry, R. B., Hazeltine, E., Kennerly, S., & Cohen, A. (2003). Bimanual interference associated with the selection of movement targets. *Journal of Experimental Psychology: Human Perception and Performance, 29*(1), 64-77.

Eliassen, J. C., Baynes, K., & Gazzaniga, M. S. (1999). Direction information coordinated via the posterior third of the corpus callosum during bimanual movements. *Experimental Brain Research, 128,* 573-577.

Feldenkrais, M. (1991). *Awareness through movement.* San Francisco: Harper.

Franz, E. A., Eliassen, J. C., Ivry, R. B., & Gazzaniga, M. S. (1996). Dissociation of spatial and temporal coupling in the bimanual movements of callosotomy patients. *Psychological Science, 7,* 306-310.

Franz, E. A., Zelaznik, H. N., Swinnen, S. S., & Walter, C. (2001). Spatial conceptual influences on the coordination of bimanual actions: When a dual task becomes a single task. *Journal of Motor Behavior, 33*(1), 103-12.

Goodman, D., & Kelso, J. A. S. (1980). Are movements prepared in part? Not under compatible (naturalized) conditions. *Journal of Experimental Psychology: General, 109,* 475-495.

Haken, H., Kelso, J. A. S., & Bunz, H. (1985). A theoretical model of phase transitions in human hand movements. *Biological Cybernetics, 51,* 347-356.

Heuer, H. (1993). Structural constraints on bimanual movements. *Psychological Research, 55,* 83-98.

Heuer, H., Kleinsorge, T., Spijkers, W., & Steglich, C. (2001). Static and phasic cross-talk effects in discrete bimanual reversal movements. *Journal of Motor Behavior, 33*(1), 67-85.

Heuer, H., Spijkers, W., Kleinsorge, T., van der Loo, H., & Steglich, C. (1998). The time course of cross-talk during the simultaneous specification of bimanual movement amplitudes. *Experimental Brain Research, 118,* 381-392.

Hoffmann, J. (1993). *Vorhersage und Erkenntnis* [Anticipation and cognition]. Goettingen: Hogrefe.

Hoffmann, J. (2003). Anticipatory behavioral control. In M. Butz, O. Sigaud, & P. Gerard (Eds.), *Anticipatory behavior in adaptive learning systems* (pp. 44-65). Heidelberg: Springer.

Hommel, B. (1998). Event files: Evidence for automatic integration of stimulus-response episodes. *Visual Cognition, 5,* 183-216.

Hommel, B., Muesseler, J., Aschersleben, G., & Prinz, W. (2001). The Theory of Event Coding (TEC): A framework for perception and action planning. *Behavioral and Brain Sciences, 24*(5), 849-878.

Ivry, R. B., Spencer, R. M., Zelaznik, H. N., & Diedrichsen, J. (2002). The cerebellum and event timing. In S. M. Highstein & W. T. Thach (Eds.), The cerebellum: Recent developments in cerebellar research. *Annals of the New York Academy of Sciences Vol. 978* (pp. 302-317). New York: New York Academy of Sciences.

Ivry, R., Diedrichsen, J., Spencer, R., Hazeltine, E., & Semjen, A. (2004). A cognitive neuroscience perspective on bimanual coordination and interference. In S. Swinnen & J. Duysens (Eds.), *Interlimb coordination.* Nowell, MA: Kluwer Academic Publishing.

Jacobs, D. (1977). *Die menschliche Bewegung* [Human movement]. Kastellaun: Aloys Henn.

James, W. (1890). *The principles of psychology* (Volumes 1-2). New York: Holt.

Kelso, J. A. S. (1981). On the oscillatory basis of movement. *Bulletin of the Psychonomic Society, 18,* 63.

Kelso, J. A. S. (1984). Phase transitions and critical behavior in human bimanual coordination. *American Journal of Physiology: Regulatory, Integrative and Comparative, 246,* R1000-R1004.

Kelso, J. A. S. (1994). The informational character of self-organized coordination dynamics. *Human Movement Science, 13,* 393-413.

Kelso, J. A. S. (1995). *Dynamic patterns. The self-organization of brain and behavior.* Cambridge, MA: MIT Press.

Kelso, J. A. S., Fink, P. W., DeLaplain, C. R., & Carson, R. G. (2001). Haptic information stabilizes and destabilizes coordination dynamics. *Proceedings of the Royal Society of London Series B - Biological Sciences, 216*(1472), 1207-1213.

Kennerly, S. W., Diedrichsen, J., Hazeltine, E., Semjen, A., & Ivry, R. B. (2002). Callosotomy patients exhibit temporal and spatial uncoupling during continuous bimanual movements. *Nature Neuroscience, 5,* 376-381.

Koehler, W. (1947). *Gestalt psychology: An introduction to new concepts in modern psychology.* New York: Liveright.

Kotchoubey, B., Schleichert, H., Lutzenberger, W., & Birbaumer, N. (1997). A new method for self-regulation of slow cortical potentials in a timed paradigm. *Applied Psychophysiology and Biofeedback, 22*(2), 77-93.

Kuebler, A., Kotchoubey, B., Ghanayim, N., Hinterberger, T., Perelmouter, J., Schauer, et al. (1998). A thought translation device for brain computer communication. *Studia Psychologica, 40*(1-2), 17-31.

Kunde, W., & Weigelt, M. (2005) Goal congruency in bimanual object manipulation. *Journal of Experimental Psychology: Human Perception and Performance, 31*(1), 145-156.

Lander, H. J., & Lange, K. (1996). Untersuchung zur Struktur- und Dimensionsanalyse begrifflich repraesentierten Wissens [Investigations on the structural and dimensional analysis of conceptually represented knowledge]. *Zeitschrift fuer Psychologie, 204,* 55-74.

Leder, H., Candrian, G., Huber, O., & Bruce, V. (2001). Configural features in the context of upright and inverted faces. *Perception, 30,* 73-83.

Lotze, H. (1852). Medicinische Psychologie oder Physiologie der Seele [Medical psychology or physiology of the mind]. Leipzig: Weidmann'sche Buchhandlung.

Mechsner, F. (2005a). [Spontaneous coordination tendencies in bimanual finger adduction and abduction]. Unpublished raw data.

Mechsner, F. (2005b). [Spontaneous coordination tendencies in bimanual finger flexion and extension]. Unpublished raw data.

Mechsner, F., Kerzel, D., Knoblich, G., & Prinz, W. (2001). Perceptual basis of bimanual coordination. *Nature, 414,* 69-73.

Mechsner, F. & Knoblich, G. (2004). Do muscles matter in bimanual coordination? *Journal of Experimental Psychology: Human Perception and Performance, 30*(3), 490–503.

Metzger, W. (1972). The phenomenal-perceptual field as a central steering mechanism. In J. R. Royce & W. W. Rozeboom (Eds.), *The psychology of knowing.* New York: Gordon and Breach.

Miller, G. A. (1956). The magical number seven, plus or minus two. Some limits on our capacity for processing information. *Psychological Review, 63,* 81-87.

Norman, D. (1981). Categorization of action slips. *Psychological Review, 88*(1), 1-15.

Oullier, O., de Guzman, G. C., Jantzen, K. J., & Kelso, J. A. S. (2003). The role of spatial configuration and homologous muscle activation in coordination between two individuals. *Journal of Sport and Exercise Psychology, 25,* S104-S105.

Povinelli, D. J. (2000). *Folk physics for apes.* Oxford: Oxford University Press.

Prinz, W. (1990). A common coding approach to perception and action. In: O. Neumann & W. Prinz (Eds.), *Relationships between perception and action: Current approaches* (pp. 167-201). Berlin: Springer.

Prinz, W. (1997). Perception and action planning. *European Journal of Cognitive Psychology, 9*(2), 129-154.

Riek, S., Carson, R. G., & Byblow, W. D. (1992). Spatial and muscular dependencies in bimanual coordination. *Journal of Human Movement Studies, 23,* 251-265.

Rock, I. (1995). *Perception.* New York: Scientific American Books.

Rosenbaum, D. A. (1980). Human movement initiation: Specification of arm, direction and extent. *Journal of Experimental Psychology: General, 109,* 444-474.

Rosenbaum, D. A. (1983). The movement precuing technique: Assumptions, applications, and extensions. In R. A. Magill (Ed.), *Memory and control of action* (pp. 231-274). NY: North-Holland.

Rosenbaum, D. A. (2002). Independence of hand movements during bimanual haptic pursuit tracking. *Abstracts of the Psychonomics Society, 7,* 23.

Rosenbaum, D. A., Kenny, S. B., & Derr, M. A. (1983). Hierarchical control of rapid movement sequences. *Journal of Experimental Psychology: Human Perception and Performance, 9,* 86-102.

Saltzman, E. L. (1995). Dynamics and coordinate systems in skilled sensorimotor activity. In R. F. Port & T. van Gelder (Eds.), *Mind as motion: Explorations in the dynamics of cognition.* Cambridge, MA: MIT Press.

Schack, T. (2002). *Zur kognitiven Architektur von Bewegungshandlungen - modelltheoretischer Zugang und experimentelle Untersuchungen* [The cognitive architecture of movements - a model theoretical approach and experimental investigations]. Unpublished Habilitation Thesis, German Sports University, Cologne, Germany.

Schack, T. & Mechsner, F. (2006). Representation of motor skills in human long-term memory. *Neuroscience Letters, 391,* 77-81.

Schmidt, R. C., Bienvenu, M., Fitzpatrick, P. A., & Amazeen, P. G. (1998). A comparison of intra- and interpersonal interlimb coordination: Coordination breakdowns and coupling strength. *Journal of Experimental Psychology: Human Perception & Performance, 24*(3), 884-990.

Schmidt, R. C., Carello C., & Turvey, M. T. (1990). Phase transitions and critical fluctuations in the visual coordination of rhythmic movements between people. *Journal of Experimental Psychology: Human Perception & Performance, 16,* 227-247.

Schmidt, R. C., & O'Brien, B. (1997). Evaluating the dynamics of unintended interpersonal coordination. *Ecological Psychology, 9*(3), 189-206.

Smetacek, V. & Mechsner, F. (2004). Making sense. *Nature, 432,* 21.

Spijkers, W., Heuer, H., Kleinsorge, T., & van der Loo, H. (1997). Preparation of bimanual movements with same and different amplitudes: Specification interference as revealed by reaction time. *Acta Psychologica, 96,* 207-227.

Spijkers, W., Heuer, H., Kleinsorge, T., & Steglich, C. (2000). The specification of movement amplitudes for the left and right hand: Evidence for transient parametric coupling from overlapping-task performance. *Journal of Experimental Psychology: Human Perception & Performance, 26,* 1091-1105.

Summers, J. J., Ford, S. K., & Todd, J. A. (1993) Practice effects on the coordination of the two hands in a bimanual tapping task. *Human Movement Science, 12,* 111-133.

Swinnen, P. S. (2002). Intermanual coordination: From behavioral principles to *neural-network interactions. Nature* Review Neuroscience, 3(5), 350-361.

Weigelt, M., Rieger, M., Mechsner, F., & Prinz, W. (in press). *Symbolic target cueing effects in bimanual coordination.* Psychological Research.

Wimmers, R. H., Beek, P. J., & van Wieringen, P. C. W. (1992). Phase transitions in rhythmic tracking movements: A case of unilateral coupling. *Human Movement Science, 11,* 217-226.

Zelaznik, H. N., & Hahn, R. (1985). Reaction time methods in the study of motor programming: The precuing of hand, digit and duration. *Journal of Motor Behavior, 17,* 190-218.

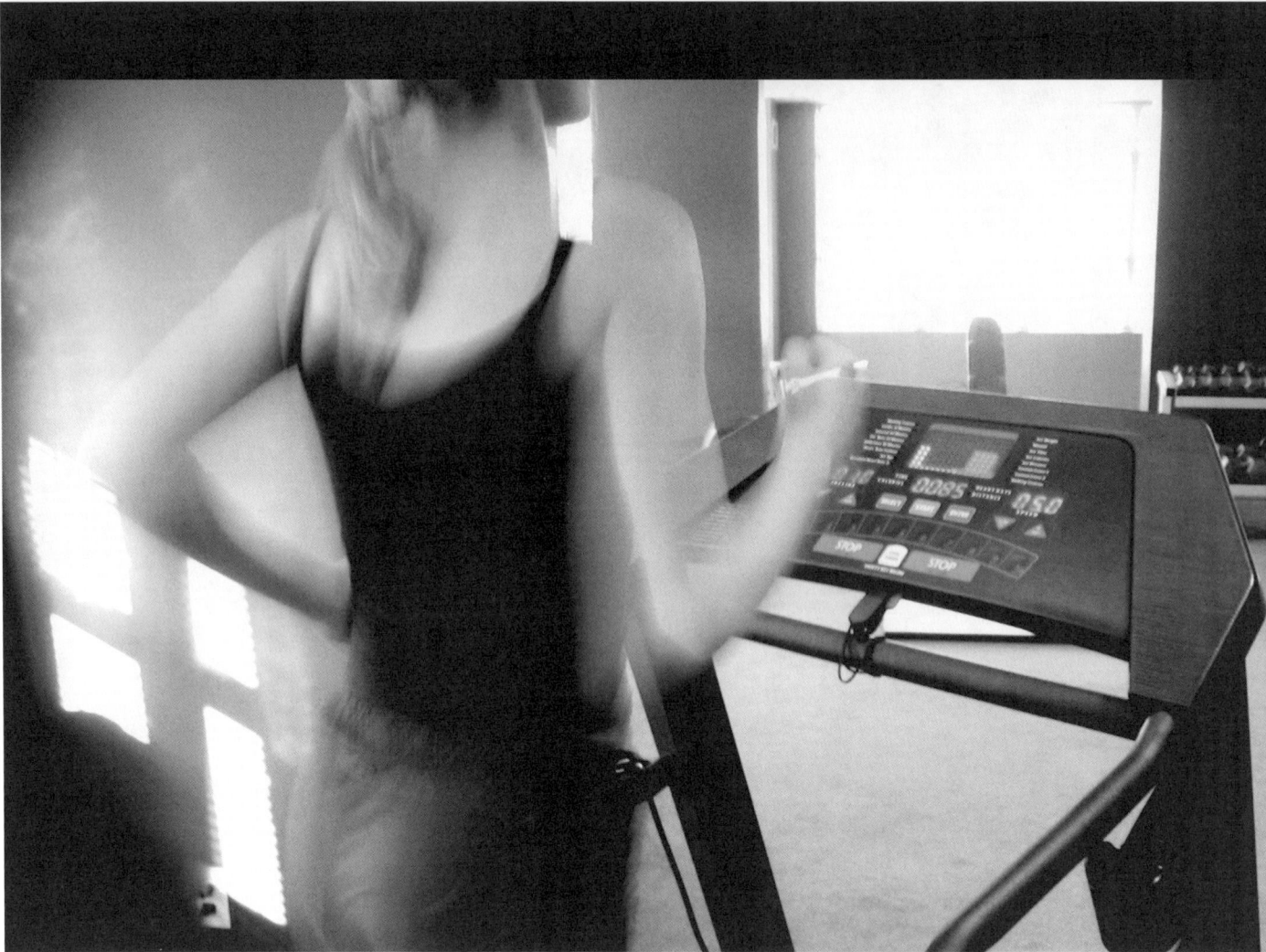

9

Cognitive Neuroscience Aspects of Sport Psychology: Brain Mechanisms Underlying Performance

BRADLEY D. HATFIELD

Sport psychologists have traditionally explained superior athletic performance with constructs like confidence, focus, and motivation, but how and why such variables influence skeletal muscle coordination is unclear. An additional approach to the study of sport performance is the application of neuroscience to understand the mechanistic links between such psychological variables and the quality of human movement. The study of neural processes presents a formidable challenge to investigators in light of the complexity of the brain and its organization, which contains more than 300 billion neurons that demand 25% of the body's energy supply while comprising just 2% of body mass. However, contemporary concepts and tools derived from neuroscience provide guidance and the means with which to unravel the mystery of the mind. Beyond the study of basic processes at the cellular and molecular biology level, the field of cognitive neuroscience seeks to understand the neural basis of the higher mental processes such as attention, motivation, and emotion, and provides insight into their influence on motor behavior (Bear, Conners & Paradiso, 2001). In addition, the field of affective neuroscience has been defined as the neurobiological study of the brain structures and processes involved in emotional experience and self-regulation (Davidson, 1988, 2002, 2004).

In order to "see" the brain at work, cognitive and affective neuroscientists employ neuroimaging tools like electroencephalography (EEG); functional magnetic resonance imaging (fMRI) and magnetoencephalography (MEG) to assess brain electrical activity, hemodynamic responses, and magnetic activity; and other peripheral psychophysiological tools such as electromyography (EMG) to assess muscle activity, electrocardiography (ECG) to assess cardiovascular processes, and skin conductance to examine sympathetic arousal. From this perspective, the purpose of the present paper is to provide concepts and summarize the results of a number of neurobiological studies to explain how an athlete's psychological state affects the quality of his or her motor performance. Particular emphasis will be focused on the brain and peripheral biophysical processes during (1) unperturbed expert performance and (2) when performing under pressure.

To begin, a fundamental concept that will guide the discussion is that of the efficiency or economy of the muscular actions of the highly skilled athlete, which can be described as graceful, fluid, and minimal in effort requirement (Hatfield & Hillman, 2001; Lay, Sparrow, Hughes, & O'Dwyer, 2002; Sparrow, 2000). In essence, the resultant limb movement of the superior athlete is highly efficient as the performer's work (i.e., moving the center of mass and the extremities in an intended or goal-directed manner) is accomplished with minimal effort within the constraints of the task demands. In this manner efficiency is simply described by: work / effort. Therefore, a high level of efficiency would imply that a given level of work is accomplished with the involvement of only those muscular and physiological processes that are essential to produce the intended work (i.e., minimal effort).

Economy of biological processes is a hallmark of highly adapted systems with fundamental examples provided by DeVries and Housh (1994), who described the efficiency of electrical activity (EEA) of skeletal muscle, as well as Daniels (1985), who described the efficiency of metabolic processes in superior endurance athletes (i.e., running economy).

The former refers to a decrease in motor unit recruitment to accomplish a given level of force production after resistance training (relative to an untrained state), while the latter refers to a lower metabolic cost of work in superior distance runners as they move through space, as indicated by reduced oxygen consumption per unit of body mass relative to their slower counterparts or competitors. As such, the work output of highly trained physiological systems is achieved with minimal energy cost. But does this principle extend to the brain and the mind of the athlete and, if so, how would it affect performance?

In an attempt to address this issue, Hatfield and Hillman (2001) described the concept of "psychomotor efficiency"—the notion that refinement or "pruning" of nonessential brain processes (such as task-irrelevant cortical association processes), is inherent in the development of expertise and emotional control and that, importantly, such a process would reduce unnecessary communication from other brain regions and potential interference with motor processes. The concept essentially posits a reduction of "neuromotor noise" in the cerebral cortex as a result of practice, thus reducing complexity and variability in motor planning and control that occur in the frontal and central regions of the forebrain, the subcortical basal ganglia, and the cerebellum. Such a state would simplify the brain and cortical processes evoked during skilled movement, increasing the probability of the athlete executing the desired or intended skeletal muscle action with economy of effort and consistency from trial to trial. Of course, this state would appear to be most beneficial to self-paced activities like golf, baseball pitching, and target shooting, but would facilitate reactive activities like open-field running in rugby and football, as the goal of any athlete is to execute the desired movement without hesitation.

The concept of psychomotor efficiency was derived from studies in exercise physiology, Bell and Fox's (1996) findings on the refinement of neural networks in the brain during development and learning, and the landmark principle of stress adaptation—the general adaptation syndrome (GAS)—introduced by Selyé (1976). Selyé described a transformational process beginning with the disruption of homeostasis, or an alarm stage, when a biological system is challenged (e.g., the need to exert muscular effort). The second stage, adaptation, refers to the long-term changes in the system accruing from repeated alarm responses (such as the training and conditioning program of an athlete) that promote a change in the architecture of tissues. Such change, as exemplified in skeletal muscle, is due to neurological adaptations and protein synthesis, primarily driven by the endocrine system, so that the muscle will then respond to the stress to which it has specifically adapted with less strain. The attenuation of strain from resistance training sessions, which is expressed symptomatically in the strength-trained athlete as lower motor unit recruitment, heart rate, and oxygen consumption during negotiation of a given workload, is an illustration of a basic developmental process that occurs in response to any repeated stressor, as the stress-induced change relates to enhanced survival and integrity of the biological system. In this case, the conditioned skeletal muscles respond to weight lifting and load bearing in a more efficient manner because of the anabolic processes triggered by the exercise bouts. In general, any biological system undergoes such change because of repeated challenges, and responds with reduced stress and strain. Of course, excessive stress results in the third stage, exhaustion, during which the adaptive capacity of the system is exceeded and the system is degraded. In an attempt to avoid such a negative catabolic state, coaches and athletes employ the principles of periodization and variations in training stress that enable peak performance while being subjected to intense training stress (Wathen, 1994). But, does such a principle of economy with sufficient levels of practice also extend to the brain?

Efficient adaptations also occur in cognitive-motor brain structures, although they differ in detail from those in peripheral physiological systems (Black, Isaacs, Anderson, Alcantara, & Greenough, 1990). Synaptic growth to facilitate adaptive cortico-cortical communication (i.e., networking between cerebral cortical regions) accompanied by critical cortico-subcortical connections occurs as a function of practice to enable intelligent movement. These changes are accompanied by the formation of internal or memory-based models (resulting from practice) that guide motor processes (Contreras-Vidal, Grossberg, & Bullock, 1997). The inhibition of nonessential neural connections likely contributes to the phenomenological experience of attention and focus. Such consolidation and pruning processes in the brain would decrease the need for effortful feature detection and elaborate cognitive analysis that characterize the novice performer and would consume attentional capacity.

Such neurological developments would likely be facilitated by environmental factors such as coaching style, as an emphasis on reinforcement (as opposed to punishment) in the context of strategic goal setting would allow the athlete to focus on intended actions as opposed to the mental elaborations of inhibiting mistakes or unintended actions. Furthermore, certain psychological qualities of the athlete like trait anxiety, intrinsic motivation, and self-efficacy would likely be critical factors for the promotion of efficient brain processes. In this manner, low trait anxiety would facilitate or cultivate the achievement of psychomotor efficiency while high trait anxiety and experiencing a coaching style with an emphasis on punishment would serve as obstacles for the achievement of such a state. Because the human mind is exceedingly complex, higher-order interactions of psychological variables may result in unexpected outcomes. For example, a highly competitive athlete may respond with heightened motivation in order to impress a critical coach. However, a conceptual model of brain processes during expert performance as described above allows for a guiding philosophical perspective that is empirically testable. Such a view, based in neuroscience, could be termed a "neurophilosophy" of expert psychomotor performance (Churchland, 1986). Although clearly relevant to the scientific or disciplinary goals of kinesiology and sport psychology, the research also holds significant implications for the coach-practitioner. That is, a concrete view of the manner in which brain or mind influences the body—a neurophilosophy of sport—can effectively guide communication between coach and athlete and increase confidence in coaching philosophy or leadership style based on comprehension of mental (i.e., brain) processes that influence the quality of muscle action and sport performance. In essence, this philosophy would stress the importance of a positive coaching style in which one would communicate instructions in a simplified goal-directed manner so as to facilitate brain development processes that would result in efficient and consistent movement/performance.

The following sections provide the evidence for such a neurophilosophy of sport as follows: (1) the basic measurement approaches used to study brain processes; (2) a summary of the evidence for the economy of cerebral cortical processes during expert motor performance; and (3) an overview of the impact of stress on the brain and motor performance.

Basic Measurement Approaches – Neuroimaging

Although a number of neuroimaging tools are available to assess the "working brain" the appropriate choice of measure depends on the investigator's question. Two major attributes of the available tools are (1) temporal resolution, which refers to the precision of a given neuroimaging technique to detect changes in brain activity as a function of time and (2) spatial resolution, which refers to the precision of a given measurement technique to localize anatomical structures or the source of brain activity during a mental operation in 3-dimensional space. Of course, the ideal neuroimaging measure would have both attributes so that very fast changes could be detected with precise localization of the neuroanatomical structures involved during the cognitive challenge. But, in reality, tools that are high in temporal resolution typically suffer from poor spatial resolution while those that are high in spatial resolution suffer from poor temporal resolution. As stated above, the tool of choice is dictated by the research question, and a given program of research may require a diversity of neuroimaging tools to examine different aspects of brain function. The following section overviews three of the primary tools available based on descriptions provided by Hatfield and Hillman (2001) and Tomporowski and Hatfield (2005).

Electroencephalography (EEG). The primary technique used to assess cerebral cortical dynamics with high temporal resolution during skilled motor behavior has been EEG. The EEG represents a time series of electrical activity or voltages sampled at high frequency (i.e., at least 100 Hz) as recorded from the scalp by placing electrodes at selected sites. There is a standard electrode placement system that specifies electrode locations based on anatomical landmarks on the head referred to as the International 10-20 system, which allows for comparison of results from various laboratories and clinical settings across laboratory settings (Jasper, 1958). The recording electrode or EEG sensor detects the transient or fluctuating summation of excitatory and inhibitory postsynaptic potentials (currents) from tens of thousands of neurons, and possibly glial cells, located below the scalp surface within the cortex of the brain, which collectively generate an electrical charge or potential. The fluctuating voltage detected by the EEG sensors is very small in magnitude and is expressed as millionths of volts or microVolts (μV). The transient continuous potentials or analog signals, changing in magnitude over time, are sampled and converted to digital values by an analog-to-digital (A-D) converter and typically amplified 20 to 50 thousand times. (Note: amplification can be much lower when the EEG is sampled with high-resolution A-D converters, which negate the need to "blow up" the signal). The sampling of the EEG needs to be at least twice the maximum frequency in the spectrum (1- 50 Hz) so as to avoid "aliasing" (or distortion of the time series); this requirement is termed the Nyquist frequency. The analog signals are then subjected to differential amplification, a process by which the resultant EEG record is actually created from the difference in voltage between the recording sites placed on the scalp over the cerebral cortex and a reference site that is typically placed on a non-brain region such as the earlobe, mastoids, or tip of the nose. The differential amplification process enables rejection of any common signals to the two sites, which are non-brain in origin, so that the amplified time series is, in fact, reflective and specific to cerebral cortical activity (i.e., common-mode rejection).

The two-dimensional EEG time series is characterized by amplitude and frequency that enable cognitive inference when consideration is given to the neuroanatomical region or location of the recording site(s). As stated above, the frequency range or spectrum of the signal extends from 1 to approximately 50 cycles per second (Hz). In essence, the raw EEG signal is composed of a mixture of frequencies. The decomposition of the complex record or EEG wave for a given time period (or epoch) is termed spectral analysis, and is accomplished mathematically by Fast Fourier Transformation (FFT). The magnitude or contribution of a given frequency to the EEG is expressed as amplitude (microvolts) or power (microvolts squared). The lower frequencies, such as the high-amplitude delta (i.e., 1-3 Hz), theta (i.e., 4-7 Hz), and alpha bands (i.e., 8-13 Hz) are generally indicative of a reduced arousal state, although recent work has associated delta with stress and theta power with sensory integration, while the higher frequencies, such as the low-amplitude beta (i.e., 13-30 Hz) and gamma bands (i.e., 36-44 Hz), are indicative of localized activation. Similar charge at the post-synaptic loci from a multitude of neurons in a given region (i.e., a column) summates and results in synchronous high-amplitude potentials. Such similarity is more likely to occur during a resting state. In contrast, activation and differential engagement of neurons results in desynchronous activity and is typically expressed as a reduction in the amplitude or power of EEG alpha. As such, the spectral decomposition of the EEG recorded from specific brain regions of interest can be employed to achieve cognitive inference.

The advantage of EEG is that it captures fast-changing events in the cerebral cortex, but it can also be used to detect communication or networking between different cortical regions by means of coherence analysis. Similarity in the spectral or frequency content of EEG recorded at different sites is indicative of cortico-cortical communication. A major limitation of EEG, however, is the problem of volume conduction or the spreading of electrical charge throughout the liquid medium of the brain. That is, the EEG signal is also detected, albeit with reduced influence, by sensors beyond those overlying the regions of interest. As such, EEG is limited as spatial resolution but superior to all other neuroimaging techniques for temporal resolution. However, the employment of dense-electrode recording arrays (typically from 64 to 256 sensors are used) along with source localization algorithms can overcome this limitation, especially if the EEG recordings are co-registered with magnetic resonance-derived images (MRI). Such an approach allows one to estimate the locus of the brain activity at a given point in time (this is termed *source reconstruction*) or to *"solve the inverse problem."* The inverse problem refers to the identification of cortical and subcortical sources of surface-recorded EEG by fitting the observed time series recorded from the scalp surface to hypothetical solutions or generators located in the brain that could account for the observed EEG by means of theoretically based algorithms.

Magnetic resonance imaging (MRI). MRI represents an anatomical or structural imaging as opposed to a functional or brain activation technique. It is a brain imaging technique whereby hydrogen atoms in brain tissue are localized by changing their atomic state by placing the subject in a powerful magnetic field. Almost all MRI scanners use detectors tuned to the radio frequencies of spinning hydrogen nuclei in water molecules. The subject's head is placed in the center of a large magnet and a radio frequency antenna coil is placed around the head for exciting and recording the magnetic resonance signal. In essence, MRI detects the energy emitted by spinning hydrogen nuclei in water molecules lined up in a strong magnetic field. To generate the images, the atoms within the various brain tissues receive a brief radio-frequency pulse tuned to their spinning frequency; they are then knocked out of alignment with the field and subsequently emit energy in an oscillatory fashion as they gradually align themselves with the field. The strength of the emitted signal depends on how many nuclei are involved in this process. This is accomplished by first aligning the body's cells in a powerful, primary magnet (strength is expressed in Tesla units) and then sending a secondary sequence of pulsed magnetic fields through the subject to detect differences in spin/resonance for different types of tissue. Greater hydrogen concentration, as a result of greater tissue density, emits a stronger signal. Importantly, hydrogen in different types of tissues (gray vs. white matter) has slightly different realignment rates, meaning that soft tissue contrast can be manipulated by changing parameter settings. In this manner, the investigator can see different types of brain tissue. The image of the gray matter of the cortex derived from cell bodies will differ from the image of the white matter tracts derived from fatty myelinated axons because of difference in water and hydrogen concentration. The obtained images of the various brain structures exhibit high spatial resolution (<1 mm).

Functional magnetic resonance imaging (fMRI). fMRI is a variant of MRI based on local activation or metabolism in brain regions. It is, therefore, a functional brain imaging technique as opposed to the purely structural conventional MRI, and is achieved by taking a high-speed series of images using MRI. In essence, haemoglobin (Hb) in the blood slightly distorts the MRI resonance properties of nearby H+ nuclei and the degree of distortion depends on whether the Hb is loaded with oxygen or not. fMR imaging enables detection of active areas of the brain—areas that are locally supplied with increased blood flow containing oxygen-rich Hb. These changes in the concentration of oxygen and blood flow lead to localized blood oxygenation level-dependent (BOLD) changes in the magnetic resonance signal. In this manner, there is a change in the response to magnetic spin signals, between oxygenated and de-oxygenated blood (the BOLD response). This difference is used to infer changes or differences in neuronal activity between experimental conditions and resting baseline states—a well-established procedure referred to as the *subtraction method*. The fluctuations in BOLD during task presentation or challenge are then detected (using the subtraction method) and image-processing techniques are used to produce maps of task-related brain activity. Importantly, the technique is safe for the subject as it uses signals intrinsic to the brain, as opposed to injection of exogenous agents; thus, repeated tests can be conducted, although limited in number when fMRI involves very powerful magnetic fields (e.g., 3 Tesla or more). Unlike EEG and magnetoencephalography (MEG), it takes several seconds for blood to move through the brain's microvasculature. As such, fMRI does provide spatially accurate images of active brain regions, for both cortical and subcortical deep structures, (spatial resolution is 2-3 mm) but its temporal resolution is relatively poor. However, one can see that the use of EEG to detect fast changing events in the cortex, along with fMRI to detect subcortical activation in structures such as the limbic system, would enable a comprehensive assessment of brain processes during skilled motor behavior. In addition, EEG can be employed during actual performance in the case of some activities like the target shooting sports as well as in virtual reality environments to simulate competitive conditions so that brain processes can be looked at in naturalistic environments. The use of fMRI is constrained such that the recording typically takes place in a closed environment in which the participant is supine and immobile, but the use of relevant tasks can provide

a wealth of complementary data to that obtained in the less restrictive EEG recording environment. For example, the study of individual differences in trait anxiety and the implications for brain processes during motor performance could be studied using both EEG and fMRI. EEG would reveal whether neuromotor noise or excessive coherence between motor and nonmotor regions was present, while fMRI could reveal the presence of hyperactivation in the limbic system (i.e., amygdala) that could further interfere with motor processes (i.e., basal ganglia).

Economy of Cortical Processes during Expert Motor Performance

The purpose of this section is to describe some of the advances that have been achieved in the application of cognitive neuroscience to sport psychology over the last 20 years, to highlight current findings regarding the neural bases of psychomotor efficiency, and to describe the manner in which stress affects brain processes and motor performance.

From a historical perspective, the application of cognitive neuroscience to sport psychology issues began with EEG studies during the preparatory period of self-paced target shooting (Hatfield, Landers, Ray, & Daniels, 1982). Marksmen provided excellent models of expert performance for psychophysiological analysis because of the intense attentional focus and emotional control required for high-level performance during a motionless task that allowed for recording of electrocortical activity with minimal artifact. Based on classic split-brain research (Gazzaniga, 1970; Sperry, 1964), the placement of recording sensors on the left and right hemispheres was routinely practiced to achieve cognitive inference from the EEG recordings. Therefore, relative activation in the language-based, left hemisphere was interpreted as explicit verbal-analytical processing while relative activation in the right hemisphere was interpreted as non-verbal, visuo-spatial processing. The relevance of this early work to applied sport psychology was based on the popular writings of Gallwey (1974) and the cognitive psychology perspective of Meichenbaum (1977) who, collectively, posited the notion of reduced self-talk during superior performance. In essence, EEG recording provided an alternative and objective approach to the interview and self-report techniques traditionally employed by sport psychologists to address the workings of the athlete's mind.

The participants in these early studies were comprised of elite marksmen and archers—Olympians, members of the United States Army Marksmanship Unit, and NCAA intercollegiate competitors. Brain activity was typically examined under non-stressed practice conditions. A consistent pattern of lateralized cerebral cortical activation was observed in a number of studies of precision target shooting performance (Bird; 1987; Hatfield et al, 1982; Hatfield, Landers, & Ray, 1984, 1987). EEG spectral power, typically in the alpha band (8-13 Hz), was contrasted between the left and right temporal regions during the aiming period of shot preparation. Because EEG alpha is inversely related to activation (Pfurtscheller, 1992) and serves as an index of cortical "idling," mental activity was inferred from consideration of (1) the functional neuroanatomy of the cortex, and (2) assessment of the relative activation of various brain regions of interest from EEG power spectral analysis. Relative to the activity observed in the right temporal region (T4) of the brain, a progressive lowering of activation was typically noted in the left temporal lobe (T3), as indicated by greater alpha power at site T3 during the aiming period leading up to the trigger pull (Hatfield et al., 1982, 1984, 1987). As stated above, left temporal activation is associated with detailed and explicit monitoring of task demands while right temporal activation is associated with visuospatial processing (Springer & Deutsch, 1998). Accordingly, the temporal EEG, alpha asymmetry observed during the aiming period of target shooting was interpreted as suppression of verbal-analytic and explicit memory processes while the maintenance of right temporal activity (i.e., as indicated by EEG alpha stability or suppression during aiming) was consistent with the maintenance of task-specific, visual-spatial processes. The observed pattern was logical in light of the well-known concept of automaticity of skill learning, an advanced stage of motor learning associated with expertise in which performers are not consciously aware of the details of their skilled movements (Fitts & Posner, 1967).

These early studies stimulated a number of subsequent EEG studies of target shooting (Deeny, Hillman, Janelle, & Hatfield, 2003; Haufler, Spalding, Santa Maria, & Hatfield, 2000, 2002; Hillman, Apparies, Janelle, & Hatfield, 2000; Janelle, Hillman, Apparies, Murray, Meili, Fallon et al., 2000; Janelle, Hillman, Apparies, & Hatfield, 2000; Kerick, Iso-Ahola, & Hatfield, 2000; Kerick, McDowell, Hung, Sanata Maria, Spalding, & Hatfield, 2001; Kerick, Douglass, & Hatfield, 2004; Loze, Collins, & Holmes, 2001; Saarela, 1999) and other self-paced psychomotor performances such as dart throwing, golf, archery, and karate (Collins, Powell, & Davies, 1990; Crews & Landers, 1993; Landers, Petruzzello, Salazar, Kubitz, Gannon, & Han, 1991; Landers, Han, Salazar, Petruzzello, Kubitz, & Gannon, 1994; Radlo, Janelle, Barba, & Frehlich, 2001; Salazar, Landers, Petruzzello, Han, Crews, & Kubitz, 1990). Typically, the investigations also involved the participation of elite athletes or experts who had been training for many years. Such highly motivated participants offered the opportunity to observe stable cerebral cortical activity patterns that had evolved over an extended period of time. The studies were typically cross-sectional in nature, involving contrasts of experts vs. novices (Haufler et al., 2000) or high skill vs. lower level skill (Hillman et al., 2000; Janelle et al., 2000), although some investigators examined changes in brain activity over time with practice (Kerick et al., 2004; Landers et al., 1994). Collectively, the results were consistent with the hypothesized simplification of neurocognitive activity with advancing skill (Hatfield, Haufler, Hung, & Spalding, 2004). That is, precision aiming was achieved in highly skilled performers with regional specificity of cortical activation.

Expert-novice contrasts of cortical dynamics. This principle was clearly supported by Haufler et al. (2000, 2002). Specifically, expert and novice marksmen were challenged with a target-shooting task as well as comparative verbal (i.e., word recognition) and spatial tasks (i.e., dot localization), with which the groups were similar in terms of experience. All three of the tasks were performed in the standing shooting position to hold any postural influence on the EEG constant. The investigators observed a remarkable reduction in cortical activation in the frontal, central, temporal, parietal, and occipital regions in the skilled group during the aiming period of the target-shooting task. The group difference was of greatest magnitude in the left temporal region, and a hemispheric asymmetry effect similar to that observed earlier by Hatfield et al. (1984) was revealed in the experts but not in the novices. As such, the experts accomplished the visuo-spatial task demands in a more efficient manner. No such group differences in cortical activation were noted between the groups when they performed the comparative cognitive tasks with which the groups were equally familiar. This finding suggests a high degree of task-specific adaptations in the brain as a result of practice. Figure 1 illustrates the reduction in cerebral cortical activity as indexed by gamma EEG power (i.e., 36 – 44 Hz), which is directly and positively related to metabolic activity, while, as predicted, no differences emerged for the spatial (Dot) and verbal tasks (Word) with which the groups were equally experienced. A more recent expert-novice contrast of target shooting performance conducted by Hung, Haufler, and Hatfield (2006), using a non-linear metric, revealed less dimensionality or reduced complexity in the EEG records of the skilled group. This finding also supports that experts negotiate task demands with activation of fewer neural resources or generators relative to beginners and clearly supports the age-old adage in coaching circles: keep it simple.

Changes in cortical dynamics with practice. Landers et al. (1994) first reported the effect of practice on cerebral cortical activation in a study of archery performance. EEG recorded from sites T3 and T4 was measured in 11 novices over a 12-week training period. Performance significantly improved over the course of instruction and was accompanied by a significant rise in T3 alpha power while no such increase was noted at T4. More recently, Kerick et al. (2004) extended this line of research and observed changes in EEG activity in a group of United States Naval Academy midshipmen who underwent 16 weeks of training in precision pistol shooting to prepare for competition. EEG was recorded from 11 sites (F3 [left frontal], Fz [midline frontal], F4 [right frontal], C3 [left central], Cz [midline central], C4 [right central], T3 [left temporal], T4 [right temporal], P3 [left parietal], Pz [midline parietal], and P4 [right parietal]) referenced to linked mastoids. The group, who had no experience with firearms training prior to the study, exhibited a significant decrease in global cortical activation during the aiming period after training, which was most pronounced

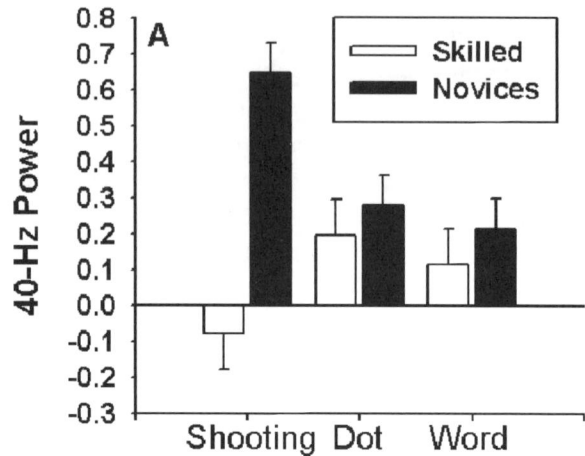

Figure 1. Comparative cerebral cortical activation (40-Hz gamma power) between experts and novices across three different tasks--shooting, visuospatial challenge (Dot), and verbal challenge (Word). Task-specific group differences are shown during shooting while no significant differences emerged for the comparative tasks.

in the left temporal region (T3). No such change in right temporal (T4) activation was noted, which implies a refinement rather than a monolithic decrease in cortical activity. Again, the general increase in event-related alpha power implies a global reduction in cortical activity and seems consistent with the phenomenological reports of highly experienced athletes that performance increasingly becomes "effortless" over time (Williams & Krane, 1998).

Cortico-cortical communication and expert shooting performance. Additional insight into the neurobiology of the skilled performance state can be attained by examination of functional interconnectivity or cortico-cortical communication between specified topographical regions of the brain. Such "networking" activity can be quantified by deriving EEG coherence estimates between selected pairs of electrodes or recording sites (Busk & Galbraith, 1975). In a recent study, Deeny et al. (2003) assessed inter-electrode coherence between motor planning (Fz) and association regions of the brain during skilled marksmanship by monitoring EEG at sites F3, F4, T3, T4, P3, Pz, and P4, as well as the motor cortex (C3, Cz, C4) and visual areas (O1 and O2). Coherence was assessed during a 4-second aiming period just prior to trigger pull in two groups of skilled marksmen who differed in ability level. The superior performance group was labeled "experts"

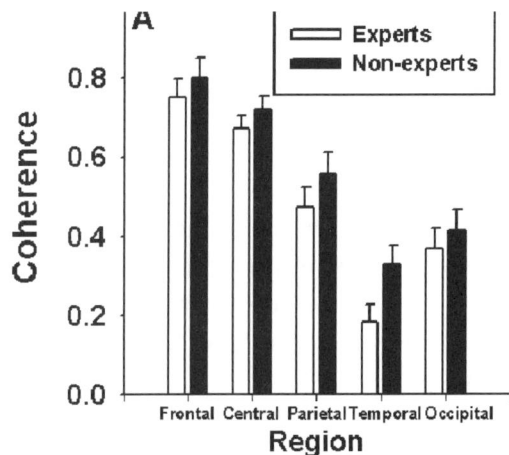

Figure 2. Comparative estimates of EEG coherence between selected brain regions and the motor planning region (Fz) in the left hemisphere for experts and skilled marksmen. The estimates are undifferentiated except at Fz-T3, which indicates a reduction in verbal-analytic influence on motor planning processes in the experts.

while the other group was labeled "skilled." An important dimension of the study was that both groups were highly experienced (approximately 18 years of experience each); however, the experts consistently scored higher under the stress of competition according to group histories, while the skilled group appeared to struggle under the pressure of competition. Figure 2 illustrates the left hemisphere Fz-F3, Fz-C3, Fz-P3, Fz-T3, and Fz-O1 coherence estimates contrasted between the two groups. A significant difference between the groups was detected for the Fz-T3 alpha band coherence, as the experts revealed significantly lower values, although no other differences were observed for either the left or right hemisphere. The same pattern of findings was also observed for beta band (13-22 Hz) coherence. The general lack of group differences in cortical networking seems reasonable as both were similarly experienced with the task and likely approached the challenge in a similar manner. However, the group difference in EEG coherence for the Fz-T3 electrode pairing was interpreted to mean that the experts were able to limit the communication between verbal-analytic and motor control processing, thereby simplifying motor planning. Consistent with the notion of psychomotor efficiency, the importance of this refined networking in the cerebral cortex is the reduction of potential interference with essential cognitive and motor functions from irrelevant associative and affective (e.g., limbic) processes. As such, the finding clearly supports a reduction in unnecessary networking between nonessential brain regions and motor planning processes to achieve superior shooting performance.

Specificity of cerebral cortical adaptations. One of the fundamental principles in exercise science is that of specific adaptation to imposed demand (SAID). This principle has received robust support in the areas of resistance and cardiovascular training and basically states that adaptations are constrained by the nature of the training stimulus. For example, high-intensity interval training promotes different cellular adaptations (i.e., greater glycolytic enzymes) than endurance training (i.e., greater capillarization of active tissue). In a recent report, DiRusso, Pitzalis, Aprile, & Spinelli (2005) extended this notion to the brain by comparing activation in the motor cortex of expert and novice marksmen who were right-handed as they prepared to generate force with their trigger finger in response to an imperative stimulus. DiRusso et al. employed a derivative of the EEG, the readiness potential (RP), to assess basic motor processes. The RP provides a precise chronometric index of the cortical activity involved in motor preparatory processes. The index is derived from averaging a number of EEG sweeps or epochs that are time-locked to repetitive stimuli (i.e., preparing for force production in response to an imperative stimulus) in order to extract signal from random background activity ("noise"). DiRusso et al. observed that the amplitudes of the resultant readiness potentials were lower in the experts and, importantly, the group difference was confined to the motor cortical region contralateral to the trained hand or trigger finger. That is, no such group differences were detected in the ipsilateral right motor cortex when the participants generated force with the index finger of the untrained left hand. Furthermore, the investigators employed dense EEG recording (as discussed earlier) in order to localize the source or location of origin of the readiness potentials. The reconstruction process did, in fact, reveal that the source of the RP was located in the premotor region, which provided anatomical validation for the study, and strongly supports the notion that SAID occurs in the brain.

EEG and the quality of motor performance. A number of studies have examined the relationship between brain activity and the quality of shooting performance. For example, Hung et al. (2006) noted that lower complexity of cortical processes was associated with superior target shooting performance. EEG measurement has also proven sensitive to detection of differences in cortical activation during the aiming period between successfully executed and rejected shots (Hillman et al., 2000; Loze et al., 2001). More specifically, exaggerated EEG alpha power was observed in expert marksmen prior to the decision to abort a shot, relative to that observed prior to trigger pull, suggesting that excessive relaxation, or a failure to regulate central arousal in an appropriate manner, leads to dysregulation of psychomotor performance. Such a notion was also supported by Salazar et al. (1990), who contrasted EEG spectral content at T3 in archers during the aiming periods associated with best and worst shots and observed higher amplitude of spectral power at 6, 12, and 28 Hz in the left hemisphere during the period prior to worst shots. Similarly, Landers et al. (1994) observed higher power for 12-Hz EEG during the worst shots in novice archers. Because the 12-Hz frequency also falls within the alpha band it would seem that such findings are more consistent with an inverted-U type relationship between performance and left temporal activation. Finally, Kerick et al. (2004) also noted a curvilinear relationship between event-related alpha power (ERAP) and pistol shooting accuracy, such that higher accuracy was associated with greater ERAP up to an optimal level, beyond which further increases in power were associated with reductions in accuracy. As such, it seems that better performance is associated with elevated but limited temporal alpha power.

In a more definitive assessment of the causal link between cortical activation and target shooting performance, Landers et al. (1994) conducted the only study published to date in which biofeedback was used to alter or experimentally manipulate brain activity in an attempt to facilitate archery performance. Accordingly, 24 pre-elite archers underwent one of three treatment conditions in which one group received a single session of "correct" feedback to reduce left hemispheric activation, a second group received "incorrect" feedback to reduce right hemispheric activity, and a third group rested and received no feedback. Comparison of pre-test and post-test performance scores revealed that only the correct feedback group improved target-shooting accuracy after treatment, while the incorrect group declined in performance. This finding is of critical importance, as it supports causal influence of cerebral cortical activity on the quality of motor behavior and provides a strong evidence for validation of the notion of refinement of cortical processes with superior performance.

Extension of EEG to the study of reactive motor tasks. In a recent effort, Kerick, Allendar, and Hatfield (2006) extended the examination of EEG to a reactive motor task during which skilled marksmen (United States marines) were required to shoot at pop-up targets in a virtual reality environment. Furthermore, cognitive load was varied by subjecting the participants to a simple task of firing at enemy-only targets as well as a task during which enemy and friendly targets required discrimination. As predicted, the higher cognitive load with the discrimination task resulted in suppression of alpha power across the cortex as well as increased theta EEG power, which indicated a heightened degree of sensory integration, likely caused by the need to monitor the environment with increased vigilance to avoid the costly mistake of friendly fire. The findings also provide convergent validation of the interpretations of the self-paced EEG studies summarized above (i.e., economy of cortical processes with expertise), as a reliable reduction in EEG alpha was noted under conditions of cognitive demand. By deduction, the synchrony of EEG alpha power noted in experts during self-paced performance does, indeed, support a reduction in the involved cognitive effort. Cerebral cortical processes have also been examined in response to other reactive task demands such as baseball hitting (Radlo et al., 2001) and the Posner cued attention paradigm in elite table tennis players (Hung, Spalding, Santa Maria, & Hatfield, 2004). These investigations were not designed to assess the notion of cerebral economy in skilled performers, but revealed distinct patterns of brain activity during attention demand in experts that were differentiated from less skilled individuals. Furthermore, the studies attest to the feasibility of EEG recording during motor performance beyond the confines of self-paced aiming tasks.

Collectively, the results of these studies suggest that superior performance is marked by mental economy—particularly that of analytical associative processes; the pruning of excessive cortico-cortical communication between such processes and motor regions underlies enhancement and consistency of psychomotor (shooting) performance, which raises the prediction that a reversal of these patterns would be observed with the imposition of stress.

Brain Processes During Psychological Stress

Importantly, few of the studies described above have manipulated psychological stress levels during the assessment of brain processes during psychomotor performance. Bear et al. (2001) summarized the neural structures involved in a system or circuit, which mediates the psychological and physiological response to stress. Generally, the stress response is orchestrated by the limbic system, but the central components of this functional circuit are the amygdalae, small almond-shaped structures located bilaterally and anterior to the hippocampi on the inferior and medial aspect of the temporal lobes. Multiple sensory pathways converge in the basal lateral nuclei of the amygdalae so that environmental events are immediately processed (Pare, Quirk, & LeDoux, 2004). Depending on the valence of the stimuli, the lateral nuclei then communicate with the central nucleus in each amygdala and subsequent connections travel to critical forebrain, brainstem, autonomic, and endocrine structures that mediate the expression of emotion (i.e., Canon's notion of the fight or flight response). More specifically, there are interconnections from the central nuclei to (1) the hypothalamus, which results in sympathetic arousal and stimulation of stress hormones via the hypothalamic-pituitary-adrenocortical (HPA) axis; (2) the periaqueductal grey, which results in motor responses; and (3) the cingulate cortex, which results in additional cortico-cortical communication with neocortical association regions such as the temporo-parietal regions. Additionally, interconnections to pontine nuclei in the reticular formation result in an increase in overall physiological arousal. In this manner, orchestrated sequelae occur in response to a stressful environment, which, collectively, can change the athlete's mental and physical state in a profound manner. For example, heart rate and cortisol levels rise, as does muscle tension, and the athlete may concomitantly experience excessive self-talk such that their attention is compromised and the execution of normally automated psychomotor skills such as marksmanship become explicitly managed—or mismanaged, that is; timing and coordination are then altered and likely reduced in quality while attention shrinks. In light of the mental and physical change alterations that accrue, the activation of the amygdalae serves as a pivotal event in the manifestation of stress and, importantly, the control of activity in the amygdalae would exact a powerful influence in terms of emotional self-regulation of the athlete's mental and physical state.

Beyond the structures and processes outlined by Bear et al. (2001) and LeDoux and colleagues (see LeDoux, 1996), a critical component of the neurobiology of fear is the executive control over limbic function and subcortical emotional circuits, which is housed anatomically in the frontal regions of the forebrain. Importantly, the anterior cortical regions have extensive anatomical connections with several subcortical limbic structures implicated in emotional behavior, particularly the amygdala (Davidson, 2002, 2004). According to the *fear circuit* model, the basic flow of events to achieve emotional control begins with activation in the dorso-lateral prefrontal cortex (DLPFC), an executive region which exerts influence over the medial frontal and orbital frontal regions that are more directly associated with emotional processes. These regions, in turn, influence the anterior cingulated cortex (ACC), which then influences and can control the activation in the amygdalae of the emotion-mediating limbic system (Pezawas et al., 2005). In this regard, the DLPFC can be thought of as a pivotal region in the critical events leading to emotional control.

In support of this notion, Richard Davidson and colleagues have generated a significant body of literature that clearly shows a positive association between left frontal activation (DLPFC) and positive affect while relative right activation is associated with negative affect (Davidson, 1988; Tomarken, Davidson, Wheeler, & Doss, 1992). Although the lateralization of frontal activation is robustly related to the valence of emotion, recent evidence points to a more fundamental association such that left frontal activation mediates approach-oriented behavior while right frontal activation is associated with avoidance or withdrawal-oriented behavior (Davidson, 2004). For example, left frontal activation is manifest during hostile behavior, which is certainly not a positive affective state, but most definitely involves approach toward an intended target. Whether positive in nature, approach-oriented, or a combination of the two dimensions, it would appear that such a neurobiological state would be highly adaptive for the athlete who must control arousal while actively engaged with challenging tasks while under great pressure.

Given that EEG alpha power is inversely related to activation (i.e., relaxation), R minus L alpha power (Log right frontal alpha power—Log left frontal alpha power), when positive, implies greater relaxation in the right region or, in other words, a state of left frontal activation. Hence, positive numbers for this metric imply left activation and executive control over emotion structures and processes. Conversely, a negative value implies greater relaxation in the left region and a lack of executive control over limbic circuits. In essence, the former implies a confident mental state while the latter implies a negative affective state. Figure 3 illustrates the frontal region and the lateralized asymmetry metric. The motivational diathesis captured by the frontal asymmetry metric (positive values imply approach motivation while negative values index withdrawal motivation) basically indexes the degree of executive control over deep brain structures involved with emotional response. Using this metric in a study of skilled marksmen, in which psychological stress was manipulated by reducing the time allotted for target shooting, Saarela (1999) observed a significant decrease in frontal asymmetry when marksmen were required to perform under the time pressure relative to a non-stress condition. Furthermore, a significant relationship between frontal asymmetry and motor performance was revealed such that lower asymmetry (i.e., relative right activation) covaried with lower shooting score (i.e., reduced accuracy).

Individual differences in emotion-related brain processes. Beyond such general cortical responses to stress, there is considerable individual variation in anxiety-related personality traits that are 40-60% heritable (Bouchard & Loehlin, 2001). That is, there are individual differences in reactivity of the amygdalae in response to stressful events based on genetic factors. Recently, it has been well documented that the promoter region of the serotonin transporter gene on chromosome is polymorphic such that those with the short allele (about 50% of population) show heightened activation of the amygdalae to emotion-eliciting stimuli, while those carrying the long allele show attenuation of fear (Hariri et al., 2002). As such, the disregulation of cortical processes with presentation of stress may be particularly problematic for carriers of the short allele of the serotonin (5-HT) transporter gene (5-HTT) during emotional challenge (Hariri et al., 2002). The polymorphism has been identified in the transcriptional control region of the 5-HTT gene such that a long promoter region (L) is associated with transcriptional efficacy while the short allele (S) is associated with transcriptional deficiency. According to Lesch et al. (1996), "genotyping of approximately 500 individuals revealed allele frequencies for the L and S types of 57% and 43% respectively, with S dominant. The genotypes are distributed according to the Hardy-Weinberg equilibrium as follows: LL – 32%, LS – 49%, and SS – 19%. As such, there is a high degree of prevalence of this anxiogenic genotype.

In this manner, the S-type allele of the 5-HTT promoter region holds significant implications for information processing and motor control and is a critical component of a proposed individual differences

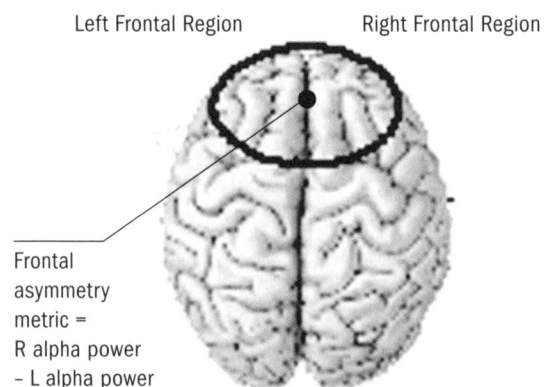

Left Frontal Region   Right Frontal Region

Frontal
asymmetry
metric =
R alpha power
– L alpha power

Figure 3. Assymetrical Activation of the Anterior Cortical Regions as Related to Emotional Responding. Positive and progressively increasing values derived from this metric equals approach task-engagement motivation. Negative and progressively decreasing values derived from this metric imply withdrawal task-avoidance motivation.

model of the stress response. A more efficient response to stress would lead to enhanced information processing, decisive decision-making, and improved coordination of motor skills (a more intelligent response to the stimuli). In essence, S carriers may be considered *stress-prone* while L carriers may be considered *stress-regulators*. This would imply that frontally mediated executive control of the fear circuit is critical for a large segment of the athlete population, as they are predisposed to be especially reactive.

Emotion and the motor loop. There are neuroimaging tools and concepts to guide the study of psychological stress on the brain and to further delineate the subtle differences in individual response, but what is also needed is a comprehensive model of stress-induced change on cognitive-motor performance. Figure 4 provides a model of the processes and outcomes underlying stress reactivity and integrates affective and cognitive activity with psychomotor performance. A central tenet is that lack of executive control over subcortical processes would result in heightened emotional influence (limbic structures) that, in turn, would disrupt higher cortical association processes resulting in alterations in the activation of the cerebral cortex and the motor loop–the fronto-basal ganglia structures that initiate and execute movement. Such disregulation interferes with attention and the connections to the motor cortex that largely control corticospinal outflow and the resultant quality of the motor unit activation (Graf-

ton, Hari, & Salenius, 2000). Excessive networking in the cortex may result in undesirable alterations in information processing as well as inconsistency of motor performance. In this manner the motor cortex becomes busy with excessive input from limbic processes via increased neocortical activity in the left hemisphere and inconsistent motor behavior will likely result (Deeny et al., 2003).

According to this model, individuals under high stress will exhibit reductions in prefrontal asymmetry (box 1) compared to a low-stress condition, implying a lack of executive control over the fronto-meso-limbic fear circuit described above. Consequently, participants will experience heightened activation of the limbic region (amygdala) (box 6). The resultant emotional reactivity, in turn, will result in EEG alpha desynchrony, particularly in the left temporal (T3) and parietal (P3) regions (box 8), along with increased cortico-cortical communication between these regions and the motor planning centers (box 4). Such disregulation of the cerebral cortex will be expressed as inconsistent input to the motor loop (boxes 2 to 5) resulting in inconsistent corticospinal output and shooting performance (motor unit activity—trigger pull—boxes 9 and 10). It is well established that attention capacity shrinks with arousal, and, consistent with this notion, the excessive cortico-cortical networking during heightened stress, as proposed here, would compromise information processing (Easterbrook, 1959). In addition, the

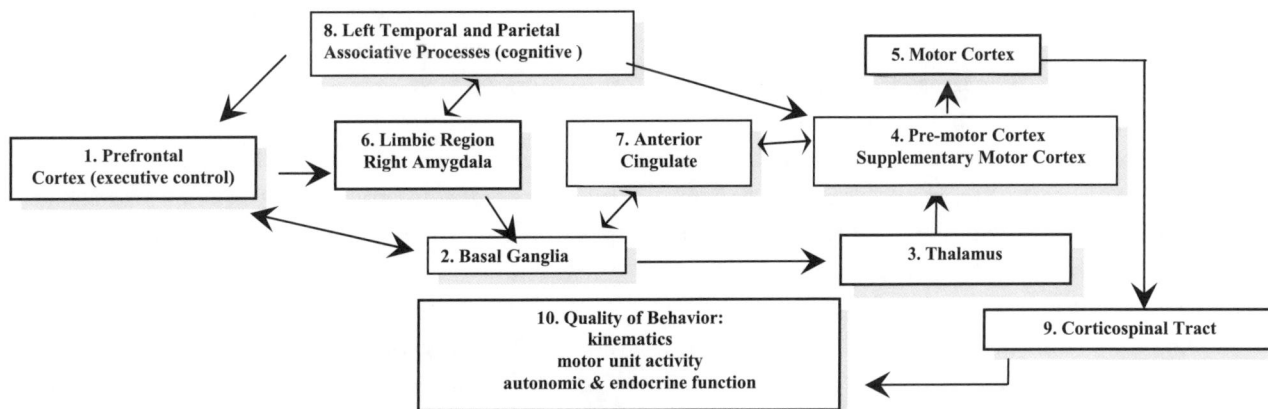

Figure 4. Cognitive Neuroscience Model of Psychomotor Performance. A schematic of critical brain regions involved in the interaction between frontal executive, emotional, motor, and cerebral cortical processes. The figure illustrates the interplay between these processes and the pivotal role of prefrontal processes to control numerous sequelae in this complex cascade of events.

experience of stress will impact peripheral cardio-vascular activity such that sympathetic autonomic activity will be increased while parasympathetic or vagal tone will be withdrawn under conditions of high stress. Endocrinological activity, as indexed by activation in the hypothalamic-pituitary-adrenal cortical axis, will become elevated and glucocorticoids such as cortisol will rise. The magnitude of change specified in the model will be related to degradation in motor performance (i.e., slower and less accurate). Importantly, the disregulation of cortical processes will be heightened in carriers of the S allele.

Partial support for the model was recently provided by Hung and colleagues (2005), who observed increased coherence between cortical association and motor planning regions when study participants were exposed to stress during a dart throwing task. However, definitive support for such a model will require sophisticated source localization strategies to examine the predicted stress-induced consequences in subcortical processes. This will require dense EEG electrode recording strategies involving a minimum of 128 channels as well as co-registration of participant EEG with structural MRI in order to solve the inverse problem with confidence. The best-fit solution is the one that minimizes the difference or error between the predicted EEG time series and the actual, or observed, EEG time series based on a number of possible sources (i.e., hypothetical neural generators). In this manner, the optimal fit, or "winning" solution, provides an estimate of the location of brain activity that is responsible for the surface EEG recordings. The solutions can be further constrained by realistic anatomical head models based on MRI images so that we have greater confidence in the possible source(s) and eliminate spurious solutions.

Neurofeedback-based intervention to control stress-related brain processes. The EEG frontal asymmetry metric provides an opportune target for neurofeedback training to enable a heightened level of executive control over emotional response and task engagement during challenge. In light of the essential need to regulate this cascade, a number of studies support the effectiveness of neurofeedback training on alterations of cortical activity in the form of specific EEG measures (Egner & Gruzelier, 2004; Rosenfeld, 2000; Rosenfeld, Baehr, Baehr, Gotlib, & Ranganath, 1996; Siniatchkin, Kropp, & Gerber,

2000). As stated above, Landers et al. (1994) conducted the only study published to date in which biofeedback (left temporal slow-wave activity) was used to alter brain activity in an attempt to facilitate target-shooting performance. After one feedback session, approximately one hour in duration, comparison of pre-test and post-test performance scores revealed that only the correct feedback group (i.e., relaxation of left temporal region) improved target-shooting accuracy while the incorrect group declined in performance. The rapidity of training effectiveness is consistent with the findings of other neuroscientists who have reported very short time periods for experience-induced synaptic change in the brain (Quinlan, Olstein, & Bear, 1999).

Although the results were intriguing, it would seem that neurofeedback to control frontal activation (i.e., R minus L alpha power) would yield broader effects on arousal regulation and, in accompaniment with an increased number of training sessions, might yield automaticity of arousal regulation under pressure as the strategy becomes better learned. Studies by Allen, Harmon-Jones, and Cavender (2001) and Baehr, Rosenfeld, and Baehr (2001) have shown that control of frontal asymmetry can be achieved in an effective manner resulting in significant alterations in emotional regulation. Importantly, the brief alterations endure for surprisingly long periods (i.e., up to 5 years).

Summary

The future appears promising for a cognitive neuroscience approach to sport psychology—but where are we going? First, the testing of conceptually based models such as the efficiency principle is imperative to guide our efforts to understand the manner by which mental processes affect neuromuscular performance. An important methodological issue is the essential requirement of inter-disciplinary study incorporating such fields as psychology, neuroscience, physics, genetics, physiology, engineering, and biomechanics. Furthermore, there is a need for more integration of sport psychology with motor control theory to further refine the predictions as well as consideration of the gene-environment (G x E) interaction. The advancement of theory in sport psychology will largely depend on developments in technology and other scientific disciplines such as mathematics (i.e., signal processing), engineering, and physics to enable the technology to see the brain at work. Expansion of knowledge beyond the traditional self-paced laboratory task protocols, such as the marksmanship task, will depend on the development of sophisticated virtual reality environments and increasing sophistication of telemetry to acquire artifact-controlled psychophysiological signals while allowing freedom of movement. Beyond the processes occurring in the brain, there is an imperative need to monitor the mind-body link and kinematic processes to discern the qualities of limb action in tandem with the underlying neurobiological or brain processes. Indeed, the study of the mind, from a kinesiological perspective, is quite limited in the absence of consideration of the moving body and muscular performance!

References

Allen, J. J. B., Harmon-Jones, E., Cavender, J. H. (2001). Manipulation of frontal EEG asymmetry through biofeedback alters self-reported emotional responses and facial EMG. *Psychophysiology, 38,* 685-693.

Baehr, E., Rosenfeld, J. P., & Baehr, R. (2001). Clinical use of an alpha asymmetry neurofeedback protocol in the treatment of mood disorders: Follow-up study one to five years post therapy. *Journal of Neurotherapy, 4,* 11-18.

Bear, M. F., Conners, B. W., & Paradiso, M. A. (2001). *Neuroscience: Exploring the brain* (2nd ed.). Baltimore, MD: Lippincott, Williams & Wilkins.

Bell, M. A., & Fox, N. A. (1996). Crawling experience is related to changes in cortical organization during infancy: Evidence from EEG coherence. *Developmental Psychobiology, 29,* 551-561.

Bird, E. I. (1987). Psychophysiological processes during rifle shooting. *International Journal of Sport Psychology, 18,* 9-18.

Black, J. E., Isaacs, K. R., Anderson, B. J., Alcantara, A. A., & Greenough, W. T. (1990). Learning causes synaptogenesis, whereas activity causes angiogenesis in cerebellar cortex of adult rats. *Proceedings of the National Academy of Science, 87,* 5568-5572.

Bouchard, T. J., & Loehlin, J. C. (2001). Genes, evolution, and personality. *Behavior Genetics, 31,* 243-273.

Busk, J., & Galbraith, G. C. (1975). EEG correlates of visual-motor practice in man. *Electroencephalography and Clinical Neurophysiology, 38,* 415-422.

Churchland, P. (1986) *Neurophilosophy: Toward a unified science of the mind/brain.* Boston, MA: MIT Press.

Collins, D., Powell, G., & Davies, I. (1990). An electroenphalographic study of hemispheric processing patterns during karate performance. *Journal of Sport and Exercise Psychology, 12,* 223-243.

Contreras-Vidal, J. L., Grossberg, S., & Bullock, D. (1997). A neural model of cerebellar learning for arm movement control: Cortico-spino-cerebellar dynamics. *Learning and Memory, 3,* 475-502.

Crews, D. J., & Landers, D. M. (1993). Electroencephalographic measures of attentional patterns prior to the golf putt. *Medicine and Science in Sports and Exercise, 25,* 116-126.

Daniels, J. T. (1985). A physiologist's view of running economy. *Medicine and Science in Sports and Exercise, 17,* 332-338.

Davidson, R. J. (1988). EEG measures of cerebral asymmetry: Conceptual and methodological issues. *International Journal of Neuroscience, 39,* 71-89.

Davidson, R. J. (2002). Anxiety and affective style: Role of prefrontal cortex and amygdala. *Biological Psychiatry, 51,* 68-80.

Davidson, R. J. (2004). What does the prefrontal cortex "do" in affect: Perspectives on EEG frontal asymmetry research. *Biological Psychology, 67,* 219-233.

Deeny, S., Hillman, C. H., Janelle, C. M., & Hatfield, B. D. (2003). Cortico-cortical communication and superior performance in skilled marksman: An EEG coherence analysis. *Journal of Sport and Exercise Psychology, 25,* 188-204.

DeVries, H. A., & Housh, T. J. (1994). *Physiology of exercise for physical education, athletics, and exercise science* (5th ed.). Dubuque, IA: Wm. C. Brown.

DiRusso, F., Pitzalis, S., Aprile, T., & Spinelli, D. (2005). Effect of practice on brain activity: An investigation in top-level rifle shooters. *Medicine and Science in Sports and Exercise, 37,* 1586-1593.

Egner, T., & Gruzelier, J. H. (2004). EEG biofeedback of low beta band components: Frequency-specific effects on variables of attention and event-related brain potentials. *Clinical Neurophysiology, 115,* 131-139.

Easterbrook, J. A. (1959). The effect of emotion on cue utilization and the organization of behavior. *Psychological Review, 66,* 183-201.

Fitts, P. M., & Posner, M. I. (1967). *Human performance.* Belmont, CA: Brooks/Cole.

Gallwey, T. (1974). *The inner game of tennis.* New York: Random House.

Gazzaniga, M. S. (1970). *The bisected brain.* New York: Appleton-Century Crofts.

Grafton, S. T., Hari, R., & Salenius, S. (2000). The human motor system. In A.W. Toga & J. C. Mazziotta (Eds.), *Brain mapping: The systems* (pp.331-363). San Diego: Academic Press.

Hariri, A. R., Mattay, V. S., Tessitore, A., Kolachana, B., Fera, F., Goldman, D., et al. (2002). Serotonin transporter genetic variation and the response of the human amygdala. *Science, 297,* 400-403.

Hatfield, B. D., & Hillman, C. H. (2001). The psychophysiology of sport: A mechanistic understanding of the psychology of superior performance. In R. N. Singer, C. H. Hausenblas, & C. M. Janelle (Eds.). *Handbook of Sport Psychology* (2nd ed., pp. 362-386). New York: John Wiley.

Hatfield, B. D., Haufler, A. J., Hung, T. M., & Spalding, T. W. (2004). Electroencephalographic (EEG) studies of skilled psychomotor performance. *Journal of Clinical Neurophysiology, 21,* 144-156.

Hatfield, B. D., Landers, D. M., & Ray, W. J. (1984). Cognitive processes during self-paced motor performance: An electroencephalographic profile of skilled marksmen. *Journal of Sport Psychology, 6,* 42-59.

Hatfield, B. D., Landers, D. M., & Ray, W. J. (1987). Cardio-vascular-CNS interactions during a self-paced, intentional attentive state: Elite marksmanship performance. *Psychophysiology, 24,* 542-549.

Hatfield, B. D., Landers, D. M., Ray, W. J., & Daniels, F. S. (1982, February). An electroencephalographic study of elite rifle shooters. *The American Marksman, 7,* 6-8.

Haufler, A. J., Spalding, T. W., Santa Maria, D. L., & Hatfield, B. D. (2000). Neuro-cognitive activity during a self-paced visuospatial task: Comparative EEG profiles in marksmen and novice shooters. *Biological Psychology, 53,* 131-160.

Haufler, A. J., Spalding, T. W., Santa Maria, D. L., & Hatfield, B. D. (2002). Erratum to "Neuro-cognitive activity during a self-paced visuospatial task: Comparative EEG profiles in marksmen and novice shooters." *Biological Psychology, 59,* 87-88.

Hillman, C. H., Apparies, R. J., Janelle, C. M., & Hatfield, B. D. (2000). An electrocortical comparison of executed and rejected shots in skilled marksmen. *Biological Psychology, 52,* 71-83.

Hung, T. M., Lin, J. H., Lo, L. C., Kao, J. F., Hung, C. L., Chen, Y. J., et al. (2005). Effects of anxiety on EEG coherence during dart throw. In T. Morris, P. Terry, S. Gordon, S. Hanrahan, L. Ievleva, G. Kolt, & P. Tremayne (Eds.), *Promoting health and performance for life: Proceedings of the ISSP 11th World Congress of Sport Psychology* [CD-ROM]. Sydney: International Society of Sport Psychology.

Hung, T. M., Spalding, T. W., Santa Maria, D. L., & Hatfield, B. D. (2004). Assessment of reactive motor performance with event-related brain potentials: Attention processes in elite table tennis players. *Journal of Sport and Exercise Psychology, 26,* 317-337.

Hung, T. M., Haufler, A. J., & Hatfield, B. D. (2006). Dimensional complexity of cerebral cortical activity during expert visuomotor performance: An examination of the psychomotor efficiency hypothesis. Manuscript submitted for publication.

Janelle C. M., Hillman C. H., Apparies R. J., & Hatfield, B. D. (2000). Concurrent measurement of EEG and visual indices of attention during rifle shooting: An exploratory case study. *International Journal of Sports Vision, 6,* 21-29.

Janelle, C. M., Hillman, C. H., Apparies, R. J., Murray, N. P., Meili, L., Fallon, E. A. et al. (2000). Expertise differences in cortical activation and gaze behavior during rifle shooting. *Journal of Sport and Exercise Psychology, 22,* 167-182.

Jasper, H. H. (1958). The ten-twenty electrode system of the International Federation. *Electroencephalography and Clinical Neurophysiology, 17,* 37-46.

Kerick, S. E., Allendar, L., & Hatfield, B. D. (2006). Cortical activity of soldiers during shooting as a function of varied task demand. Manuscript submitted for publication.

Kerick, S. E., Douglass, L., & Hatfield, B. D. (2004). Cerebral cortical adaptations associated with visuomotor practice. *Medicine and Science in Sport and Exercise, 36,* 118-129.

Kerick, S. E., Iso-Ahola, S. E., & Hatfield, B. D. (2000). Psychological momentum in target shooting: Cortical, cognitive-affective, and behavioral responses. *Journal of Sport and Exercise Psychology, 22,* 1-20.

Kerick, S. E., McDowell, K., Hung, T. M., Santa Maria, D. L., Spalding, T. W., & Hatfield, B. D. (2001). The role of the left temporal region under the cognitive motor demands of shooting in skilled marksmen. *Biological Psychology, 58,* 263-277.

Landers, D. M., Han, M. W., Salazar, W., Petruzzello, S. J., Kubitz, K. A., & Gannon, T. L. (1994). Effects of learning on electroencephalographic and electrocardiographic patterns in novice archers. *International Journal of Sport Psychology, 25,* 313-330.

Landers, D. M., Petruzzello, S. J., Salazar, W., Kubitz, K. A., Gannon, T. L., & Han, M. (1991). The influence of electrocortical biofeedback on performance in pre-elite archers. *Medicine and Science in Sports and Exercise, 23,* 123-129.

Lay, B. S., Sparrow, W. A., Hughes, K. M., & O'Dwyer, N. J. (2002). Practice effects on coordination and control, metabolic energy expenditure, and muscle activation. *Human Movement Science, 21,* 807-830.

LeDoux, J. (1996). *The emotional brain.* New York: Simon & Schuster.

Lesch, K., Bengel, D., Heils, A., Sabol, S., Greenberg, B. D., Petri, S., et al.(1996). Association of anxiety-related traits with a polymorphism in the serotonin transporter gene regulatory region. *Science, 274,* 1527-1531.

Loze, G. M., Collins, D., & Holmes, P. S. (2001). Pre-shot EEG alpha-power reactivity during expert air-pistol shooting: A comparison of best and worst shots. *Journal of Sports Sciences, 19,* 727-733.

Meichenbaum, D. (1977). *Cognitive behavior modification.* New York: Plenum Press.

Pare, D., Quirk, G. J., & LeDoux, J. E. (2004). New vistas on amygdala networks in conditioned fear. *Journal of Neurophysiology, 92,* 1-9.

Pezawas, L., Meyer-Lindenberg, A., Drabant, E. M., Verchinski, B. A., Munoz, K. E., Kolachana, B. S., et al. (2005). 5-HTTLPR polymorphism impacts human cingulated-amygdala interactions: A genetic susceptibility mechanism for depression. *Nature Neuroscience, 8,* 828-834.

Pfurtscheller, G. (1992). Event-related synchronization (ERS): An electrophysiological correlate of cortical areas at rest. *Electroencephalography and Clinical Neurophysiology, 83,* 62-69.

Quinlan, E. M., Olstein, D. H., & Bear, M. F. (1999). Bidirectional, experience-dependent regulation of N-methyl-D-aspartate receptor subunit composition in the rat visual cortex during postnatal development. *Proceedings of the National Academy of Science, 96,* 12876-12880.

Radlo, S. J., Janelle, C. M., Barba, D. A., & Frehlich, S. G. (2001). Perceptual decision making for baseball pitch recognition: Using P300 latency and amplitude to index attentional processing. *Research Quarterly for Exercise and Sport, 72,* 22-31.

Rosenfeld, J. P. (2000). An EEG biofeedback protocol for affective disorders. *Clinical Electroencephalography, 31.*

Rosenfeld, J. P., Baehr, E., Baehr, R., Gotlib, I. H., & Ranganath, C. (1996). Preliminary evidence that daily changes in frontal alpha asymmetry correlate with changes in affect in therapy sessions. *International Journal of Psychophysiology, 23,* 137-141.

Saarela, P. I. (1999). The effects of mental stress on cerebral hemispheric asymmetry and psychomotor performance in skilled marksmen. Unpublished doctoral dissertation, University of Maryland.

Salazar, W., Landers, D. M., Petruzzello, S. J., Han, M. W., Crews, D. J., Kubitz, K. A. (1990). Hemispheric asymmetry, cardiac response, and performance in elite archers. *Research Quarterly for Exercise and Sport, 61,* 351-359.

Selyé, H. (1976). *The stress of life.* New York: McGraw-Hill.

Siniatchkin, M., Kropp, P., & Gerber, W. (2000). Neuro-feed-back—The significance of reinforcement and the search for an appropriate strategy for the success of self-regulation. *Applied Psychophysiology and Biofeedback, 25,* 167-175.

Sparrow, W. A. (2000). *Energetics of human activity.* Champaign, IL: Human Kinetics.

Sperry, R. W. (1964). The great cerebral commissure. *Scientific American, 210,* 42-52.

Springer, S. P., & Deutsch, G. (1998). *Left brain, right brain: Perspectives from cognitive neuroscience.* New York: W.H. Freeman.

Tomarken, A. J., Davidson, R. J., Wheeler, R. E., & Doss, R. C. (1992). Individual differences in anterior brain asymmetry and fundamental dimensions of emotion. *Journal of Personality and Social Psychology, 62,* 676-687.

Tomporowski, P., & Hatfield, B. D. (2005). Effects of exercise on neurocognitive functions. *International Journal of Sport and Exercise Psychology, 3,* 263-279.

Wathen, D. (1994). Periodization: Concepts and applications. In T. R. Baechle (Ed.), *Essentials of strength training and conditioning* (pp. 459-472). Champaign, IL: Human Kinetics.

Williams, J. M., & Krane, V. (1998). Psychological characteristics of peak performance. In J. M. Williams (Ed.), *Applied sport psychology* (pp. 158-170). Mountain View, CA: Mayfield.

Section V
Motor Skill and Expert Performance

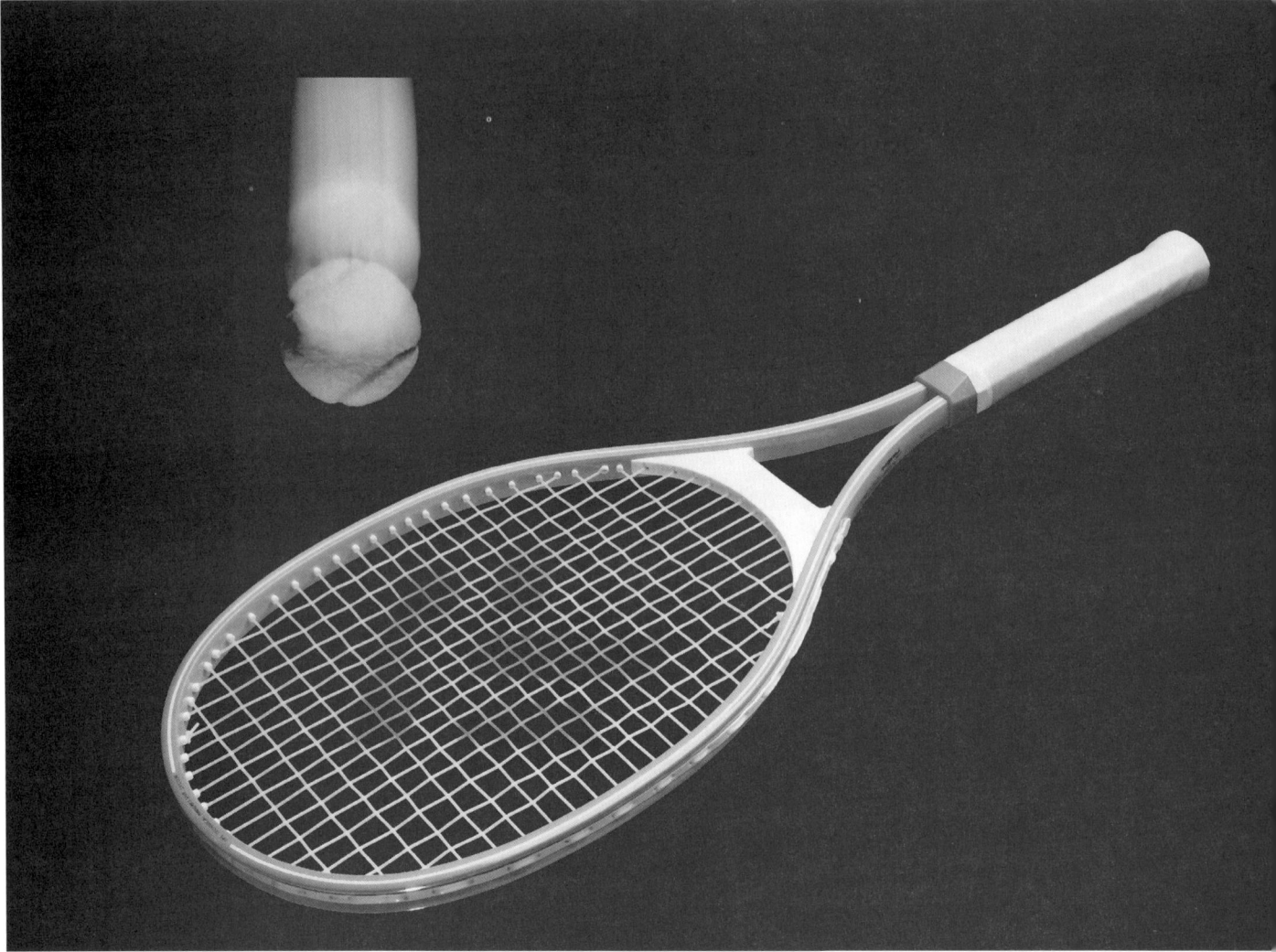

10

Issues in Motor Learning for Instructional Strategies

KARL M. NEWELL AND S. LEE HONG

Change in Motor Learning: A Coordination and Control Perspective

In this paper, we will outline an approach to some of the central issues that pertain to the nature of change in the learning and performance of physical activities in education and sport settings. The formulation of the issues discussed is driven by both the needs of the applied settings and the recent laboratory research conducted on motor learning and control. Full accounts of the relevant theory and practice of each issue are provided with the general and specific references that follow.

Theoretical Background to Discussion
Before outlining key issues and questions for consideration, we want to briefly mention that the meta-

phor that has driven and organized research for the learning and performance of motor skills has changed over the 100 years of the study of motor learning. The last 25 years have seen the introduction of, and now emphasis on, the self-organization construct within the movement domain (Kelso, 1995; Kugler, Kelso, & Turvey, 1980, 1982; Kugler & Turvey, 1987; Turvey, 1990) as a shift away from the computer metaphor. The self-organizing approach to human movement arose from the introduction of Bernstein's (1967) *degrees of freedom* and *redundancy* problems, which highlighted the importance of coordination in the control of the many degrees of freedom of the motor system. This theoretical framework focuses on the organization of the dynamics of the motor system at multiple levels of analysis over multiple time-scales of change (Newell, Liu, & Mayer-Kress, 2001).

A view of the motor system as self-organizing,

ISSUES IN MOTOR LEARNING FOR INSTRUCTIONAL STRATEGIES   141 dynamic, and constantly evolving has yet to be integrated into the field of physical education and sport coaching, as it has often been considered as little more than metaphorical because there has been limited direct application of the concepts to sport and physical education settings. However, this theoretical framework holds different propositions for learning and performance than the traditional theories of reflex chaining, learning theory, motor programs, and schema. The cognitive metaphors of motor program and schema have tended to dominate perspectives about instructional strategies and motor skill learning. We plan to capture key elements of the new approach to motor learning, along with their implications for physical education and sport, through a dynamical systems perspective on the role of practice and learning for change in physical activity. We also seek to provide practical applications for the dynamical systems theories presented here.

Physical activity requires the organization of a system with many degrees of freedom, a good proportion of which may be redundant to satisfy the immediate task demands of the activity or sport in question (Bernstein, 1967). Having many degrees of freedom—namely muscles, joints, and limb segments—poses the problem of control and coordination during skilled performance. Some of these degrees of freedom can be considered redundant when more than a single configuration or movement pattern allows for the achievement of the movement goal. It should be noted that the special demands of high-level performance in sport tend to reduce the redundancy problem, and, arguably, in some instances may eliminate it. The organization and reorganization of the learning system involves a mapping of information and movement dynamics to produce stable, yet continually evolving dynamical solutions to satisfy the relevant task constraints. The learner passes through a spiral of stability-instability-stability, both within the progressions over time of learning a particular skill and in the natural embedding of different activities into daily life.

We now begin to unpack these briefly introduced general assumptions of current theory by amplifying their impact through questions about the role of practice in learning and performance in physical education and sport. The theoretical background to the issues and discussion is more fully outlined in papers from our laboratory (Newell, 1991, 1996; Newell, Kugler, van Emmerik, & McDonald, 1989; Newell, Liu, & Mayer-Kress, 2001, 2003, 2005; Newell & McDonald, 1994; Newell & Valvano, 1998).

What Is the Nature of the Change in Performance over Time?

Performance in a physical education or sport activity is the product of a continually evolving dynamical organization of the human system. The dynamics for the performance of a particular skill are embedded in a broader set of dynamical organizations and reorganizations that support the conduct of all activities of daily living. The broad organization of the dynamics of human performance has been evolving since conception of the individual, as the evolving changes in the structural and functional (i.e., anatomical and physiological) constraints provide natural patterns of organization to the system dynamics as the individual interacts with its environment. These natural organizations tend to hold more dynamical stability than other patterns of movement performance.

Motor learning over the life span involves the continual evolution of the system dynamics and the ebb and flow of stable and unstable solutions to task demands. Learning involves change in the qualitative organization of movement dynamics, which naturally involves periods of performance instability at various levels of analysis. Thus, learning requires the establishment of new stable patterns of dynamics that can be brought together over a sufficient time scale to realize the demands of either a new task to be learned, or the continued improvement in the performance of a given task. Within this theoretical framework, the macroscopic, structural variables (order parameters) *enslave* the *microscopic* variables (e.g., muscle fibers, joints), which function within *coordinative structures*. The enslaving of microscopic variables by the macroscopic variables results in a situation where the behaviors of the former can be described by the latter.

A good example of this enslaving principle is the tactical structure used to coordinate a team of soccer players. With 10 field players, their actions must be coordinated to achieve both offensive and defensive agenda. As such, the coordinative structures in this situation are the tactical systems of play, e.g., 4-4-2, 5-3-2. These structural variables serve to reduce the

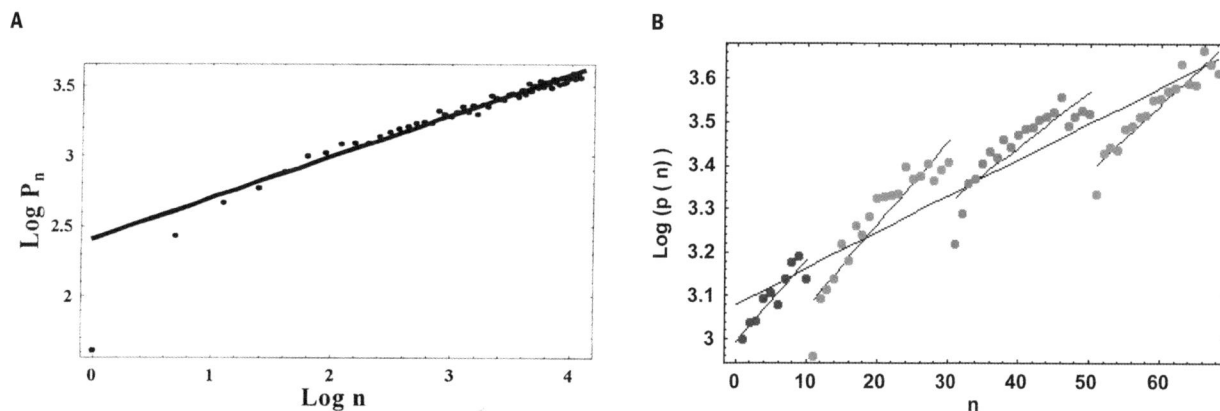

Figure 1. A. The original Snoddy (1926) power law for the mirror tracing data; B. A two time scale exponential function fitted to the same mirror tracing data (adapted from Mayer-Kress, Newell, & Liu, 1998).

independence of the actions of each of the players and allow the coach to more easily direct play as a whole. As far as the rules of the game are concerned, all of the field players are able to perform identical tasks and can be considered redundant to one another, just as in the motor system. Yet, each player possesses individual strengths and weaknesses that make them more viable options for certain offensive or defensive tasks. Thus, the organization pattern can be described by a set of structural variables (such as midfield, attack, and defense) that emerge from the movements of the players on a field with respect to one another. The players (or microscopic variables) are still enslaved by the greater structure of the team tactics, for example, having four midfielders or a sweeper. In terms of human movement, the many muscles and limb segments can be controlled through a few independent degrees of freedom, with their structured behaviors manifested as coordination patterns.

There are multiple time scales to the qualitative change in the learning and performance of physical skills. Motor learning is concerned primarily with those changes to performance that are relatively persistent over days, weeks, and years (such as those evident in the study of learning curves); however, there are many influences on performance and a large number are on short time scales, reflecting trial to trial and even within-trial variation. These time scales can be linked to the nature of the stable dynamics supporting performance and the transitions between the evolving stable modes of performance.

The received position as to the nature (function) of change in motor learning is that it is a power law, although the apparently contrasting propositions of qualitative stages to learning have also been proposed. The power law holds that there are multiple (technically infinite) time scales of change in performance over time, with the amount of improvement decreasing with increasing practice time; it is a rule of diminishing returns. Recent research, however, confirms the long-held observation that the averaging of data can mask the interpretation of the pattern of change in performance over time. Moreover, the current practice of using computerized curve-fitting functions that focus only on the r^2-values can lead to poor decisions about the nature of the change in learning. As an example, consider Figure 1 where we show that the first demonstration of a power in motor learning by Snoddy (1926) is actually more closely approximated by a small limited set of two characteristic time scales.

Thus, there is qualitative and quantitative change in performance over time that is driven by an embedded set of systems, each with its own time scale of change. It has been proposed recently that there is not one function of the change in performance over time, as is held by the power law. The emergence of change in learning is driven by many factors that arise from the confluence of constraints from the organism, environment, and task, and the nature of dynamics that need to be produced to satisfy the task demands. Thus, different tasks can have different functions of change, particularly when they are only considered in the short term of practice (which they usually are). This naturally leads to an inquiry as to how these changes occur.

Learning as Searching

Changes in performance over time are elicited by deterministic and stochastic (chance) influences on the evolving movement dynamics. Teachers of physical activities try to enhance the probability of systematic change in performance over time through planned interventions in the form of instructional strategies for learning, for example, by using part-practice, where the whole movement is broken up into its component parts. Beyond instructor interventions, *searching* arises from the natural exploration of the perceptual-motor workspace and specific strategic approach taken by the instructor and performer to the change in the movement dynamics over time. Searching affords information about the interaction of the performer with the environment and the nature of the underlying supporting dynamics for action. Searching also allows an individual performer to learn the stability boundaries of the current movement pattern by testing the limits within which a given movement pattern is able to sustain the achievement of the desired goal. The motion of the body-environment interaction provides information about this relationship, and searching provides the vehicle for picking up that information. This information for searching can arise in principle from all sensory systems, though the use of vision and proprioception appears primary in most motor learning situations.

Searching can take place within a trial or a current performance and between trials in an attempt to produce a more task relevant outcome on the next trial. It has been postulated that during the acquisition of skill, learners use a small set of search principles that are dependent on the constraints placed upon the learner by the task and environment (Newell, 1986). Instructors can play an important role here to channel the search of the learner toward motor solutions of the movement goal in a way that may not be readily identified by the individual.

Learning requires the search beyond the boundaries of a stable coordination mode or movement pattern while functioning in a changing environment in order to attempt an unformed (unstable) coordina-tion pattern for a given task demand. Infants naturally pass these boundaries when, for example, they fall over many times while learning to stand. The apparent act of failing at the task provides information about the stability boundaries to the action. And, even at more advanced stages of learning, there are benefits that arise from a suboptimal performance, where the correction of minor errors may lead to large improvements in performance. The effectiveness of searching, which is a continuous process in learning, will depend on the willingness of the learner to engage in such exploration. This is one of the opportunities for intervention available to the instructor; stressing psychological aspects of learning, such as motivation and self-efficacy, will eventually encourage the learner to explore the limits of his or her current movement solutions.

Teachers need to consider ways in which to guide a performer toward the dissolution of a relatively successful dynamic and alter the coordination pattern in the search for a movement pattern that will temporarily be unstable and probably less rewarding during task performance, but will eventually lead to more stable achievements of the task goal. This challenge forms the basis for instructional issues, such as whole-part and progressive stages learning, and the nature of the to-be-learned movement pattern for the task at hand. Problems can arise when learners are consistently performing the task with a coordination pattern that affords only modest, but repeatable, outcome results. This is often the critical period in which the performer must decide whether the construction of a new, potentially more rewarding movement pattern is worth the effort and resulting drop in performance during the period of instability that inevitably arises in transitioning from one coordination pattern to another.

Learning transpires through searching, and the evolution and dissolution of the stable dynamical regions of coordination modes for a given task. We need to understand more about the nature of the relevant information that facilitates the search and the transitions of the stable modes of performance. Learning then is realized in part by either discovering or searching for the dynamic laws of movement organization in action.

A major problem in understanding the notion of learning through searching is the determination of the information that learners use to conduct and facilitate the search. The ecological approach to perception and action, proposed by Gibson (1979), has laid the foundation for new ways to consider this question, but little progress has been made in this important area with direct applications to learning the skills necessary for sport or physical activity. Gibson's approach is important to skill acquisition because it is focused directly on action as a means of interacting with the environment. As such, objects and events within the environment provide sources of direct perceptual information in the form of *affordances* to the performer, which provide the performer with an estimate of the "do-ability" of a given action. This concept of affordances proposes that the information is not obtained from the environment through symbolic representations, but rather, through the actions or behaviors that are "afforded" by the objects and events in the environment. For example, when a soccer or basketball player is making an attempt to dribble past an opponent, he or she bases the type of feint employed on the positions of the defenders and speed of their approach relative to his or her own. The question of the information relevant for action is an important issue for instructors, who should base the information provided to the learner on the principle that information is naturally accumulated during the learning process.

Degrees of Freedom and
Redundancy in the Coordination Solution

The ability of the human sensori-motor system to realize a task goal with different coordination solutions has led to several proposals over the years of the largely similar ideas of motor equivalence, equifinality, redundancy, degeneracy, and abundance. These ideas all propose that more than a single movement pattern can potentially serve as means of achieving a movement goal. We will use the notions of degrees of freedom and redundancy from Bernstein (1967) as examples, because they are most widely accepted in the field of motor learning and control. The large number of component mechanisms of the organism (torso, limbs, muscles, motor units, and so on) naturally leads to the idea that task outcomes can be realized in more than one way from a system with many degrees of freedom. For example, at the level of joint space, there are about 120 degrees of free-

dom (potential independent planes of motion of the torso and limb segments), and the number of degrees of freedom increases dramatically as one considers the problem at micro-levels of the system.

Beyond the problem of possessing a high number of degrees of freedom, many of these degrees of freedom are also redundant, meaning that more than a single combination of behaviors of these degrees of freedom can be employed as a means of generating a motor solution for a given task. Using the grasping and raising of a cup, this redundancy can be seen even in a simple 3-link representation of the arm and hand (Figure 2). Clearly, all four joint configurations presented are viable solutions to the problem, but different solutions will be employed, depending on the context in which the behavior is being performed.

The history of the study of motor skill learning is such that to a large degree, the degrees of freedom problem has been ignored. A major reason for this may be due to the default action of choosing tasks for study with arguably only one biomechanical degree of freedom (e.g., elbow flexion tasks), or more generally when tasks are selected where the performer can already perform the coordination mode. Over the last 20 years or so, however, there has been a concerted effort to study the coordination and control of the many degrees of freedom of whole body activities more typically associated with the tasks of physical education and sport.

Recently, a study has emphasized the need to understand coordination of the torso and limb segments in the execution of a task (Hong & Newell, 2006). To a large extent, this work centers on the study of the degree of common variance in the motion at joint angles and limb segments with a view to determining if the individual behaviors of the system's many degrees of freedom can be compressed into a functional unit or units, reducing the number of degrees of freedom that require control during the execution of the task. In the context of motor learning and development, the issue gets expanded into a question of whether or not there is a change, over time and through the course of practice, in the compression of the individual degrees of freedom into these coordinative structures or patterns.

Mainly, studies to date show that the strength of the coordination of the individual degrees of freedom

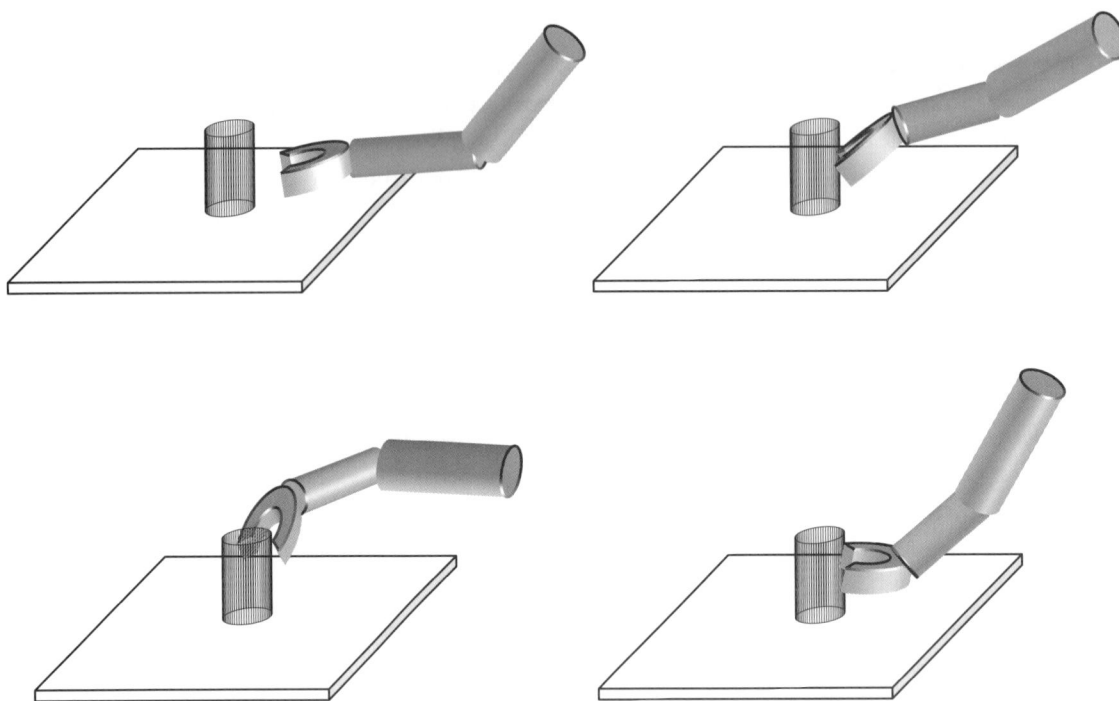

Figure 2. Schematic 3-link illustration of reaching options toward a glass. Note the redundant options that result in a stable solution, allowing the performer to achieve the goal of grasping and raising the glass.

that the motor system possesses is driven to a degree by the constraints placed upon the action by the desired outcome (Newell, 1996). For example, the motions of the limb segments require fewer independent dimensions of action in the highly coordinated act of walking than they do in the act of kicking a soccer ball in the context of a game. Understanding the functional organization of these coordination modes and their evolution with learning is currently receiving attention in research.

The redundancy of the motor system can be witnessed when qualitatively different coordination patterns can be employed to satisfy similar task demands. For example, during the game of soccer, passes can be made with various surfaces of the foot, e.g., the instep, inside, and outside of the foot. Different patterns of movement trajectories might all satisfy the ball being delivered successfully to a team mate, but the selection of the appropriate movement pattern will depend on the context created by specific game situations. These expressions of redundancy are afforded by the many degrees of freedom of the organism (as noted earlier), the breadth of goal-satisfying conditions (to varying degrees) in the

task solution (for example, the bandwidth of acceptance in a target task), and the constraints that are present in the environment. These constraints can serve to either increase or decrease the amount of redundancy by altering the number of goal-equivalent motor solutions. Thus, the confluence of constraints (Figure 3) serves to realize different degrees of redundancy in motor control that need to be exploited by the learner of motor skills. In Bernstein's (1967) terms, the expression of skill is essentially that of the mastery of redundant degrees of freedom.

The redundancy of the coordination solution gives rise to the idea that the search principles outlined previously may be made on certain behavioral dimensions of the overall motor solution and not others. Thus, the constraints on the action may channel the search differentially as a way to reduce the effective degrees of freedom and the problems of control, while at the same time arriving at a task solution. With such insights into the human action system, the instructor can channel the search strategies by tightening or relaxing the constraints already placed on the performer. A long-standing technique of reducing/occluding vision of the ball during both

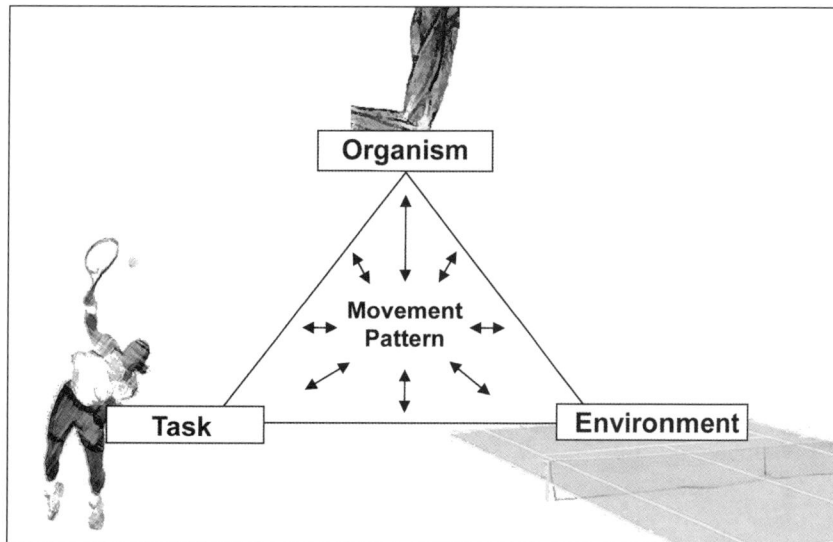

Figure 3. Illustration of the constraints placed upon the movement by the task, organism, and environment.

basketball and soccer dribbling is a form of increased environmental constraint. The instructor could also relax a task constraint by allowing soccer players to pass the ball by hand as a means of teaching off-the-ball movement. Advances in our understanding of this central degrees-of-freedom problem to motor learning and development will provide fresh insights for the teaching of whole body activities in physical education and sport.

Augmented Information and Channeling the Search for Task Relevant Stable Solutions

Augmented information is that which is not intrinsically available to the learner when learning and performing the task. It is added to information normally available in the organism-environment interaction during practice of the task. Increasing technological developments make the distinction of natural (intrinsic) and augmented information a fine line and a matter of definition, particularly in person-machine interactions, where information that is construed as augmented can one day be permanently built into the system of future machine designs to, in essence, provide natural information the next day. There are a number of different types of augmented information and media through which such information can be conveyed.

There appear to be at least three categories of augmented information that are used to facilitate motor learning and performance: prescriptive information, information feedback, and transition information. These three can be considered in a common augmented information framework in which the augmented information provides the support for facilitating the search of the perceptual-motor workspace, the construction of attractor dynamics, and the realization of the task goals.

Prescriptive information. Augmented information that is prescriptive provides information about the to-be-achieved end-state movement kinematics and task outcome. The information can specify the relative, absolute, and common motion components of a to-be-achieved coordination and control solution to the task demands. This information, or elements of it, is most typically conveyed by oral instructions and/or a demonstration of a behavioral outcome of a to-be-achieved coordination and control solution. The demonstration may be via some medium, such as film or videotape, or it can be a live demonstration by an instructor.

The presentation of prescriptive augmented information for the acquisition of movement skills is a common occurrence in activities of dance, sport, and music. This is based upon the intuitive perspective that this category of information is effective for learning, and that "a picture is worth a thousand words." The empirical evidence in support of such a proposition is not as compelling as the intuition, which suggests subtle interactions between the effects of this category of information, the nature of the skill, and the skill level of the performer.

Information feedback. This category of augmented information provides information about some past state or states of the movement dynamics produced by the learner in an evolving movement sequence or on a just-completed movement trial. The information feedback could be provided about any absolute, relative, or common motion property, but there are principles about the most useful information to provide. Concurrent information feedback provides information about prior states of the ongoing movement sequence. Terminal information feedback provides information about earlier movement properties or their consequences (movement outcome) upon completion of the trial.

A major challenge lies in choosing the appropriate type of information feedback at each stage of learning. Information feedback has been shown to be a variable that strongly influences the learning and performance of movement skills (Newell, Morris, & Scully, 1985). In the learning of one or two degree-of-freedom movement tasks the emerging principle is that the degrees of freedom contained in the information should match the degrees of freedom requiring constraint in the task. Deciding which type of information feedback is appropriate for learning whole-body actions is more profound because many informational properties of the action may be considered.

In tasks requiring the coordination of many biomechanical degrees of freedom, it is the case that information feedback is often not very direct about the nature of the change that needs to be made on the next trial. The consequence is that in many task situations information feedback does not constrain the search sufficiently for the learning of new coordination modes, leading to less effective and efficient learning than has been apparent in investigations of the learning of single-limb tasks under the same information feedback conditions. This suggests the use of more *feedforward* augmented information that provides predictive information regarding a movement, in order to facilitate the acquisition of a new coordination mode.

Transition information. A category of augmented information that has not been studied sys-

tematically is that of transition information. This is information that relates directly to the change in the coordination and control solution that needs to occur at some future time in the ongoing trial or on the next trial in a learning sequence. This type of information appears to be particularly useful in the acquisition of a new set of relative motions or movement form for the task at hand. Transition information is that which specifies a to-be-achieved property of a coordination and control solution that should be searched for in the upcoming movement trial, but in the act of realizing that goal, a transition to another coordination and control solution emerges. Thus, transition information is not prescriptive information in that it is not prescribing the to-be-achieved end-state dynamics of the to-be-learned movement skill, and it is not information feedback in that it does not provide information about past movement states and their goals realized. Rather, it provides information *directly* about the change in movement coordination and control, as opposed to both prescriptive or feedback information.

Theoretically, transition information is a control parameter that facilitates the search through the perceptual-motor workspace for the realization of a task relevant coordination and control solution, and it may appear unrelated to the to-be-achieved end-state dynamics. Kernodle and Carlton (1992) tested the effect of different kinds of augmented information on the acquisition of throwing a sponge ball as far and as accurately as possible. For measures of the form of the movement pattern and of the distance thrown, results showed that transition information was more useful than information feedback, attentional focusing, and knowledge of results. Figure 4 shows the key information category effects over practice trials and days.

A key issue for a theory of motor learning is the integration of the concept of information into the Bernstein coordination problem and the changing regulation of redundant degrees of freedom. The categories of augmented information described earlier provide different forms of information to the learner and support the information naturally available for motor learning and control in the organism-environment interaction. These categories of augmented and natural information are rarely considered in a cohesive theoretical framework, but they can be usefully

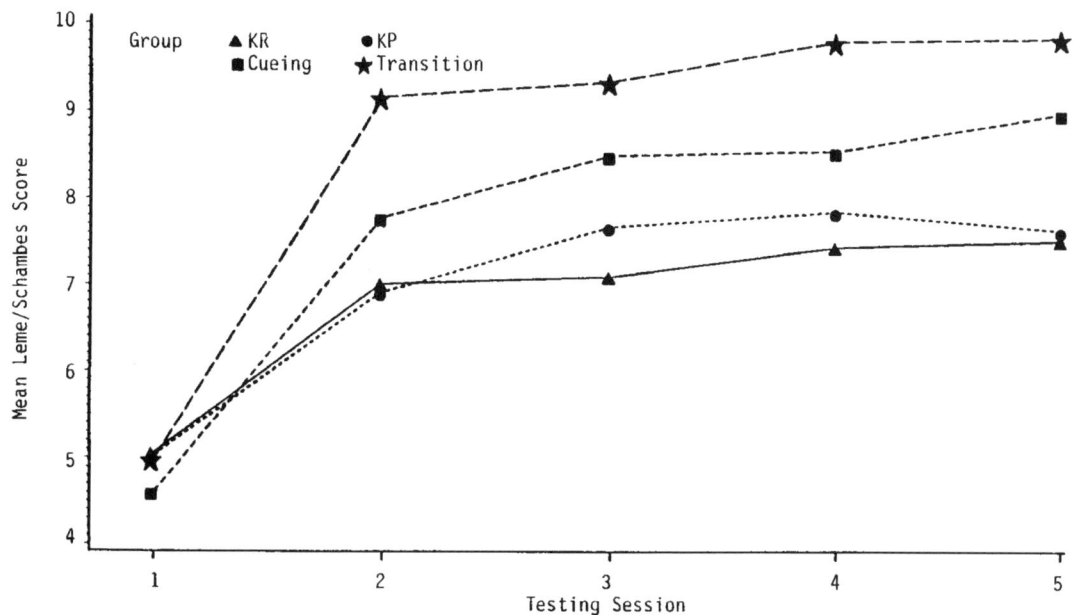

Figure 4. The mean throwing score as a function of augmented information condition (from Kernodle & Carlton, 1992).

viewed as information that facilitates the search for task relevant coordination and control solutions. The respective categories of information provide different types and degrees of constraint on the search behavior and the emergent channeling of the task relevant movement dynamics. In practice, instructors tend to intertwine the use of these categories according to the nature of the task and the skill level of the performer in order to facilitate motor learning.

In general, augmented information acts as an environmental constraint to action. The different categories of information provide varying boundary conditions to the search through the perceptual-motor workspace in the realization of new task goals. Information facilitates exploratory behavior in motor learning and is an integral part of coming to terms with Bernstein's problems of learning to regulate redundant degrees of freedom. The view of practice as "repetition without repetition," as its role in the exploration of the workspace, in actuality leads the learner to attempt the task with different movements on each subsequent trial.

Practice Schedules and Search Strategies in Learning

A long-standing problem in motor skill learning is the establishment of the most appropriate schedule of practice for the activity at hand. This problem is usually viewed under what is called *massed* and *distributed* practice schedules (Schmidt & Lee, 2005). Practice is considered to be massed if there are no rest periods or breaks between practice trials; it is considered to be distributed if the time that passes between the trials is equal to or greater than that of the trial length itself. On the surface, there may seem to be little difference between these two practice schedules, but there are many issues involved in the construction of the "ideal" practice session for a particular task. For example, differences in the duration of a practice trial, the physiological demands of the task, and also the role that rest and fatigue play in learning must be taken into account.

The idea that learning reflects an evolving set of dynamical relations extends to studies of the cortical organization and activity that arises from use and disuse over time. Recent research has shown that the homunculus layout of effector connections in the motor cortex can be reconfigured as a consequence of use and disuse (Merzenich, 1998). This striking finding adds further evidence to the view that long-term, persistent changes to even the neural connections occur with sufficient practice.

Regular and sustained physical practice, therefore, is essential to preserving the effectiveness of the system output in particular tasks, although mental practice can also induce system changes. The limits to increased performance within a given practice session may be due to the problems of fatigue and the generation of inappropriate movement patterns, and the loss of attention in task execution through motivational losses. Practice does not make perfect as the old adage holds, but it is essential in the pursuit of high performance. Deliberate practice in a task with attentional effort is not mere repetition of the movement and activity; rather, it involves learning the ability to adapt to the constantly changing physiological demands, the constraints of the environment, and the limits to the physiological capacity of the organism itself.

A key issue, the solution to which remains unknown at this time, is the role that fatigue may play in skill learning. It is possible that fatigue serves to force the learner to explore originally unstable, possibly less rewarding patterns of movement. Another possibility is that fatigue generates a sufficient amount of instability within the motor system that causes the stable attractor pattern to be driven through a "phase transition," an abrupt shift toward a different, potentially undesirable pattern of coordination in terms of the task outcome. This is an area of research that has yet to receive sufficient focus, especially since many of the tasks employed in the study of motor learning serve little purpose as activities of daily living. In the context of sport, when skills practiced under typically inert conditions must be transferred to competitive situations, fatigue may also play a role. This raises an important question as to whether the specificity of the practice of motor skills must also encompass the physiological demands of the sport. These transfer of learning situations generally arise when practice involves the repetition of drills such as passing or footwork in an attempt to transfer these into the context of the competitive game.

Finally, given that the degree of redundancy is influenced by the confluence of constraints to action, it follows that the task demands of different sports skills will afford the potential for greater or fewer viable solutions to a given motor problem. The greater the task demands, in terms of requiring a performance outcome that is closer to a performer's maximal performance, the more the region of redundant solutions is narrowed. Indeed, it follows that

the exhibition of the true maximum performance of an individual at a given moment in time, in events like jumping and throwing and other track and field events, may in principle hold no redundant solutions. On the other hand, it may be that even the highly skilled performer never reaches this level of performance. These conjectures reflect the ways in which task constraints may influence the potential redundancy in the coordination solution.

Summary of Perspective

There is nothing as basic as a good applied question and nothing as applied as a good basic theory. The problem of practice in the acquisition of skill captures the essence of this statement. Motor learning is not about acquiring symbolic representations for action. Rather, it is about being able to temporarily map environmental information to movement dynamics in the assembly of a task relevant coordination solution, where each subsequent performance of the task is influenced by the dynamics of previous engagements in activity as well as the local constraints. The outline to the issues of change and learning addressed here, although only representing a beginning sketch, provides a coherent basis for a more principled consideration of the role of practice in physical activity.

References

Bernstein, N. (1967). *The co-ordination and regulation of movements.* New York: Pergamon.

Gibson, J. J. (1979). *The senses considered as perceptual systems.* Boston: Houghton Mifflin.

Kelso, J. A. S. (1995). *Dynamic patterns: The self-organization of brain and behavior.* Cambridge, MA: MIT Press.

Hong, S. L., & Newell, K. M. (2006). Change in the organization of degrees of freedom with learning. *Journal of Motor Behavior, 38,* 88-100.

Kernodle, M. W., & Carlton, L. G. (1992). Information feedback and the learning of multiple-degree-of-freedom activities. *Journal of Motor Behavior, 24,* 187-196.

Kugler, P. N., & Turvey, M. T. (1987). *Information, natural law, and the self-assembly of rhythmic movement: Theoretical and experimental investigations.* Hillsdale, NJ: Erlbaum.

Kugler, P. N., Kelso, J. A. S., & Turvey, M. T. (1980). On the concept of coordinative structures as dissipative structures: I. Theoretical lines of convergence. In G. E. Stelmach & J. Reqiun (Eds.), *Tutorials in motor behavior* (pp. 1-49). New York: North-Holland.

Kugler, P. N., Kelso, J. A. S., & Turvey, M. T. (1982). On the control and coordination of naturally developing systems. In J. A. S. Kelso & J. E. Clark (Eds.), *The development of movement control and co-ordination* (pp. 5-78). New York: Wiley.

Mayer-Kress, G. J., Newell, K. M., & Liu, Y-T. (1998). What can we learn from learning curves? *InterJournal, 246.*

Merzenich, M. (1998). Long-term change of mind. *Science, 282,* 1062-1063.

Newell, K. M. (1986). Constraints on the development of coordination. In M. Wade & H. T. A. Whiting (Eds.), *Motor development in children: Aspects of coordination and control* (pp. 341-360). Dordrecht, Germany: Martinus Nijhoff.

Newell, K. M. (1991). Motor skill acquisition. *Annual Review of Psychology, 42,* 213-237.

Newell, K. M. (1996). Change in movement and skill: Learning, retention, and transfer. In M. Latash & M. Turvey (Eds.), *Dexerity and its development* (pp. 393-432). Hillsdale, NJ: Erlbaum.

Newell, K. M., & McDonald, P. V. (1994). Learning to coordinate redundant biomechanical degrees of freedom. In S. Swinnen, H. Heuer, J. Massion, & P. Casaer (Eds,), *Interlimb coordination: Neural, dynamical, and cognitive constraints* (pp.515-536). New York: Academic Press.

Newell, K. M., & Valvano, J. (1998). Therapeutic intervention as a constraint in learning and relearning movement skills. *Scandinavian Journal of Occupational Therapy, 5,* 51-57.

Newell, K. M., Kugler, P. N., van Emmerik, R. E. A., & McDonald, P. V. (1989). Search strategies and the acquisition of coordination. In S. A. *Wallace (Ed.), Perspectives* on the coordination of movement (pp. 85-122). Amsterdam: North-Holland.

Newell, K. M., Liu, Y-T., & Mayer-Kress, G. (2003). A dynamical systems interpretation of epigenetic landscapes for infant motor development. *Infant Development and Behavior, 26,* 449-472.

Newell, K. M., Liu, Y-T., & Mayer-Kress, G. (2005). Learning in the brain-computer interface: Insights about degrees of freedom and degeneracy in a landscape model of motor learning. *Cognitive Processing, 6,* 37-47.

Newell, K. M., Liu, Y-T., & Mayer-Kress, G. (2001). Time scales in motor learning and development. *Psychological Review, 108,* 57-82.

Newell, K. M., Morris, L. R., & Scully, D. M. (1985). Augmented information and the acquisition of skill in physical activity. *Exercise and Sport Sciences Reviews, 13,* 235-262.

Schmidt, R.A., & Lee, T. D. (2005). *Motor control and learning (4th. Edition): A behavioral emphasis.* Champaign, IL: Human Kinetics.

Snoddy, G. S. (1926). Learning and stability. *Journal of Applied Psychology, 10,* 1-36.

Turvey, M. T. (1990). Coordination. *American Psychologist, 45,* 938-953.

Acknowledgments

This work was supported by National Science Foundation grants 0114568 and 0518845.

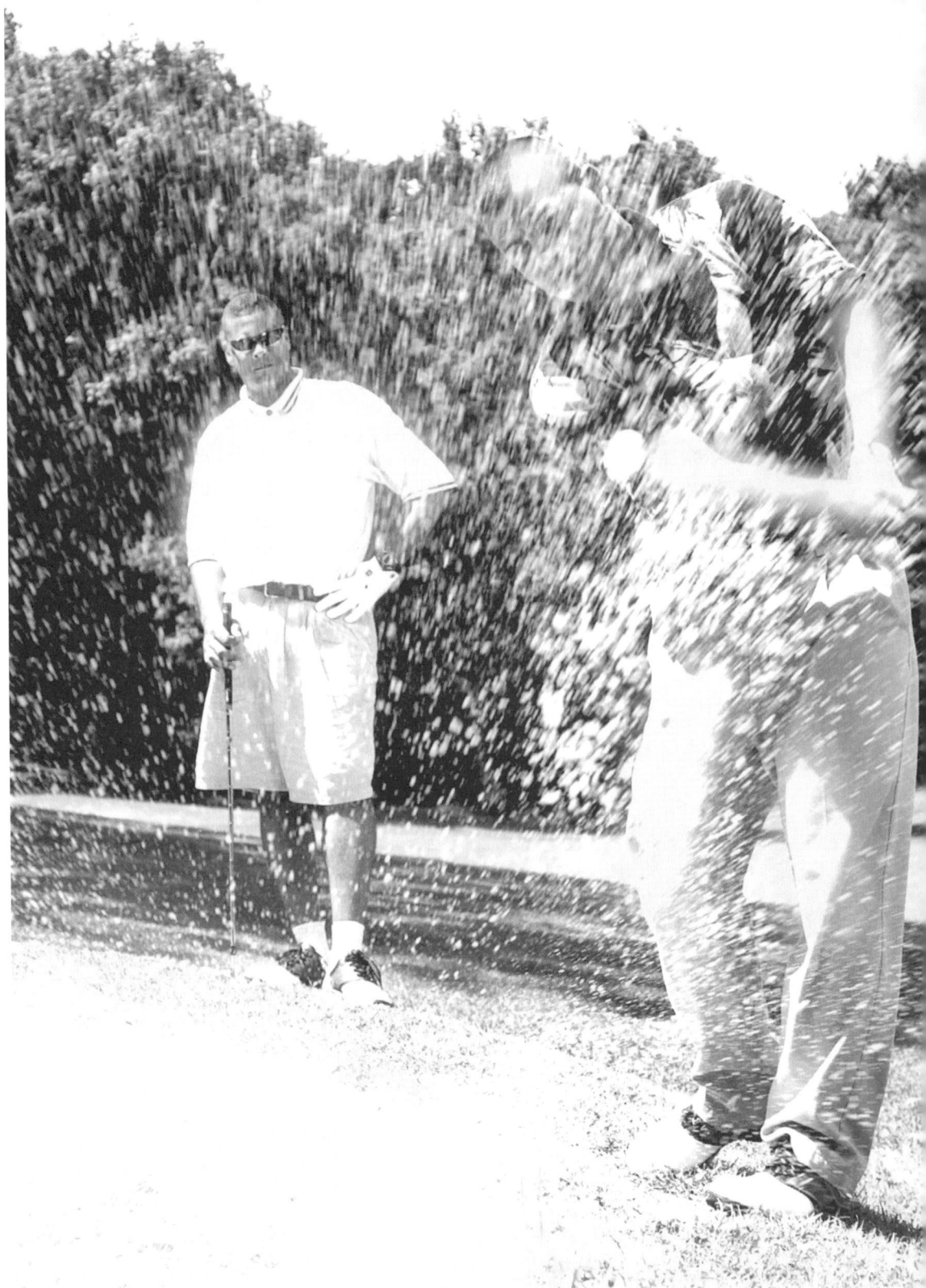

Courtesy of Lance Cpl. Christopher Roberts/U.S. Marine Corp

11

Understanding Skilled Performance: Memory, Attention, and Choking under Pressure

SIAN L. BEILOCK

Life is full of difficult tasks, ranging from playing a round of golf, to taking a college entrance exam, to giving a talk in front of your friends and colleagues. One thing that we as psychologists try to understand is the mental processes that support such skills. However, it is not just psychologists who are interested in the cognitive mechanisms that govern successful skill execution. In commenting on hitting a baseball for example, the famous Yogi Berra once said this: "How can you hit and think at the same time?" Yogi's words of wisdom suggest that thinking too much about on-line execution can be detrimental to performance. Whereas this notion might apply to the high-level hitting performance of a baseball expert, it may not extend across all levels of skill expertise or to all task types. In this chapter, I will discuss several lines of research that my colleagues and I have conducted in an attempt to shed light on differences in the attentional mechanisms governing execution across skill levels and task domains. Moreover, I will explicate how we have been using these differences in the executive control structures governing performance as a means to understand the execution failures that ensue when the attentional demands of performance are not met.

Theories of Skill Acquisition and Automaticity

The essence of Yogi Berra's quote, "How can you hit and think at the same time?" is reflected in skill acquisition and automaticity theories of high level performance. In essence, highly practiced, well-learned skills are thought to be controlled by procedural knowledge that operates largely outside of working memory (Anderson, 1993). This is in contrast to novice skill execution, which is based on declarative knowledge held in working memory and attended to in a step-by-step fashion (Fitts & Posner, 1967; Proctor & Dutta, 1995). These proposed differences in the attentional demands of novice and skilled performance reflect the idea that performance proceeds through identifiably different learning phases, characterized by both qualitative changes in the cognitive substrate governing execution and changes in performance itself.

Fitts and Posner's (1967) three-stage model of skill acquisition suggests that early in learning, novices use explicit cognitive processes to control execution in a step-by-step fashion. Because of the involvement of conscious cognitive processes, this initial stage of skill learning has been termed the *cognitive phase*. After learners understand the nature of the task, they are thought to enter an *associative phase* in which the need to consciously control real-time performance diminishes and the performer begins to develop associations between specific stimulus situations and corresponding action responses. With extended practice, performance reaches the *autonomous phase*. In this final stage of skill learning, execution is believed to be based on an automatic task representation in which conscious attentional control is no longer required to execute a particular action when confronted by a specific stimulus situation.

Although Fitts and Posner's (1967) characterization of skill level differences has been extremely influential to the study of human skill acquisition, it should be noted that their framework is mostly descriptive. Nonetheless, it does allow one to form explicit hypotheses regarding differences in the attentional demands of novice and expert performance and the memory structures associated with performance at different levels of skill learning. Importantly, these differences can be empirically verified. In the first line of work described below, my colleagues and I have attempted to test the above-mentioned hypotheses regarding differences in the attentional substrate governing novice and expert performance (Beilock, Wierenga, & Carr, 2002). Our

method involved three lines of evidence and the sensorimotor task of golf putting as our test bed.

Attention, Memory, and Control of Novice and Experienced Performance

The first comparison involved the generic knowledge and episodic memories of experienced and novice performers. *Generic* knowledge captures schema-like or prescriptive information about how a skill is typically done, whereas *episodic* knowledge captures a specific memory, an autobiographical record of a particular performance. We predicted that experienced golfers would give longer, more detailed generic descriptions of the steps involved in a typical or "generic" putt compared to the accounts given by novices. After all, experienced golfers have spent thousands of hours honing their sport skill. Such practice opportunities should provide them with an opportunity to acquire a large amount of general knowledge about how their skill is typically performed (Beilock & Carr, 2001). In contrast, if on-line, well-learned golf putting is supported by procedural knowledge (as theories of automaticity and skill acquisition would predict), experienced golfers may well give shorter, less detailed episodic recollections of any particular putt in comparison to less skilled golfers. Because proceduralization reduces the need to attend to the specific processes by which skill execution unfolds, experienced golfers' episodic recollections of step-by-step real-time performance should be impoverished. This logic is driven by demonstrations that the successful explicit retrieval of information from memory is dependent on attention to this material at the time of encoding (Craik, Govoni, Naveh-Benjamin, & Anderson, 1996; Naveh-Benjamin, Craik, Guez, & Dori, 1998). Thus, if experienced golfers are not explicitly attending to on-line performance, their memories for the specific execution processes that supported performance may suffer.

The second comparison involved the attentional demands of single versus dual-task performance. Putting performance in a single-task, isolated environment was compared to performance in a dual-task condition in which individuals performed a series of putts while simultaneously engaging in a secondary auditory monitoring task (participants monitored a series of words for a specified target word). Upon hearing the target word, individuals repeated it out loud. A recognition memory test for a subset of the distractor words heard while putting was administered after the dual-task was complete. Dual-task putting, word monitoring performance, and recognition memory for words heard while putting were used as measures of the attentional requirements involved in the golf putting task.

If well-learned putting does not require constant on-line attentional control, then the addition of a secondary monitoring task should not harm putting performance in comparison to single-task conditions. Furthermore, because experienced golfers' attentional resources should not be overly taxed by the putting task, they should have attention available to devote to the secondary task. As a result, both their target detection performance and their recognition memory for words heard while putting should be similar to that based on an auditory monitoring task performed in isolation as a baseline measure (i.e., when participants are not simultaneously performing a putting task). In contrast, novel skill execution that must be attended in real time should be differentially impacted by secondary task demands. The addition of a secondary monitoring task should not only harm novice putting performance, but should also result in poorer recognition memory for words heard while putting in comparison to the performance of either of these tasks in isolation. Novices should not be able to devote adequate attention to the monitoring task when simultaneously performing the putting task, and vice versa.

The third comparison involved our "funny putter" manipulation. My colleagues and I compared putting performance and memory protocols for experienced and novice golfers under both single-task and dual-task conditions. A subset of our novice and experienced golfers used a normal, regular putter while performing in this experiment. Another group of novices and experienced golfers used an altered "funny putter." The funny putter consisted of a regular putter head attached to an "s" shaped and arbitrarily weighted putter shaft. The design of the funny putter was intended to require experienced golfers to alter their well-practiced putting form in order to compensate for the distorted club, forcing them to al-

locate attention to the new skill execution processes. If the novel, funny putter requires experienced performers to alter skill execution processes, they should be forced to attend to task control in a step-by-step fashion in much the same way as individuals in less-practiced states. As a result, experienced golfers using the funny putter may no longer be able to attend to multiple tasks simultaneously. This would result in a decrease in dual-task putting performance and/or secondary auditory monitoring performance and recognition memory. Although the addition of novel task constraints via the funny putter may hinder performance, use of the tool should direct one's attention back to controlling the step-by-step execution of the primary task at hand, which in turn may enhance the experienced golfers' memories of how their skills unfolded. In contrast, novice performers should not be affected by the funny putter in the same way as more experienced golfers. Because novices have not yet adapted to putting under normal conditions, performance should not be drastically influenced by an altered putting environment. That is, to the novice, all putters are funny.

Eighty-four novice and experienced golfers participated in this study. Novice participants ($n = 42$) had no previous golf experience. Experienced participants ($n = 42$) were local high school and college students with 2 or more years of high school varsity golf experience or a Professional Golfers' Association (PGA) handicap less than 8. Individuals were randomly assigned within skill level to either a regular putter or funny putter condition in a 2 (novice golfer, experienced golfer) x 2 (regular putter, funny putter) experimental design, with 21 participants in each group.

All participants took part in the same experimental procedure. Individuals first took 2 blocks of 20 putts followed by a generic memory questionnaire. The first block was designed to familiarize participants with the putting task and served as a pre-test measure of performance. The second block served as the single-task condition. Next, participants completed a word monitoring task in which they listened for a target word embedded in a series of words being played from a tape recorder, and upon hearing the target, repeated it aloud. The monitoring task was followed immediately by a short arithmetic task. The purpose of this task was to eliminate recency effects associated with the word list in the monitoring task. A recognition memory test for a subset of the words presented in the single-task word monitoring condition was then administered. Participants next performed a dual-task putting and word monitoring task followed by an episodic memory questionnaire. Finally, participants completed a second arithmetic task after which they received another recognition memory test based on a subset of the words presented during the dual-task putting and word monitoring condition.

Thus, all participants, regardless of skill level or putter type, went through the exact same experimental procedure. We can now look to putting performance, recognition memory for words heard while putting, and generic and episodic memory protocols to explore differences in the on-line attentional demands of golf putting performance at different levels of expertise

In terms of putting performance, as can be seen in Figure 1, both novice groups (regular and funny putter), as well as experienced golfers using the funny putter showed performance decrements from the single-task to the dual-task putting condition. In contrast, experienced golfers using the regular putter continued to improve in putting accuracy from the single to dual-task condition.

There were no significant differences in target word identification across novice and experienced golfers for either the single-task auditory monitoring task or the dual-task auditory monitoring condition. This is likely due to the fact that target word identification failure occurred relatively infrequently across both conditions. In terms of recognition memory for words heard while putting, however, differences similar to those observed in primary putting performance are evident. As seen in Figure 2, both of the novice groups and the experienced golfers using the funny putter showed decrements in recognition memory (A) for words heard while putting, in comparison to a single-task word recognition test given as a base-line measure. The experienced golfers using the regular putter did not show this decrement in word recognition performance.

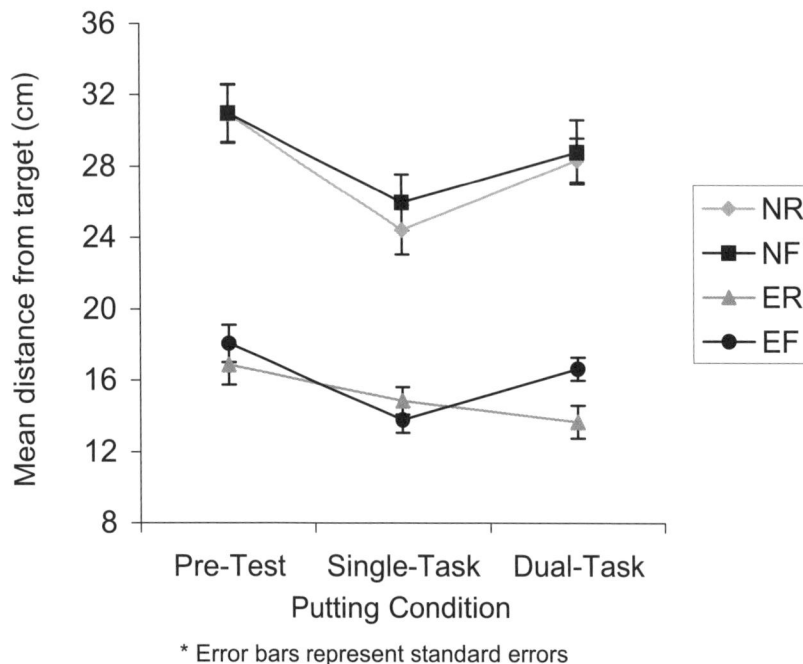

* Error bars represent standard errors

Figure 1. Mean distance (cm) from the target that the ball stopped after each putt in the pre-test, single-task, and dual-task conditions for the novices using the regular putter (NR), the novices using the funny putter (NF), the experts using the regular putter (ER), and the experts using the funny putter (EF). Reprinted from Beilock, S.L., Wierenga, S.A., & Carr, T.H. (2002). Expertise, attention, and memory in sensorimotor skill execution: Impact of novel task constraints on dual-task performance and episodic memory. *The Quarterly Journal of Experimental Psychology: Human Experimental Psychology, 55,* 1211-1240.

Thus, as illustrated by both putting performance and word recognition data, performing in a dual-task environment harmed novice golfers and experienced golfers using the funny putter, but did not disrupt putting performance or word recognition ability in experienced golfers putting under normal conditions. These results suggest that expertise leads to the encoding of task components in a proceduralized form that supports effective real-time performance, without the need for constant on-line attentional control. As a result, experienced golfers, performing under normal, practiced conditions, are better able than novices to allocate a portion of their attention to other stimuli and task demands if the situation requires it. However, these experienced golfers should be less able to allocate attention to and remember the step-by-step details of their performance. We can look to the generic and episodic memory protocols as a means to address this question.

As seen in Figure 3, protocol data showed that novice golfers produced short generic descriptions and longer episodic recollections. The type of putter did not influence novices' protocols. This is to be expected, given that the novices were not experienced with either putter type. Experienced golfers using the regular putter produced an opposite pattern. Their generic descriptions were longer than those of the novices, reflecting golf expertise. Additionally, regular putter experts gave shorter episodic recollections in comparison to their generic descriptions and also in comparison to novices' episodic recollections. This impoverished episodic recollection demonstrates what Beilock and Carr (2001) have termed "expertise-induced amnesia." Although the extensive generic knowledge of experts may be declaratively accessible during off-line reflection, it does not appear to be accessed during real-time performance controlled by automated procedural knowledge. In contrast, experienced golfers using the funny putter did not show impoverished episodic recollection. These experts provided the most elaborate generic and episodic protocols, and their episodic recollections were longer than their generic descriptions, as opposed to those produced by the regular

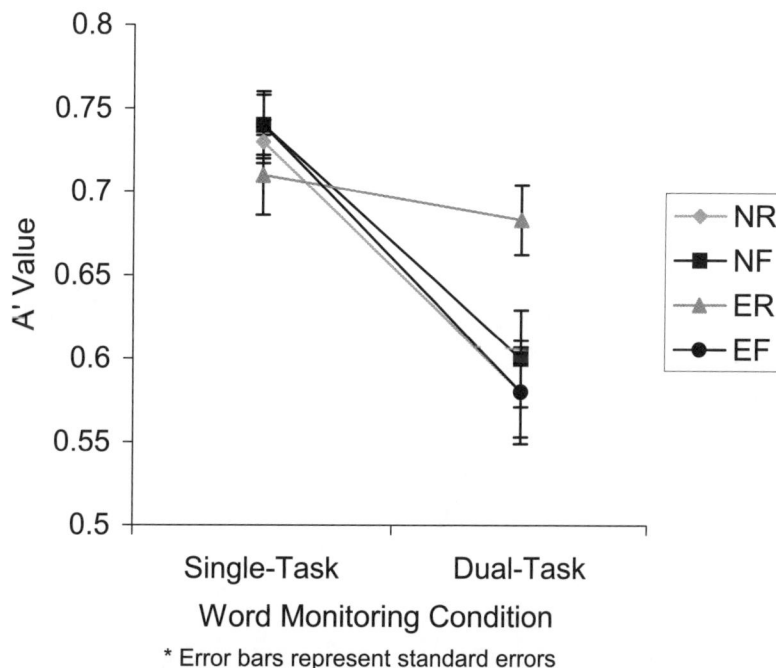

Figure 2. Mean A' value for the single-task and dual-task recognition memory tests for the novices using the regular putter (NR), the novices using the funny putter (NF), the experts using the regular putter (ER), and the experts using the funny putter (EF). Reprinted from Beilock, S.L., Wierenga, S.A., & Carr, T.H. (2002). Expertise, attention, and memory in sensorimotor skill execution: Impact of novel task constraints on dual-task performance and episodic memory. *The Quarterly Journal of Experimental Psychology: Human Experimental Psychology, 55,* 1211-1240.

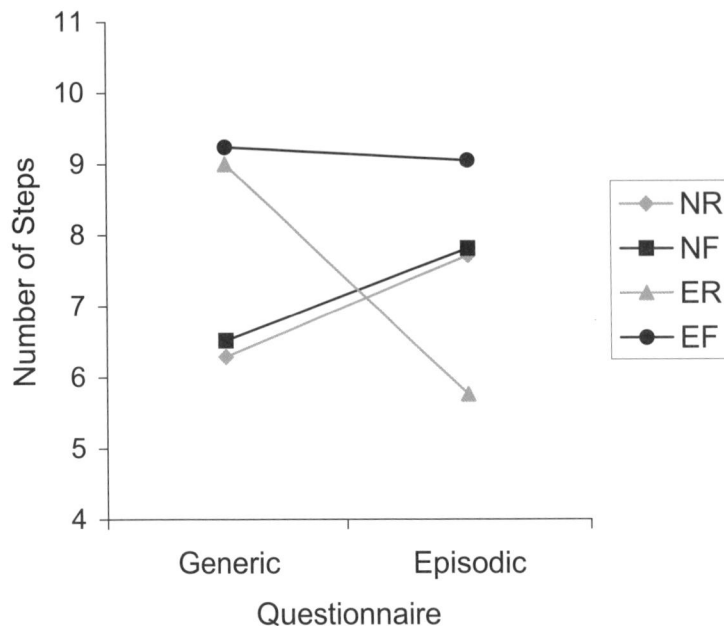

Figure 3. Mean number of steps for the generic and episodic questionnaires for the novices using the regular putter (NR), the novices using the funny putter (NF), the experts using the regular putter (ER), and the experts using the funny putter (EF). Reprinted from Beilock, S.L., Wierenga, S.A., & Carr, T.H. (2002). Expertise, attention, and memory in sensorimotor skill execution: Impact of novel task constraints on dual-task performance and episodic memory. *The Quarterly Journal of Experimental Psychology: Human Experimental Psychology, 55,* 1211-1240.

putter experts. Thus, when a proceduralized skill is disrupted by the imposition of novel task demands, expertise-induced amnesia disappears. Furthermore, when experts start attending to task performance, their expert knowledge allows them to remember more of what they are attending to than novices.

Although examining the overall number of steps reported in the memory protocols lends some insight into what our golfers were attending to during on-line execution and, thus, what they were able to explicitly retrieve after the fact, one way to more specifically address this issue is to look at the types of golf-related steps participants reported in their generic and episodic memory protocols. To achieve this goal, we divided protocol steps into three categories. Assessment or planning referred to deciding how to take a particular putt and what properties the putt ought to have. Examples are "I looked to see how far from the target I was," "there is little or no break in the putt," "look at the contour of the green," and "mentally create a line of sight" (from the ball to the hole or target). Mechanics or execution referred to the components of the mechanical act that implements the putt. Examples are "grip the

putter," "take the putter back," and "follow through as far as putter was taken back," all of which deal with the effectors and the kinesthetic movements of the effectors required to implement a putt. Ball destinations or outcomes referred to where the ball stopped or landed.

Because the altered weight and shape of the funny putter was designed to directly affect the mechanical aspect of the putting task in the present study, one might imagine the most striking differences in memory protocols would be observed as a function of putter type and expertise in the reporting of mechanical steps. This is precisely what occurred. Experienced golfers using the funny putter gave somewhat more mechanics steps in their episodic protocol in comparison to their generic description. In contrast, experienced golfers using the regular putter gave significantly fewer. Thus, both sets of golfers gave varied accounts of the mechanical properties involved in their putting performance in a manner consistent with the fact that one group used a tool designed to specifically alter how one attends to the mechanics of putting. The novices using regular and funny putters did not differ in their mechanics accounts. Both groups gave more detailed mechanical descriptions in their episodic, in comparison to generic, protocols. Because novices must attend to execution in a step-by-step fashion, this explicit on-line attentional control affords them the ability to remember how their execution actually unfolded. For a detailed description of protocol reports, see Beilock et al. (2002).

This experiment documents a particular property of the cognitive substrate of sensorimotor skill execution—namely, the declarative accessibility, or openness to introspection and report, of skill processes and procedures at different levels of expertise. Inferences can be made from experienced and novice golfers' generic and episodic memory representations concerning the underlying control structures driving real-time performance. Specifically, the real-time control structures supporting performance differ as a function of skill level. Novice performances are attended to on-line. Experienced skill execution (especially mechanical instantiation) does not mandate step-by-step attentional control, as long as experienced golfers are operating in a normal environment with normal task tools. These conclusions are relevant to understanding expertise, and may also lend insight into performance decrements in situations (e.g., high pressure situations) that tend to force attention to performance in ways that may be non-optimal, especially for highly skilled performers. The next section, detailing the cognitive mechanisms governing suboptimal performance in high-pressure situations, addresses just this issue.

Choking under Pressure

The desire to perform as well as possible in situations with a high degree of perceived importance is thought to create performance pressure (Baumeister, 1984; Hardy, Mullen, & Jones, 1996). Paradoxically, despite the fact that *performance pressure* often results from aspirations to function at an optimal level, pressure-packed situations are where suboptimal skill execution may be most visible. The term *choking under pressure* has been used to describe this phenomenon. Choking is defined as performing more poorly than expected given one's skill level, and is thought to occur across many diverse task domains where incentives for optimal performance

are at a maximum (Beilock & Carr, 2001; Lewis & Linder, 1997; Masters, 1992; Wang, Marchant, & Morris, 2004).

Although documenting instances of choking under pressure (in both laboratory and real world settings) provides insight into the conditions under which this type of skill failure occurs, it is an understanding of the cognitive mechanisms governing pressure-induced failure that will truly advance our knowledge of the choking phenomenon. Moreover, a clear picture of choking processes sets the stage for the development of training regimens designed to alleviate these unwanted performance failures. The obvious question then is "Why does choking under pressure occur?"

The following sections outline two of the main attentional theories that have been used to account for performance decrements under pressure and the empirical research my colleagues and I have conducted in an attempt to test these accounts of less-than-optimal performance. It should be noted that, although the majority of this research focuses on how high-demand situations change the deployment of attentional resources during on-line execution, there is also work examining the physiological and biomechanical processes associated with less-than-optimal performance. A full account of these processes is outside the scope of the current work. For a detailed review, see Beilock and Gray (in press).

Explicit Monitoring Theories

Explicit monitoring theories suggest that pressure situations raise self-consciousness and anxiety about performing correctly (Baumeister, 1984). This focus on the self is thought to prompt individuals to turn their attention inward on the specific processes of performance in an attempt to exert more explicit monitoring and control than would be applied in a non-pressure situation (Baumeister, 1984; Beilock & Carr, 2001; Lewis & Linder, 1997). Such explicit attention to step-by-step skill processes and procedures is thought to disrupt well-learned or proceduralized performance processes that normally run largely outside of conscious awareness (Beilock, Bertenthal, McCoy, & Carr, 2004; Kimble & Perlmuter, 1970; Langer & Imber, 1979). Masters' (1992) *reinvestment theory* suggests that the specific mechanism governing explicit monitoring is "dechunking."

Pressure-induced attention to execution causes an integrated or proceduralized control structure that normally runs off without interruptions to be broken back down into a sequence of smaller, independent units—similar to how the performance was organized early in learning.

Recently, researchers have conducted a number of studies to examine the attentional correlates of suboptimal performance under pressure in high level sensorimotor skills using explicit monitoring theories as a guideline. Many of these studies do not involve pressure at all, but attempt to mimic the attentional demands that pressure might induce. The logic here is that if researchers can discover the types of attentional manipulations that compromise performance, they can then use this evidence to begin to infer how pressure might exert its impact.

Beilock, Carr, MacMahon, and Starkes (2002) directly manipulated the attentional focus of experienced soccer players while they were performing a soccer dribbling task. Experienced soccer players dribbled the ball through a series of cones while performing either a secondary auditory monitoring task (designed to distract attention away from execution—similar to the auditory monitoring task used in Beilock et al.'s (2002) golf putting work mentioned earlier) or a skill-focused task in which individuals monitored the side of the foot that most recently contacted the ball (designed to draw attention to a component process of performance, mimicking the proposed mechanism of explicit monitoring theories). Performing in a dual-task environment did not harm the dribbling skill of experienced soccer players in comparison to a single-task practice condition used as a baseline. When the soccer players were instructed to attend to performance (i.e., monitoring the side of the foot that most recently contacted the ball), their dribbling skill deteriorated in comparison to both the dual-task condition and a single-task baseline. Consistent with explicit monitoring theories of choking, step-by-step attention to skill processes and procedures appears to harm well-learned performance.

Supporting evidence regarding the differential impact of distraction versus skill-focused attention has also been obtained from a different kind of manipulation: speed versus accuracy performance instructions. Beilock et al. (2004) found that simply limiting the opportunity for skill-focused, explicit monitoring through instructions to perform a putting task rapidly improved the performance of experienced golfers, relative to a condition in which the same golfers were told to take as much time as they needed to be accurate. The impact of this manipulation was phenomenologically noticeable. Several golfers reported that the speed instructions aided their performance by keeping them from thinking too much about execution.

Although these types of attention studies lend indirect insight into the cognitive mechanisms driving skill failure in high stakes situations, it is also possible to more directly assess the impact of pressure to perform at a high level on skill execution. In a recent study, Gray (2004) directly investigated the effects of performance pressure on baseball batting in highly skilled Division I Intercollegiate baseball players. Individuals performed a virtual batting task in a pre-test situation and were then split into two groups. Batters in the "pressure group" were instructed that they had been paired with one other batter in the study and they would receive a monetary reward if both of them could increase their total number of hits in the next block of trials by a designated amount. Batters in this group were further instructed that their teammate had already successfully reached the criterion for reward. Thus, both social pressure and monetary incentives were used to induce feelings of performance pressure in the baseball players (a manipulation first used by Beilock & Carr in 2001). Batters in a second, "control group," were given no further information. Both groups (i.e., pressure and control) then continued to perform the virtual batting task (i.e., in a post-test).

Batters in the pressure group exhibited clear choking effects. Mean temporal batting errors were significantly higher following the pressure manipulation in comparison to previously. Not only did these batters fail to reach the incentive criterion, their performance under pressure was actually worse than their baseline performance—direct evidence of choking. In terms of batters in the control group, there was no significant difference between mean temporal errors in the two blocks of trials. The most interesting result, however, comes from evidence documenting how the pressure situation changed the attentional focus of the baseball players. While performing in the post-test, both the pressure and control participants were asked to judge the direction their bat was moving at specified intervals. In the pressure group there was a significant decrease in the percentage of judgment errors in this task in comparison to a pre-test used as a baseline. This decrease was not seen for control group participants. This result indicates that the pressure caused batters to turn their attention inwards and explicitly monitor their swing execution. Although this pressure-induced change in attentional deployment resulted in more accurate skill-focused judgments, it also appeared to disrupt automated execution processes, resulting in less-than-optimal batting performance.

Explicit monitoring theories of choking under pressure suggest that suboptimal performance of a well-learned skill under pressure results from an attempt to exert explicit monitoring and control on proceduralized knowledge that is best run-off as an uninterrupted and unanalyzed structure (Baumeister, 1984; Beilock & Carr, 2001; Beilock et al., 2002; Lewis & Linder, 1997; Masters, 1992). Thus, high-level skills based on an automated or proceduralized skill representation may be more susceptible to the negative consequences of performance pressure than less practiced performances. This is due to the fact that the former operate largely outside of working memory, and pressure-induced attention should most strongly disrupt processes that are normally devoid of step-by-step attentional control.

Beilock and Carr (2001) have found support for the notion that well-learned, but not novice, sensorimotor skill execution is susceptible to performance decrements under pressure via this mechanism of inappropriate explicit monitoring or execution focus. Participants learned a golf putting skill to a high level and were exposed to a high-pressure situation both early and late in practice. Early in practice, pressure to do well did not harm performance. At later stages of learning, performance decrements under pressure emerged. Thus, it appears that the proceduralized performances of experts are negatively affected by performance pressure. Novice skill execution, however, is not harmed by pressure-induced attention to execution, because less skilled performance is already explicitly attended to in real time. This finding is consistent with Marchant and Wang's (2001) assertion that most of the evidence for choking under

pressure has been derived from well-learned sensorimotor tasks that automate via proceduralization with extended practice (see also, Wang, Marchant, Morris, & Gibbs, 2004).

All of this evidence suggests that explicit monitoring theories account quite well for the choking phenomenon. One might notice, however, that a majority of the skills used in the research mentioned here were well-learned sensorimotor skills that are thought to run largely outside of working memory with extended practice (Fitts & Posner, 1967; Keele, 1986; Proctor & Dutta, 1995). Working memory is a short-term memory system that is involved in the control, regulation, and active maintenance of a limited amount of information with immediate relevance to the task at hand (Miyake & Shah, 1999). Although the types of well-learned sensorimotor skills that have been studied so far (e.g., a well-learned golf putt on a straight, flat green) may not rely heavily on working memory, there are sports skills that likely utilize working memory resources. This applies, in particular, to skills that involve holding and manipulating information on line, such as the types of decision making and strategizing that are important components of high level performance (e.g., reading a complex green, strategizing about an upcoming move). Thus, it is an open question as to how skills that *do* rely heavily on working memory fare in a demanding high pressure situation. It seems unlikely that such skills would fail because of pressure-induced attention to execution, as these skills are presumably already attended to on line. Thus, are there other mechanisms by which such skills might fail?

Distraction Theories

If we look to literature in which heavily working memory-demanding skills have been tested (e.g., the test-taking and math anxiety literature), most individuals believe pressure-induced distraction underlies such unwanted performance decrements (as opposed to the type of pressure-induced over-attention that explicit monitoring theories support). Specifically, *distraction theories* propose that pressure influences task performance by creating a distracting environment that compromises the working memory resources available for primary task performance. Distraction-based accounts of suboptimal performance suggest that performance pressure shifts attentional focus to task-irrelevant cues, such as worries about the situation and its consequences. This shift of focus changes what was single-task performance into a dual-task situation in which controlling the task at hand and worrying about the situation compete for the limited working memory resources of the performer.

The most notable arguments for the distraction hypothesis come from research involving academic test anxiety (Ashcraft & Kirk, 2001; Eysenck, 1979; Wine, 1971). Individuals who become highly anxious during test situations, and consequently perform at a suboptimal level, are thought to divide their attention between task-relevant and task-irrelevant thoughts more so than those who do not become overly anxious in high pressure situations (Wine, 1971).

Additional support for a distraction account of choking comes from recent work specifically examining the impact of performance pressure on cognitive task performance. Beilock, Kulp, Holt, and Carr (2004) had individuals perform easy math problems, as well as those that placed heavy demands on working memory, in both low and high pressure situations. The high pressure scenario was based on several sources of pressure that commonly exist across skill domains—monetary incentives, peer pressure, and social evaluation. Although it is an empirical question as to exactly how these different sources of pressure exert their influence, the purpose of the study was to capture the real-world phenomenon of choking. Thus, we created a pressure scenario that incorporated as many components of high pressure performance as possible. In athletics, for example, performance is frequently scrutinized by others, there are often monetary consequences for winning and losing, and team success is dependent on the performance of individual athletes, which may generate peer pressure to perform at an optimal level. In academic arenas, monetary consequences for test performance are manifested in terms of scholarships, and future educational opportunities and social evaluation of performance come from mentors, teachers, and peers.

Beilock, Kulp et al. (2004) found that pressure does indeed cause individuals to worry. Moreover, only those math problems that were strongly reliant on the working memory resources that such worries are thought to consume caused signs of failure

under pressure. Thus, there is evidence that pressure can compromise working memory resources, causing failure in tasks that rely heavily on this system. Support comes from working-memory-intensive math problem solving under pressure (Beilock, Kulp et al., 2004). There is also added support in terms of susceptibility to choking under pressure as a function of working memory capacity.

In particular, my colleague and I have examined the relation between pressure-induced performance decrements in mathematical problem solving and individual differences in working memory capacity (Beilock & Carr, 2005). As mentioned earlier, working memory at heart involves control, regulation, and active maintenance of a limited amount of information with immediate relevance to the task at hand (Miyake & Shah, 1999). Some people have more of this ability (high working memory individuals) and some have less (low working memory individuals). In this work, individuals lower or higher in working memory performed both easy and difficult math problems under low pressure and high pressure conditions. The pressure condition was created by implementing the same scenario described in the Beilock, Kulp et al. (2004) research previously outlined.

As can be seen in Figure 4, decrements under pressure were limited to difficult problems that made the largest demands on working memory, as one might expect. Surprisingly, however, only individuals high in working memory capacity showed these decrements. Individuals lower in working memory capacity performed less well on high-demand problems in the absence of pressure, but did not decline from their established (though significantly lower) level of achievement when pressure was applied. Under normal conditions, high working memory individuals outperform low working memory individuals because they have superior attentional allocation capacities of these types. When such attentional capacity is compromised, the advantage for high working memory individuals disappears. Thus, this work provides support for a distraction-based account of performance pressure by demonstrating systematic differences in susceptibility to performance pressure as a function of individual differences in working memory capacity. That is, to the extent that pressure can operate by impacting the working memory resources available for performance, it follows that

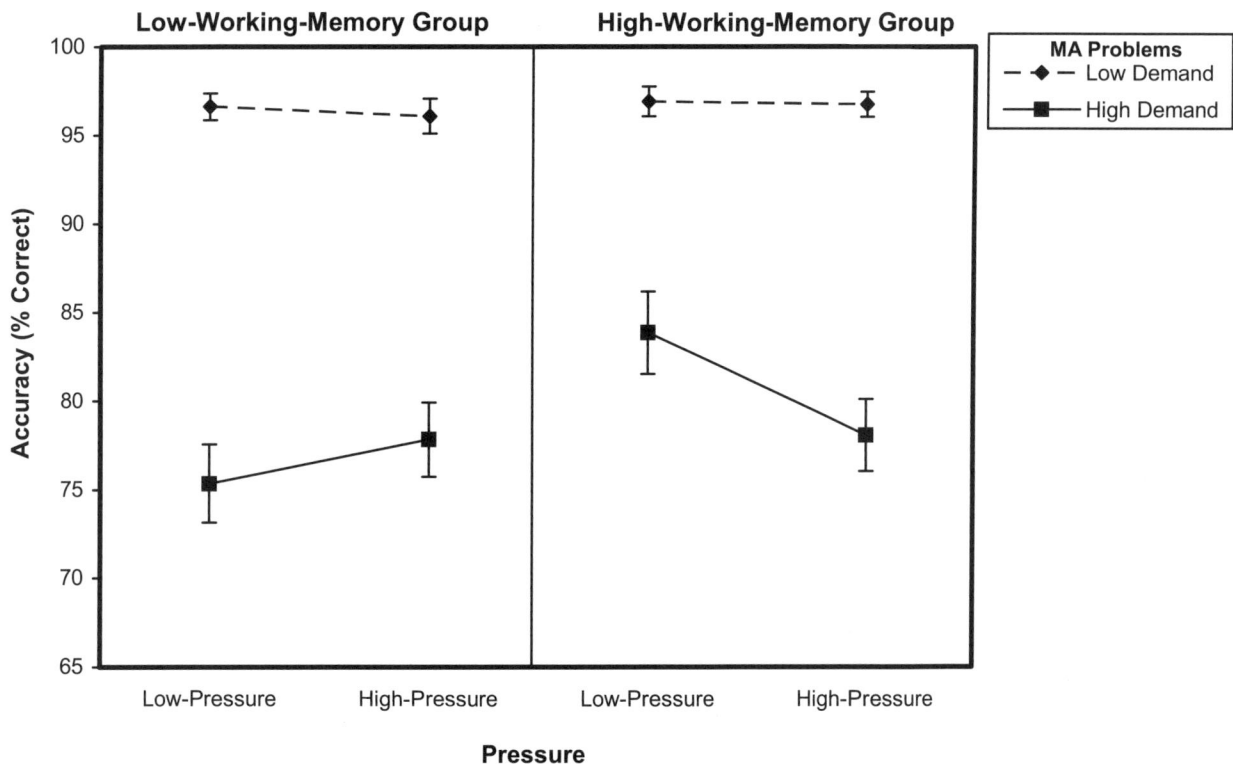

Figure 4. Mean accuracy (upper graph) and mean reaction time (lower graph) for the low-working-memory group (left panel) and for the high-working-memory group (right panel) for the easy (low demand) and difficult (high demand) math problems in the low-pressure and high-pressure tests. Error bars represent standard errors. Reprinted from Beilock, S.L., & Carr, T.H. (2005). When high-powered people fail: Working memory and "choking under pressure" in math. *Psychological Science, 16,* 101-105.

individual differences in this resource should moderate the impact of pressure on performance.

Performance Pressure's Dual Impact

Explicit monitoring and distraction theories essentially make opposite predictions regarding how pressure exerts its impact. Distraction theories suggest that pressure shifts needed attention away from execution; explicit monitoring theories suggest that pressure shifts too much attention to skill execution processes. Can both theories be correct?

Beilock, Kulp, et al. (2004) have suggested that performance pressure creates two effects that alter how attention is allocated to execution: (1) Pressure induces worries about the situation and its consequences, thereby reducing working memory capacity available for performance, as distraction theories would propose. (2) At the same time, pressure prompts individuals to attempt to control execution in order to ensure optimal performance, in line with explicit monitoring theories. This suggests that how

a skill fails is dependent on performance representation and implementation.

Tasks that require executive control of a sequence of steps or maintenance of intermediate products may fail via pressure-induced consumption of working memory (e.g., complex math tasks, sport strategizing). In contrast, tasks that automate via proceduralization should fail when attention is drawn to step-by-step execution (e.g., a well-learned and repeatedly executed golf putt). It is important to note that it does not seem to be merely a cognitive versus motor distinction that predicts how a skill will fail under pressure. That is, just because one is performing an academically based, cognitive task does not mean this task will show signs of failure via pressure-induced distraction. Likewise, sports skills do not necessarily fail via pressure-induced explicit monitoring. Rather, it appears to be the manner in which skills utilize on-line attentional resources that dictates how they will fail (though this is often related to skill domain).

Thus, sports skills that make heavy demands on working memory, such as strategizing, problem solving, and decision making (i.e., skills that involve considering multiple options simultaneously and updating information in real time) will likely fail as a result of pressure-induced working memory consumption—similar to a working-memory-dependent academic task. These skills, however, will be relatively impervious to attempts at focusing one's remaining attention on step-by-step control that is also induced by pressure. In contrast, sensorimotor skills that run largely outside of working memory will fail when pressure-induced attention disrupts automated control processes—and not because the overall capacity of working memory has been reduced. Of course, future work is needed to fully understand how pressure situations exert their impact across the entire range of skills for which important performances sometimes result in disappointing outcomes.

Conclusion

In conclusion, in this chapter I have presented two different lines of work that focus on the acquisition and maintenance of complex skills. The first line utilizes differences in the memory structures and on-line attentional demands of novice and expert sensorimotor skill execution (e.g., golf putting) to develop an account of the real-time control structures supporting motor skill performance across levels of learning. This work was followed by a presentation of my recent research examining the executive control processes supporting higher level cognitive tasks (e.g., mathematical problem solving) in demanding and high pressure situations. Together, these two lines of work demonstrate how task type and skill level differences in the attentional demands governing performance can be used to understand the nature of successful skill execution and why, at times, it fails to occur. Thus, if one brings the chapter back full circle to Yogi Berra's quote presented in the first paragraph (i.e., "How can you hit and think at the same time?"), the answer seems to be that it depends—it depends on the skill level of the performer and the cognitive demands of the skill being performed.

References

Anderson, J. R. (1993). *Rules of mind*. Hillsdale, NJ: Erlbaum.

Ashcraft, M. H., & Kirk, E. P. (2001). The relationships among working memory, math anxiety, and performance. *Journal of Experimental Psychology: General, 130*, 224-237.

Baumeister, R. F. (1984). Choking under pressure: Self-consciousness and paradoxical effects of incentives on skillful performance. *Journal of Personality and Social Psychology, 46*, 610-620.

Beilock, S. L., Bertenthal, B. I., McCoy, A. M., & Carr, T. H. (2004). Haste does not always make waste: Expertise, direction of attention, and speed versus accuracy in performing sensorimotor skills. *Psychonomic Bulletin & Review, 11*, 373-379.

Beilock, S. L. & Carr, T. H. (2001). On the fragility of skilled performance: What governs choking under pressure? *Journal of Experimental Psychology: General, 130*, 701-725.

Beilock, S. L., & Carr, T. H. (2005). When high-powered people fail: Working memory and "choking under pressure" in math. *Psychological Science, 16*, 101-105.

Beilock, S. L., Carr, T. H., MacMahon, C., & Starkes, J. L. (2002). When paying attention becomes counterproductive: Impact of divided versus skill-focused attention on novice and experienced performance of sensorimotor skills. *Journal of Experimental Psychology: Applied, 8*, 6-16.

Beilock, S. L., & Gray, R. (in press). Why do athletes "choke" under pressure? In G. Tenenbaum and B. Eklund (Eds.), *Handbook of sport psychology* (3rd ed.). Wiley.

Beilock, S. L., Kulp, C. A., Holt, L. E., & Carr, T. H. (2004). More on the fragility of performance: Choking under pressure in mathematical problem solving. *Journal of Experimental Psychology: General, 133*, 584-600.

Beilock, S. L., Wierenga, S. A., & Carr, T. H. (2002). Expertise, attention, and memory in sensorimotor skill execution: Impact of novel task constraints on dual-task performance and episodic memory. *The Quarterly Journal of Experimental Psychology: Human Experimental Psychology, 55*, 1211-1240.

Craik F. I. M., Govoni R., Naveh-Benjamin M., & Anderson N. D. (1996). The effects of divided attention on encoding and retrieval processes in human memory. *Journal of Experimental Psychology: General, 125*, 159-180.

Eysenck, M. W. (1979). Anxiety learning and memory: A reconceptualization. *Journal of Research in Personality, 13*, 363-385.

Fitts, P. M., & Posner, M. I. (1967). *Human performance*. Belmont, CA: Brooks/Cole.

Gray, R. (2004). Attending to the execution of a complex sensori-motor skill: Expertise differences, choking and slumps. *Journal of Experimental Psychology: Applied, 10*, 42-54.

Hardy, L., Mullen, R., & Jones, G. (1996). Knowledge and conscious control of motor actions under stress. *British Journal of Psychology, 87*, 621-636.

Keele, S. W. (1986). Motor control. In K. R. Boff, L. Kaufman, & J. P. Thomas (Eds.), *Handbook of perception and human performance* (Vol. 7). New York: Wiley.

Kimble, G. A., & Perlmuter, L. C. (1970). The problem of volition. *Psychological Review, 77*, 361-384.

Langer, E., & Imber, G. (1979). When practice makes imperfect:

Debilitating effects of overlearning. *Journal of Personality and Social Psychology, 37,* 2014-2024.

Lewis, B., & Linder, D. (1997). Thinking about choking? Attentional processes and paradoxical performance. *Personality and Social Psychology Bulletin, 23,* 937-944.

Marchant, D. B., & Wang, J. (2001). Choking: Current issues in theory and practice. Paper presented at the 10th World Congress of Sport Psychology, Skiathos Island, Greece.

Masters, R. S. W. (1992). Knowledge, knerves and know-how: The role of explicit versus implicit knowledge in the breakdown of a complex motor skill under pressure. *British Journal of Psychology, 83,* 343-358.

Miyake, A., & Shah, P. (1999). Toward unified theories of working memory: Emerging general consensus, unresolved theoretical issues, and future research directions. In A. Miyake & P. Shah (Eds.), *Models of working memory: Mechanisms of active maintenance and executive control* (pp. 442-481). New York: Cambridge University Press.

Naveh-Benjamin, M., Craik, F .I. M., Guez, J., & Dori, H. (1998). Effects of divided attention on encoding and retrieval processes in human memory: Further support for an asymmetry. *Journal of Experimental Psychology: Learning, Memory, and Cognition, 24,* 1091-1104.

Proctor, R. W., & Dutta, A. (1995). *Skill acquisition and human performance.* Thousand Oaks, CA: Sage.

Wang, J., Marchant, D. B., & Morris, T. (2004). Coping style and susceptibility to choking under pressure. *Journal of Sport Behavior, 27,* 75-92.

Wang, J., Marchant, D., Morris, T., & Gibbs, P. (2004). Self-consciousness and trait anxiety as predictors of choking in sport. *Journal of Science in Medicine and Sport, 7,* 174-185.

Wine, J. (1971). Test anxiety and direction of attention. *Psychological Bulletin, 76,* 92-104.

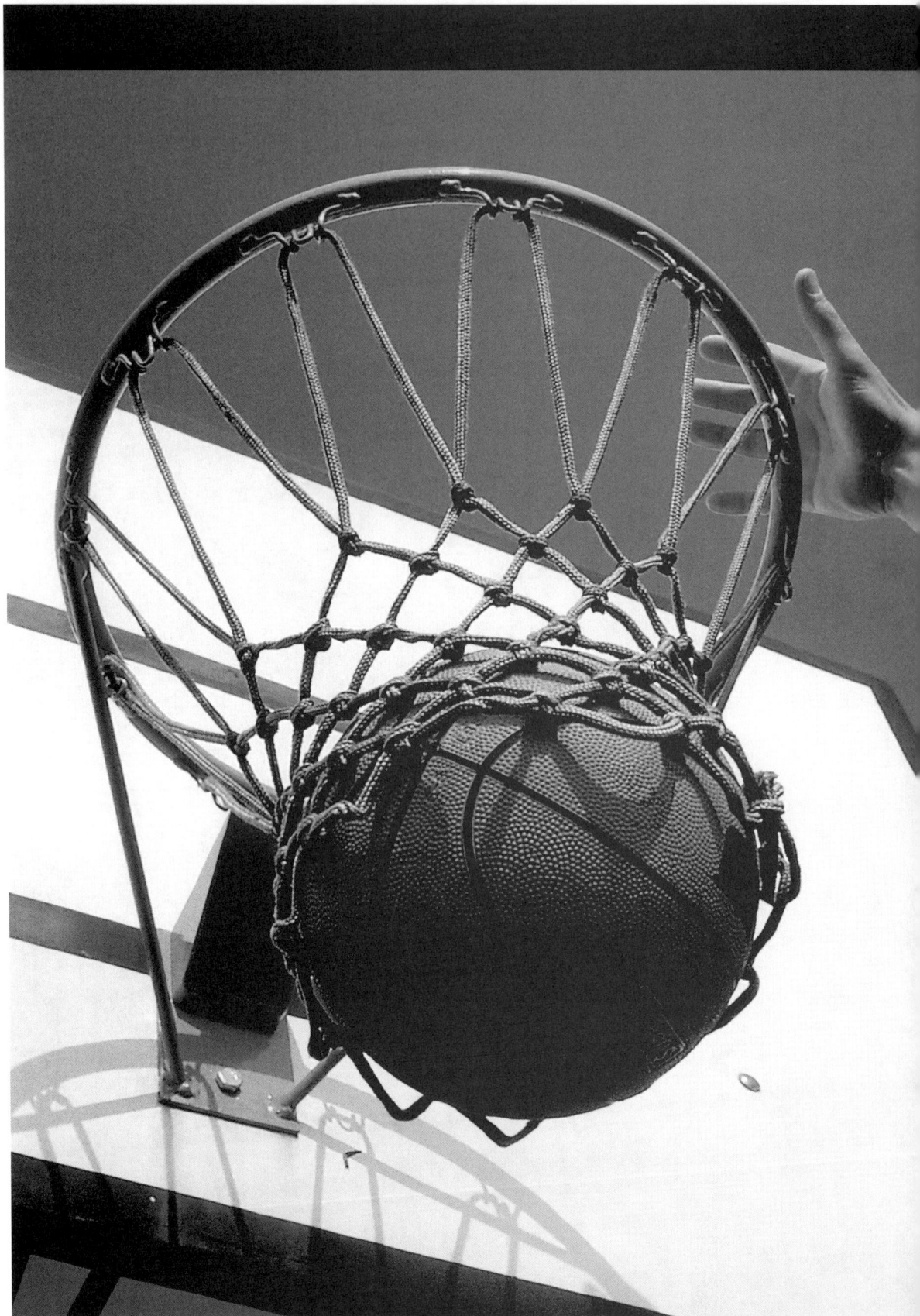

12

Epilogue to *Sport and Exercise Psychology: International Perspectives*

PETER TERRY, SANDY GORDON, AND TONY MORRIS

Introduction

In August 2005, after several years of preparation, the plans finally became reality. Almost 600 delegates from over 50 countries descended on the Darling Harbour Convention Centre, in the heart of the beautiful city of Sydney, Australia, to attend the 11th ISSP World Congress of Sport Psychology, *Promoting Health and Performance for Life*. For five stimulating days, sport and exercise psychologists from around the world came together, ostensibly to share their research findings and practitioner experiences and to hold business meetings, but in reality to do much more—to engage in impromptu seminars over lunch, to plan research collaborations, to so-

cialize together, and to forge lifelong friendships. In short, they came to strengthen the worldwide sport psychology community. Even the sometimes fickle Sydney weather put on a big, sunny smile befitting the occasion.

This chapter has been written to serve three purposes; firstly, to provide a brief commentary on the contributions to this book of the keynote and invited presenters; secondly, to document the principal events over the period of ISSP 2005, including the highlights of the scientific and social programs; and thirdly, to evaluate the strengths and weaknesses of the 11th World Congress, using both quantitative and qualitative delegate feedback data plus our own impressions of the event.

Contributions by Keynote and Invited Presenters

Most of those who have contributed chapters to this book were chosen as keynote speakers at ISSP 2005 for the simple reason that they are seen as world leaders in their field. As such, they were selected by the ISSP Managing Council to provide scholarly critiques of research or reviews in their particular areas of expertise. This book therefore represents a state-of-the-art collection of writings on the psychology of sport from a very wide range of perspectives. As noted in Chapter 1, the chapters in this book, based on invited presentations, are organized in a thematic sequence, starting with theory and research in sport psychology, moving on to sport psychology practice, then psychology of exercise, cognitive psychology and psychophysiology, and, finally, motor skill and expert performance. There are two chapters in each thematic section.

Following our introductory chapter, Dr. Carol Dweck, professor of psychology at Stanford University and the opening keynote presenter at ISSP 2005, provided a broad but insightful overview of the characteristics of a sporting champion in Chapter 2. Dweck opined that champion athletes differ from others at least in part because of their mindset. Her *entity* and *incremental* self-theories of intelligence provide a fascinating perspective on how champions tend to think, feel, and behave. Her arguments are well supported by results of research she and her colleagues have conducted to investigate how well these two self-theories—entity and incremental—can explain different levels of goal achievement behavior, effort, coping, and confidence. Dweck also discussed the constructs of potential and talent, acknowledging their importance in athlete development but concluding that mindset is of at least equal importance. Perhaps the most significant conclusion to be drawn from the research of Dweck and others referred to in the chapter is that mindset can be learned. The idea that sport psychologists, coaches, and parents are able to socialize a desire for learning, perseverance, and commitment, while subsequently promoting confidence and enjoyment, seems a particularly attractive and compelling proposition.

In Chapter 3, ISSP Young Investigator award winner, Dr. F. Hülya Aşçi of Başkent University in Ankara, Turkey, shared her understanding of the physical self, which is regarded by health promotion researchers as an important outcome, correlate, and antecedent of physical activity behavior. She first presented a concise account of different approaches and methodologies that have been used to examine physical self from both multidimensional and hierarchical perspectives. She then presented a review of the attempts that have been made to develop instruments that could be used to measure physical self across different cultures and summarized the difficulties experienced. Finally, Aşçi concluded with a review of interventions designed to examine the relationship between exercise and physical self. The take-home message for sport and exercise psychologists, as well as health promotion researchers, is that interventions using exercise have the potential to influence the development of the physical self and such changes enhance overall self-evaluation and sense of well-being.

Moving onto sport psychology practice, in the fourth chapter, Dr. Sandy Gordon and his colleagues from the School of Human Movement and Exercise Science at the University of Western Australia argued that applied sport psychology researchers often fail to ground their investigations within theoretical or conceptual models. Subsequently, using mental toughness as an example, they described a Personal Construct Psychology (PCP) framework that could be used to study any desirable psychological attribute in exercise or sport settings. Specifically, they described a model of the PCP experience cycle and illustrated how a PCP interview protocol could be employed to understand as well as to identify and develop mental toughness. The case for grounding investigations of psychological attributes in exercise and sport settings in theory is clearly presented, as is the application of such an approach to investigate a buzz topic in sport: mental toughness.

Sport psychology practitioners will appreciate gaining insight into the lessons learned by Dr. Ken Ravizza, professor in the Department of Kinesiology at California State University (Fullerton), and Dr. Traci Statler, assistant professor at California State University (San Bernardino), during their extensive consulting experiences. In Chapter 5, they used a consultant-as-model approach to illustrate how the mental skills that athletes are asked to refine and develop should also be used by consultants to improve their own performance. Ravizza and Statler shared valuable tips for establishing a successful practice, such as the development of a personal philosophy for consulting, the recognition of personal strengths and weaknesses, and the creation of long-term strategies to maintain the desire to learn. Applying peak performance strategies in preparation for the consulting role, maintaining a present focus, and using performance routines were also recommended. Ravizza and Statler provided many examples from their personal experiences, which served to enhance both the authenticity, as well as the impact, of the advice offered.

In Chapter 6 Dr. Nanette Mutrie, professor of exercise and sport psychology at the University of Strathclyde in Scotland, began the Psychology of Exercise section with a discussion of the exercise psychologist's vital role in the increasing global awareness of the health benefits of physical activity before going on to address the training methods for exercise psychologists. In addition to using traditional theoretical frameworks and evidence-based interventions in the training of health promotion professionals, Mutrie also encouraged colleagues to consider complementary frameworks from positive psychology, suggesting that this would promote new partnerships with health and environmental psychologists and a change in the sole emphasis on physical health to also include mental health. In conclusion, Mutrie challenged the international sport and exercise psychology community by questioning the adequacy and appropriateness of current provisions for professional training in a field of enquiry that she claimed may be better served by the title "physical activity and sport psychology."

In Chapter 7, Dr. Dan Landers, Regents Professor of kinesiology at Arizona State University, and Dr. Brandon Alderman, assistant professor in the Division of Kinesiology and Health at the University of Wyoming, provided a rigorous evaluation of the efficacy of exercise compared to other methods of treating anxiety and depression disorders. In particular, they addressed the vexed questions of whether there is sufficient evidence to conclude that the effects of exercise on anxiety/depression are causal, whether exercise combined with other treatments is superior to exercise alone, whether exercise has better compliance compared to drugs and therapy, and whether exercise has fewer health risks and more health benefits than other treatments. The evidence they presented provides a compelling case for a more widespread application of exercise by the medical community as a first-line treatment for mental health issues.

The next contributor, Dr. Franz Mechsner, senior researcher at the world-famous Max Planck Institute for Human Cognitive and Brain Sciences, provided the eighth chapter, the first on cognitive psychology and psychophysiology. Mechsner presented his position in the long-running debate surrounding whether or not movement is controlled by precise and detailed instructions from the brain for the action of every muscle, or if movement can be conceived as being directly controlled by goals or intentions in the brain in the same way a driver steers a car without ever knowing what specific messages are sent from the steering wheel to the road wheels. Mechsner argued cogently for a psychological account of the control of voluntary movement. He supported his persuasive theorizing with an impressive list of studies, many conducted by him and his colleagues. Mostly, these studies involved seemingly simple variations of the apparently trivial action of finger wiggling. Mechsner's results, however, have far-reaching implications. They showed that "automatic" patterns of finger wiggling (called symmetrical movement) persisted regardless of the orientation of the hands, thus supporting a perceptual-conceptual basis for this movement, which cannot be explained by the movement of homologous muscles. Mechsner's important work on the way we translate thoughts into actions has been eloquently summarized in his seminal chapter.

In Chapter 9, Dr. Brad Hatfield, professor of sport psychology in the Department of Kinesiology at the University of Maryland, provided a detailed and comprehensive overview of the cognitive neuroscience aspects of sport and exercise psychology, focusing in particular on the brain mechanisms that underlie expert performance. After reviewing the pros and cons of various methods by which brain activity can be monitored, measured, and represented, and presenting the key theoretical principles in the area, Hatfield explained some of the neurological characteristics of the expert performer and compared the brain activity typical of superior and inferior performances. This chapter provides an excellent introduction for those readers previously unfamiliar with neuroscience and a comprehensive resource for those with pre-existing knowledge of the area.

The motor skill and expert performance section opened with Chapter 10, contributed by Dr. Karl Newell, professor of kinesiology and biobehavioral health at Pennsylvania State University. He addressed the considerable challenge of integrating a dynamical systems approach with traditional research into learning and feedback in the sport and motor skills domains. The different conceptual and meta-language characteristics of these two approaches make for a complex yet absorbing read. Newell and co-author S. Lee Hong focused their discussions especially on the qualitative and quantitative changes in motor performance that occur over time and throughout the lifespan, the crucial role of augmented information during motor learning and performance, and the thorny problem of establishing optimum practice schedules.

In Chapter 11, ISSP Young Investigator award winner for 2005, Dr. Sian Beilock from the Department of Psychology at Chicago University, addressed factors influencing the acquisition and maintenance of complex skills. In particular, she explained how memory and attentional processes combine to become real-time control structures supporting motor skill performance across different levels of learning, and discussed how skilled performance breaks down in demanding and high pressure situations—the so-called choking phenomenon. Her explanations of the memory and attentional failures underpinning the sudden breakdown of different types of sports skills make fascinating reading for theoreticians and practitioners alike, as do the ingenious studies she has undertaken with colleagues to test her propositions.

ISSP 2005 Program of Events

Pre-Congress Events

Like many international conferences, the ISSP World Congress got under way well in advance of the Opening Ceremony. As a prelude to the main event, two very popular pre-congress events were staged throughout August 14th and the morning of the fif-

teenth. Dr. Dan Gould (U.S.A) kicked off the Pre-Congress Workshops with a presentation entitled, *Mental Training: Lessons Learned by Moving from the Ball Field to the Boardroom and Back,* which proved to be a sell-out. Other invited workshops in this popular series included Dr. Kerry Mummery (Australia) and Dr. Grant Schofield (New Zealand) on *Promoting Physical Activity at the Community Level: Lessons from the 10,000 Steps Rockhampton Project;* Dr. Ken Ravizza (U.S.A.), Dr. Istvan Gorgenyi (Australia), and Dr. Patsy Tremayne (Australia) on *Coaching the Mental Game;* and finally, Dr. Tony Grant (Australia) on *Applied Positive Psychology and Executive Coaching,* an area that has experienced meteoric expansion globally over the past few years.

The second event was part of a long-standing World Congress tradition of staging free workshops for students, named in honor of the former ISSP President, the late Dr. Denis Glencross. Several members of the ISSP Managing Council volunteered their time to put on a series of well-attended and enthusiastically received presentations, including Dr. Judy Van Raalte (U.S.A.) on *Applied Sport Psychology Services: Getting Started;* Dr. Bola Ikulayo (Nigeria) on *Theoretical Frameworks in Sport Psychology*; Dr. Dorothee Alfermann (Germany) on *Career Coaching in Sport*; Dr. Ronnie Lidor (Israel) on *Teaching Beginners Pre-Performance Routines*; and Dr. Natalia Stambulova (Sweden) on *Empowering Athletes in Crises-Transitions.* An almost palpable buzz was carried forward to the Congress itself by more than 50 student delegates who attended the "Glencross" Workshops, generated as much by meeting and interacting with one another as by involvement in the workshops.

Moreover, even before these Pre-Congress Workshops were held, the international spirit of the event had been aroused. The College of Sport Psychologists of the Australian Psychological Society (APS), one of the co-hosts of ISSP 2005, re-vitalized its Visiting Scholar Scheme to coincide with the Congress. The College invited Dr. Ken Ravizza of California State University at Fullerton, an ISSP 2005 keynote speaker, to repeat his very successful tour of Australia in 2003 by once again filling the role of visiting scholar. Ravizza, with his anecdote-packed presentations and energetic style, proved a very popular choice among the academic and sporting communities alike. Although he was not able to visit all the major Australian cities, the residents of Sydney, Adelaide, and Melbourne certainly enjoyed the benefit of his entertaining presence.

Day 1 – Opening Ceremony

With most delegates now registered, the Congress formally started at 6 p.m. on Monday, August 15th, with a Welcome Reception and Opening Ceremony at a Sydney dockside venue overlooking the Harbour at Cockle Bay. The general level of excitement at the Opening Ceremony created a noise level that almost drowned out the speeches. Thankfully the assembled throng calmed down just long enough to hear ISSP President, Dr. Keith Henschen, declare the Congress open; APS President, Ms. Amanda Gordon, welcome the delegates on behalf of the broader psychology community in Australia; and APS College of Sport Psychologists President, Dr. Peter Terry, present a special award to Mr. Jeffrey Bond, Head of Psychology at the Australian Institute of Sport for 21 years, for his exceptional contributions to the sport psychology profession. Bond also became the inaugural recipient of the APS Colleges' Award of Distinction. The formal part of the evening concluded with another welcome, this time from the Chair of the Organizing Committee, Dr. Tony Morris.

On subsequent days, the Scientific Program followed a consistent pattern. Presentations commenced at 8 A.M. each day with three concurrent 90-minute symposia in which high-quality papers focused around a specific theme were presented consecutively, followed by a 60-minute keynote address held in the impressive 2000-seat auditorium, and then morning tea. Another three concurrent 90-minute sessions, either symposia or free oral papers, were held before lunch. In the afternoon, three concurrent 90-minute sessions were followed by a second 60-minute keynote address and then three concurrent 60-minute workshops, except on the last two days when the final session was taken up with the ISSP General Assembly and Closing Ceremony, respectively. Posters were on display throughout the day in a central location. The Scientific Program wrapped up at 6 P.M. each evening; a schedule that made for very full days and, as with most conferences, stamina proved a valuable asset.

Overall, the scientific program included a total of 594 presentations comprised of eight keynote addresses and two invited presentations to which this book is principally devoted; plus 25 symposia of between four and nine papers each, 42 free oral presentations, seven workshops, one forum, and 398 poster presentations.

Day 2

The morning of Tuesday, August 16th, started with concurrent symposia convened by Dr. Patsy Tremayne (Australia) on *Consulting Across Domains* and Dr. Natalia Stambulova (Sweden) on *Career Transitions*, plus free oral presentations on the theme of motivation, featuring presenters from Singapore, Taiwan, the U.K., and the U.S.A. This was followed by the eagerly-awaited first keynote address from Dr. Carol Dweck of Stanford University on *Self-Theories: The Mindset of a Champion*.

Further symposia convened before lunch, with Dr. Robert Vallerand's (Canada) *Passion in Sport* and Dr. Janet Starkes' (Canada) *Skilled Performance in Masters Athletes*, plus free orals—*Perceptual and Motor Skill*—featuring presenters from Australia, France, Germany, and the U.S.A. In the afternoon, concurrent symposia were held, convened by Dr. Peter Terry (Australia) on *Mood and Sport Performance,* Dr. Bonnie Berger (U.S.A.) on *Increasing Physical Activity,* and Dr. Panteleimon Ekkekakis (U.S.A.) on *Affect in Acute Exercise.*

These were followed by the second keynote address of the day, delivered by Dr. Nanette Mutrie of Strathclyde University in Scotland on *Applied Exercise Psychology - Promoting Activity and Evaluating Outcomes*. To round up the day's presentations, workshops on the topics of resonance, coaching, and parenting were provided by delegates from Canada, Denmark, and the U.S.A., respectively. Pleasingly, the first two keynote presenters, in common with other keynote presenters on subsequent days, generated substantial media interest and were in great demand for press and radio interviews.

The social program continued apace during the evening with the ISSP Official Dinner Cruise. More than 120 delegates boarded the Captain Cook Cruiser at 7:30 P.M., before setting off for a spectacular tour around majestic Sydney Harbour against a glittering backdrop of the city at night. It was an unforgettable evening for those present and a wonderful opportunity to meet colleagues from around the world in a relaxed, informal setting.

Day 3

Wednesday August 17th started with concurrent symposia convened by Dr. Frank Gardner (U.S.A.) on *Professional Development and Supervision* and Dr. Ronnie Lidor (Israel) on *Cognitive Strategies in Learning and Performance,* plus free oral presentations on exercise psychology, featuring delegates from Australia, Holland, Hong Kong, South Korea, and the U.K. This was followed by the morning keynote address from Dr. Sandy Gordon of the University of Western Australia, *Identification and Development of Mental Toughness,* which included examples from his applied work in international cricket.

Dr. Gordon continued after morning tea with a symposium on the same subject that also included experts from Canada, India, and the U.S.A.; concurrently, Dr. Gershon Tenebaum (U.S.A.) convened a symposium on *Expert Performance* and free orals on various themes were delivered by presenters from Australia, New Zealand, Sweden, and U.S.A. In the afternoon, concurrent symposia were convened: Dr. Dieter Hackfort (Germany) on *Action-Theory Approach,* Dr. Luci Teixeira-Salmela (Brazil) on *Physical Activity and Ageing,* and Dr. Gayelene Clews (Australia) on *Alcohol in Sport.* These were followed by Dr. Brad Hatfield's (University of Maryland) keynote address, titled *Cognitive Neuroscience Aspects of Sport Psychology: Brain Mechanisms Underlying Performance,* and concurrent workshops on the rarely visited topics of psychology of ballroom dancing, psychological safety, and the erotic in consulting were provided by delegates from Australia, Finland, and Australia, respectively.

The evening saw delegates spill out from the Convention Centre for welcome respite from the day's academic proceedings, engaging in informal cultural and social interchange over drinks at the myriad bars and restaurants for which Darling Harbour is rightly famous. The next day, one or two early morning presenters occasionally showed the wear and tear of the previous evening's festivities, but generally everyone came through unscathed and re-invigorated.

Day 4

The penultimate morning started with concurrent symposia, convened by Dr. Cliff Mallett (Australia) on *Coach Development and Education* and Dr. Duarte Araujo (Portugal) on *Sport Tasks,* plus free orals on the themes *Professional Practice* and *Drugs* given by presenters from Australia, the U.K., and the U.S.A. The symposia were followed by the morning keynote, in which Dr. Franz Mechsner, from the Max Planck Institute in Munich (Germany) presented on *A Psychological Approach to Voluntary Movements: Issues, Problems, and Controversies.*

More symposia followed late morning, convened by Dr. Jean Côté (Canada) on *Youth Sports;* Dr. Mike Weed (U.K.) on *Sport, Health, and Exercise;* and a forum convened by Dr. Wilson Readinger (U.S.A.) on *Recognition-Primed Decision Making in Sport.* The afternoon keynote address featured Dr. Daniel Landers of Arizona State University, with a presentation titled *Exercise Relative to Other Treatments for Reduction of Anxiety/Depression: Overcoming the Principle of Least Effort.*

Keynote presenter, Dr. Franz Mechsner (Germany), then provided a workshop on *A Psychological Approach to Voluntary Movements: Issues, Problems and Controversies,* which ran concurrent to a symposium convened by Dr. Dorothy Alfermann (Germany) on *Physical Self-Concept,* and free oral presentations, featuring delegates from Australia, Greece, Hungary, Taiwan, and the U.K.

The ISSP General Assembly was held from 4:30 to 6 P.M. on the afternoon of Thursday, August 18th. This gathering saw the election of new officers for ISSP, including a new President, Dr. Dieter Hackfort. In addition, some of the Managing Council members stood down, having completed their terms of office, and others stepped up, having just been elected to serve by the ISSP membership. Later during the evening, the "culture vultures" among the delegates took advantage of the fact that the Sydney Opera House—one of the great architectural icons of the world—was within walking distance of the Congress, and dressed up in their finest outfits to attend Puccini's La Bôhème.

Day 5

The final day of the Congress got under way with concurrent symposia, convened by John Salmela (Brazil) on *Parental Involvement in Sport* and Rich Masters (Hong Kong) on *Implicit Learning*, plus free orals on the theme of emotions, presented by delegates from Malaysia, Turkey, and the U.S.A.

Next up was Dr. Karl Newell, of Penn State University, with a keynote presentation titled *Change in Motor Learning: A Coordination and Control Perspective*. His session was followed by presentations from the ISSP Early Career awardees; Dr Sian Beilock of Chicago University on *From Novice to Expert Performance: Memory, Attention, and "Choking Under Pressure"* and Dr. F. Hülya Aşçi of Başkent University in Turkey on *Physical Self: Its Examination from Cultural and Mental Wellbeing Perspectives*. A symposium convened by Bruce Abernethy (Hong Kong) on *Expert Performance* was presented concurrently to the Early Career presentations, alongside free oral presentations on the psychology of injury, which featured presenters from Australia, Sweden, and the U.K.

In the afternoon, further symposia were presented, convened by Tony Morris (Australia) on *Flow in Sport,* Phillip Tomorowski (U.S.A.) on *Exercise and Cognition*, and Elizabeth Shoenfelt (U.S.A.) on *Team Building.* The scientific program was wrapped up by the final keynote address, given in entertaining fashion by the inimitable Dr. Ken Ravizza, of California State University at Fullerton, on *Lessons Learned from Sport Psychology Consulting*. It proved a fitting way to round off a busy five days of the latest developments in the world of sport psychology.

ISSP 2005 was a truly international event with delegates from at least five continents. Not surprisingly, the largest contingent came from host nation Australia and close neighbor New Zealand, with sizeable numbers also attending from Japan, Taiwan, the U.K., and the U.S.A. However, other attendees came from Africa, in particular, Botswana, Morocco, Nigeria, and South Africa; from the Americas, especially Argentina, Brazil, Canada, and Mexico; from all over Asia, notably China, Hong Kong, India, Indonesia, Iran, Malaysia, the Philippines, Singapore, and Thailand; and from Europe, including Belgium, Croatia, Czech Republic, Denmark, Finland, France, Germany, Greece, Holland, Hungary, Ireland, Italy, Norway, Poland, Portugal, Slovenia, Spain, Sweden, Switzerland, and Turkey.

ISSP 2005 Delegate Feedback

Quantitative and qualitative feedback data were obtained from 50 delegates, although the extent to which the feedback they provided was representative of all the delegates is, of course, unknown. Descriptive statistics for the quantitative aspects of the feedback are summarized in Table 1. With reference to the organization of the Congress, delegates praised the "fantastic range of topics" and the "excellent staff at the reception desk," but 19 delegates (38%) wanted more applied presentations, 19 (38%) expressed disappointment with the catering arrangements, seven (14%) wanted an extra concurrent session, and four (8%) felt that Velcro strips should have been provided by the organizers.

Additional comments, from one or two delegates each, suggested more presentations on exercise psychology, involvement of more athletes and coaches in presentations, earlier notification of abstract acceptance, single day registration, a later start to the day's proceedings, Congress t-shirts for sale, on-site Internet facilities, extending the Congress by one day, and uploading posters, slides, and comments to a weblog to facilitate digital downloads.

The quality of the poster presentations was rated higher than the oral presentations. Nine respondents (18%) expressed the opinion that more time should have been allocated to the posters. The use of cards displaying times when poster presenters would be available and the availability of poster handouts were both identified as excellent ideas. Most respondents praised the Darling Harbour Convention Centre as a venue, although five (10%) commented that the auditorium was too large and/or too formal for the event. The speaker preparation room and audio-visual facilities also received favorable comment. The social program received the least favorable ratings by delegates. Nine respondents (18%) wanted more *free* social activities. At least three of these respondents identified themselves as students who could not afford the price of the social events offered.

Table 1. Delegate Feedback (*N* = 50) on the 11th ISSP World Congress of Sport Psychology

Item	Poor	Good	VG	Exc	*M*	*SD*
Organization	8	30	10	2	2.12	0.72
Oral Presentations	3	24	20	3	2.46	0.71
Poster Presentations	0	19	25	6	2.74	0.66
Keynote Presentations	5	22	20	3	2.42	0.76
Venue	5	11	17	15	2.76	1.12
Social Program	26	15	24	1	1.44	0.84

Note. VG = very good; Exc = excellent

One aspect of this World Congress that was both notable and inspirational was the energetic involvement of the many graduate students from around the world. The poster sessions, in particular, had a vibrancy and quality of presentation that is rarely matched at such conferences. The sheer youthful enthusiasm evident throughout the Congress augurs particularly well for the future health of the profession and the success of future ISSP events.

Conclusions

Collectively, the Proceedings CD-ROM and this book provide a permanent record of the 11th ISSP World Congress of Sport Psychology, which embraced the theme, "Promoting Health and Performance for Life." The generations of sport psychology researchers and practitioners to come, who will uncover new knowledge and perhaps understand things far better than we do today, will have in this text a record of the contemporary knowledge base in 2005 against which to judge the progress they have made.

As the sun finally set on ISSP 2005, so the mantle of responsibility passed to the organizers of the next ISSP World Congress, in the historic city of Marrakesh in Morocco during 2009. On behalf of all those involved in the planning and delivery of ISSP 2005, especially our fellow members of the Organizing Committee, Drs. Lydia Ievleva, Stephanie Hanrahan, Greg Kolt, and Patsy Tremayne, we would like to conclude by thanking the International Society of Sport Psychology, its then President, Dr. Keith Henschen, and members of its Managing Council, for allowing the Australian Psychological Society and the APS College of Sport Psychologists the honor of co-hosting such a prestigious and memorable event. We hope to meet up with you in 2009, and to see you "Down Under" again some day.

Index

About the Editors

Tony Morris

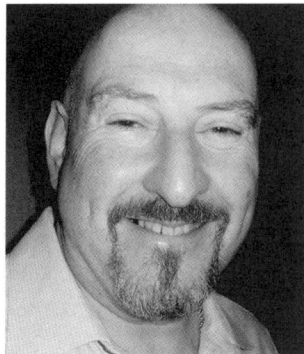

Tony Morris is a professor of sport, exercise, and health psychology at Victoria University. He was born in Leeds, England, and has lived in Melbourne, Australia, for 17 years. Trained in psychology, with a PhD in education, he previously worked in motor learning and sport psychology for eight years in the UK. Tony has published seven books and monographs, four as editor and three as author, and has authored more than 150 book chapters, journal articles, and refereed conference proceedings papers. In the UK, he helped form the British Association of Sports Sciences (BASS, now BASES) and was its second Honorary Secretary. He led the development of the Australian College of Sport Psychologists and was its inaugural chair. He has been a member of the Managing Council of the Asian South Pacific Association of Sport Psychology (ASPASP) since 1995, was Secretary General from 1996 to 1998, and has been President of ASPASP since 1998. He was a member of the Managing Council of the International Society of Sport Psychology (ISSP) from 1997 to 2005, when he was Chair of the Organizing Committee for the 11th ISSP World Congress of Sport Psychology. Tony has worked with many research students, having graduated more than 20 doctoral students. His primary areas of research interest include the application of psychological skills and techniques across all aspects of sport and physical activity and the involvement of physical activity in the prevention and treatment of illness, especially in chronic illness and disability. He has worked with athletes and teams at a range of levels, including international performers. He has presented approximately 100 invited lectures around the world, including more than 10 keynote presentations at international conferences.

Peter Terry

Peter Terry is a professor, the head of psychology, and the Professorial Research Fellow at the University of Southern Queensland. Born in London, Peter completed an honors degree in movement studies and English, and a postgraduate certificate in physical education from London University, before earning an MA in sport psychology from the University of Victoria in Canada and a PhD in psychology from the University of Kent. He taught in the Department of Sport Sciences at Brunel University for 16 years, eventually becoming professor of sport psychology in 1997 before moving to Australia in 2000. Author of more than 150 publications and presenter of more than 100 conference papers, he is a Fellow of the British Association of Sport and Exercise Sciences and is immediate past President of the Australian Psychological Society's College of Sport Psychologists. His research interests include mood and emotions, mental training, and psychometrics. Peter has worked with hundreds of international and professional athletes as an applied practitioner, including Olympic medallists in nine sports. He was Great Britain team psychologist for bobsled at the 1992 (Albertville), 1994 (Lillehammer) and 1998 (Nagano) Olympic Winter Games, for tennis at the 1992 Olympic Summer Games in Barcelona, a headquarters psychologist at the 1996 Olympic Games in Atlanta, and team psychologist for shooting at the 2000 (Sydney) and 2004 (Athens) Olympic Games. He has helped guide the development of athlete support over many years for the British Olympic Association, the Queensland Academy of Sport, the Women's Tennis Association, and several countries within the Asia-Pacific region.

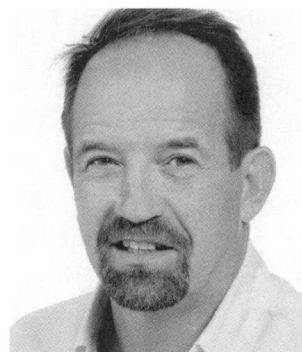

Sandy Gordon

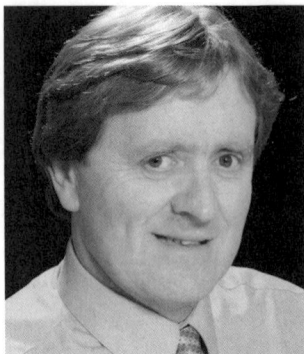

Sandy Gordon is a senior lecturer in the School of Human Movement and Exercise Science at The University of Western Australia (Perth), where he teaches sport and exercise psychology and coaching psychology. He was born in Huntly, Scotland, and received a physical education diploma at Jordanhill College in Glasgow. Upon graduation he taught physical education at Hazlehead Academy in Aberdeen for two years. Subsequently, he completed an advanced DipEd and MEd eegree through part-time study, during a six-year period teaching in the Department of Physical Education at Aberdeen University. In 1981 and 1986, respectively, he graduated with an MA and PhD in sport psychology from the University of Alberta in Canada before moving to Australia in 1987. He has authored or co-authored more than 80 book chapters and journal articles, and has presented more than 100 conference papers, a third of which were as an invited keynote speaker. In addition to mental toughness, his current research interests include resilience in sport, emotional labor in the service of professional sport, and the psycho-immunological aspects of sport injury. He is a Registered Sport Psychologist, Fellow Member of the Australian Psychological Society (APS), and past National Chair of the APS College of Sport Psychologists. He serves on three editorial boards and regularly reviews for several other periodicals that publish applied sport psychology research. Sandy has contributed to coach education programs in more than 10 countries in addition to Australia and has extensive consulting experience in the performing arts and business, as well as sport.

About the Authors

Brandon Alderman, PhD

Brandon Alderman, PhD, is an assistant professor in the Division of Kinesiology and Health at the University of Wyoming. His research interests include the effects of acute and chronic exercise on stress, psychological and physiological mechanisms underlying the mental health benefits of exercise, and youth physical activity.

F. Hülya Aşçı, PhD

F. Hülya Aşçi, PhD, is an associate professor in sport sciences at Başkent University in Ankara, Turkey. Her research interests include physical self-perception, exercise and psychological well-being, and psychometric issues.

Sian L. Beilock, PhD

Sian L. Beilock, PhD, is an assistant professor in the Department of Psychology at the University of Chicago. She received a double PhD in kinesiology and psychology from Michigan State University in 2003. These dual degrees reflect her interest in examining the cognitive and neural processes governing skilled performance and its failure across different task types, performance environments, and levels of expertise.

Timothy Chambers

Timothy Chambers is completing doctoral studies in the School of Human Movement and Exercise Science, at The University of Western Australia. His research employs a Personal Construct Psychology framework and aims to better understand and develop resilience among swimmers and swimming coaches. Other research interests include performance and applied sport psychology for endurance sports.

Carol S. Dweck, PhD

Carol S. Dweck, PhD, is the Lewis and Virginia Eaton Professor of Psychology at Stanford University. She is a leading researcher in the area of motivation, specializing in the beliefs and goals that enhance motivation and maximize performance. Her book, *Self-Theories,*

was named book of the year by the World Education Foundation, and her latest book, *Mindset,* was recently published by Random House.

Daniel Gucciardi

Daniel Gucciardi is completing doctoral studies in the School of Human Movement and Exercise Science, at The University of Western Australia. His research, which is driven by a Personal Construct Psychology framework, is seeking to identify, understand, and develop mental toughness among Australian Rules footballers. Other research interests include performance and applied sport psychology.

Bradley D. Hatfield, PhD

Bradley D. Hatfield, PhD, is a professor of sport psychology in the Department of Kinesiology at the University of Maryland. His research interests include the use of psychophysiological methods to assess the effects of exercise on mental health.

S. Lee Hong

S. Lee Hong is completing doctoral studies in kinesiology at Pennsylvania State University. His research interests include motor control, learning, and development from dynamical systems perspectives.

Daniel M. Landers, PhD

Daniel M. Landers, PhD, is the Regents' Professor in the Department of Kinesiology at Arizona State University. His research interests include examination of the effects of exercise on (a) relaxation/mood alteration, including anxiety and depression; (b) ability to cope with psychosocial stressors, (c) quality and quantity of sleep, and (d) cognitive functioning.

Franz Mechsner, PhD

Franz Mechsner, PhD, is a senior lecturer in the Department of Psychology and Sport Science at Northumbria University in Newcastle Upon Tyne, United Kingdom. He began as a novelist and science journalist for 15 years, and in following years he investigated psychological factors in human movement control at the Max Planck Institute for Psychological Research in Munich, Germany, at the Hanse Institute for Advanced Study in Delmenhorst, Germany, and at the Leibniz Research Center for Occupational Health in Dortmund, Germany.

Nanette Mutrie, PhD

Nanette Mutrie, PhD, is a professor of exercise and sport psychology at the University of Strathclyde, Glasgow, Scotland. She is also the director of the Scottish Physical Activity Collaboration (http://www.sparcoll.org.uk). Her research interests include the promotion of walking for sedentary and clinical populations and exercise as elements of cancer rehabilitation.

Karl M. Newell, PhD

Karl M. Newell, PhD, is a professor of kinesiology and biobehavioral health and is the Associate Dean for Research and Graduate Education at Pennsylvania State University. His research interests include coordination, control, and skill of normal and abnormal human movement across the life-span; development of coordination; acquisition of skill; information and movement dynamics; mental retardation and motor skills; and drug exercise influences on movement control.

Kenneth H. Ravizza, PhD

Kenneth H. Ravizza, PhD, is a professor in the Department of Kinesiology at California State University, Fullerton. His research interests include examining the nature of peak performance in human movement activities.

Traci A. Statler, PhD

Traci A. Statler, PhD, is an assistant professor in the Department of Kinesiology at California State University, San Bernardino. Her research interests include the attainment of excellence as it relates to applied sport psychology consulting; the psychological dynamics of sport injury, focusing on developing educational training modules to better prepare certified athletic trainers to deal with these issues; and the many factors that shape the world of collegiate athletes, with the aim of improving their overall collegiate experience.